Legal, Ethical, and Management Aspects of the Dental Care System

W9-DDE-701

Legal, Ethical, and Management Aspects of the Dental Care System

Irene R. Woodall, R.D.H., Ph.D.

Adjunct Associate Professor, Department of Dental Care Systems, School of Dental Medicine, University of Pennsylvania, Philadelphia, Pennsylvania and Clinical Associate Professor, Department of Applied Dentistry, School of Dentistry, University of Colorado, Denver, Colorado

with contributions in the areas of quality assurance, financial management, collective bargaining, and insurance from

J. Marvin Bentley, Ph.D.

Assistant Professor, Department of Dental Care Systems, School of Dental Medicine, University of Pennsylvania, Philadelphia, Pennsylvania

THIRD EDITION

with **32** illustrations

The C. V. Mosby Company

ST. LOUIS · WASHINGTON D.C. · TORONTO   1987

MOSBY

A TRADITION OF PUBLISHING EXCELLENCE

Editor: Darlene Barela Cooke
Assistant editor: Donna Saya Sokolowski
Editing/Production: Publication Services
Book design: Kay M. Kramer

THIRD EDITION

Copyright © 1987 by the C.V. Mosby Company

All rights reserved. No part of this publication may be reproduced, stored in a retrieval system, or transmitted, in any form or by any means, electronic, mechanical, photocopying, recording, or otherwise, without prior written permission from the publisher.

Previous editions copyrighted 1977, 1983

Printed in the United States of America

The C.V. Mosby Company
11830 Westline Industrial Drive, St. Louis, Missouri 63146

Library of Congress Cataloging-in-Publication Data

Woodall, Irene R. (Irene Rita), 1946-
    Legal, ethical, and management aspects of the
dental care system.

    Includes bibliographies and index.
    1. Dentistry—Practice.   2. Dental auxiliary
personnel.   3. Dental care—United States.   4. Dental
laws and legislation—United States.   5. Dental ethics.
I. Bentley, J. Marvin.   II. Title.   [DNLM: 1. Dental
Care—United States.   2. Ethics, Dental.   3. Legislation,
Dental—United States.   4. Practice management, Dental.
WU 77 W881L]
RK58.W67   1987   617.6′0068   86-12863
ISBN 0-8016-5625-7

C/D/D   9 8 7 6   02/A/272

Once again
to
Conrad Woodall
and our children
Charlotte Claire and **Amanda Marie**
for the light in their eyes, the love in their hearts
and the joy and peace they bring me

Foreword

When I wrote the foreword to the second edition I importuned the reader that understanding change is crucial to coping with the enormous upheaval occurring in the profession. Since then the rate of change has increased, the forces affecting what all of us do have grown, the options concerning dental health care delivery and reimbursement have multiplied and the stresses, perceived or real, of trying to provide dental health services are such that feeling overwhelmed is more the norm than the exception. And, of course, the doomsayers are having a field day! Dental caries is a disease of the past (it isn't), fewer patients see dentists (not so), and incomes are plateauing or decreasing (actually, on average, incomes of dental professionals have increased each year since this book was written). But as the philosophers might say—perception is reality, no matter the facts. We tend to believe what we want to believe regardless of the evidence and we tend to disregard anything contrary to what we think is real or factual, again, regardless of the evidence. Habitual opinion becomes our fact.

The trick in all this is to separate fact from fiction and at least to identify what is happening so that you can chart your own course rather than being swept away by events. The need for dental care has not abated. Most of the people in the United States still do not seek routine dental care and a virtually untapped market exists in the form of the older person, the fastest growing segment of our society. Physically and mentally disabled people as well as the homebound go without *any*

dental care. At the same time many dentists complain of too few patients.

The fundamental difference between success now and in the past is that we have to compete. We have to convert the enormous unmet need for dental care into demand. We have to market our practices. We have to manage effectively and efficiently. We have to create practice environments that make it pleasant for both dental provider and consumer. We have to understand the human, technical, financial and management issues of dental health care delivery. And that is what *"Legal, Ethical and Management Aspects of the Dental Care System"* is all about.

This book can help you wend your way through the maze of strategies used to control your own destiny. In very clear language Dr. Woodall demonstrates, as I said in the foreword to the second edition, "how to get the job done." Deciding what you want (goals) and devising ways to achieve them is a central theme. Being effective, efficient, and knowledgeable is another central message. And, as in the previous edition, Dr. Woodall stresses the importance of working with people as the essence of getting things done.

There are many changes in this edition that reflect the changes that have occurred in what confronts you in practice. What has not changed is the easy to read, understand, and use format of the book. The questions at the end of each chapter serve to emphasize the more fundamental points, an important feature retained from the previous edition. Finally, the great care and concern for clarity that characterized the second edition remains intact. *"Legal, Ethical and Management Aspects of the Dental Care System"* has been a labor of love for Dr. Woodall and the quality of writing reflects it.

Sheldon Rovin, DDS, MS
Professor & Chairperson,
Department of Dental Care Systems,
School of Dental Medicine,
University of Pennsylvania;
Associate Director, Leonard Davis
Institute and National Health
Care Management Center,
Wharton School, University of Pennsylvania

Preface

This book is written for students and for clinicians whose careers will be affected by changes in dentistry, dental hygiene, policymaking, ethics, the economy, the law, modes of practice management, and personal and professional needs. In other words, it is intended for dental health care professionals who expect to have a continuing career in the decades ahead. Most of the text is written for hygienists, dentists, and dental assistants, with a few chapters more applicable to dental auxiliaries and dental hygiene, specifically.

The messages and tone of the book have changed dramatically since it was first introduced ten years ago. The issues have shifted, the directions for career development have expanded and grown in complexity, and the overall outlook for dental hygiene and dentistry in general has changed with forces internal and external to the professions. Therefore, there are major revisions in this edition. Some chapters seemed passé and have been eliminated; an entire new section emphasizing skills in practice management has been developed; and new approaches to continuing problems are suggested.

The strategy for using the book is nearly the same. It can become a basis for healthy debate or discussion in the classroom, at study clubs and component meetings, and among informal groups of interested professionals. An ideal use would be for groups of dentists and hygienists to use the text as a stimulus for discussion and a dialogue. One or more chapters can be designated for outside reading, and one of the suggested group activities can be selected to create a forum for discussion or to help the group use the information included in the chapters.

Dental health care delivery is at a critical point in its development. Professionals' responses to the issues will help determine its growth, its usefulness to a public in need of quality dental care, and its financial viability. It therefore makes very good sense that professionals know what those issues are, recognize how others view and respond to them, and develop an informed opinion from which to take action and from which to listen to the inevitable changes the future will bring.

Irene R. Woodall

Acknowledgements

This third edition was made possible, in part, by many of the people who supported the second edition. High on the list is Con Woodall, who prepared the index and made numerous contributions to the logistics and content development of several chapters making the revision both fun and easier to accomplish. Right with him are Lotte and Mandy Woodall who withheld their justifiable criticism of how I was spending my time and provided me with two very important reasons to complete the task and get on with the joys of motherhood. Other supporters from before include Marvin Bentley, Chris Smith, and Shel Rovin.

I am deeply indebted to Darlene Cooke and Donna Sokolowski, editors at C.V. Mosby, for their continuing moral and substantive support.

My new environment brought many new colleagues into the action. They include Tom Berry, Larry Domer, Jane Engele, Lynn Brown, Michelle Morgan, Diane Sawczyn, Larry Frederick, Barb Jones, Cheryl and Geoff Smith, Linda Snider, Sue Washburn, Renee Colman, Vonnie Henery, and many more of my friends and colleagues who helped me with photography, finding information, keeping my mind intact, and cheering my progress. A special thank you to all of you. And thanks again to my trusty TRS-80 Model II for miracles worked.

Acknowledgments

Contents

Legal, Ethical, and Management Aspects of the Dental Care System

PART ONE

Dental health professionals—defining roles, relationships, and requirements

The decades of the 1960s and 1970s were times of great change in dental care delivery. New technology was introduced, efficiency and ergonomic considerations received attention, and mechanisms for reimbursement for services were expanded beyond the fee-for-service standard to include insurance, prepayment plans, and variations of those arrangements.

One of the most important developments was analysis of the scope of functions that could be safely and logically delegated to clinicians other than dentists. Dental hygienists and dental assistants learned and provided a much wider array of services. New categories of dental health professionals were introduced, including expanded duty dental assistants (EDDAs) and expanded function dental assistants (EFDAs). Dental regulatory laws were changed in varying ways to accommodate the innovations in the majority of licensing jurisdictions.

The 1980s, with their early struggles with spiraling monetary inflation and diminishing dental disease, saw a greater focus on alternative financial arrangements, professional marketing, "lean" practice management strategies, and retrenchment regarding the use of expanded-function personnel. Hygienists, in particular, began looking more seriously at alternative ways to define the dental team and the financial relationships between hygienists and dentists to permit hygienists to function independent of the employer-employee arrangement. Some describe the situation as recalcitrance, others see it as long overdue assertion of basic rights, and others see it as an essential move for maintaining dental hygiene as a viable profession with many career pathways and opportunities for growth.

This section provides group members with ways to assess and clarify their own and others' beliefs and attitudes regarding dentistry, dental hygiene, dental assisting, and the dental team as a whole. It provides a history of the dental team and a primer on current issues in educational requirements and credentials. It addresses the issue of quality of care and how it affects the profession and consumers. Overall, this section sets the stage for the issues and ideas presented in the remaining sections.

CHAPTER 1

The issues, beliefs, and attitudes
in dental health care delivery

OBJECTIVES: The reader will be able to:

1. List personal experiences from the following viewpoints that have helped shape his/her perceptions of dental health care providers:
   a. As a patient.
   b. As a beginning student.
   c. As a clinician (either in school or in practice).
2. Discuss how technological change, economic and political forces, and changing life-styles may affect the "security" of a well-defined occupational role in the years ahead.
3. Participate in a values clarification process by
   a. identifying at least six descriptive statements regarding dental health care providers with which he/she agrees.
   b. forming a partnership (dyad) with another person whose six descriptive statements are compatible.
   c. forming a group of four with another dyad, whose collective descriptive statements are compatible with the partnership's.
   d. describing why each statement is agreed on and ranking the group of statements according to their "importance."
   e. sharing the choices and ranking with other groups.
4. Participate in active listening.
5. Identify how others' perceptions of dental health care providers differ from his/her own and explain why the others have chosen different points of view or beliefs.
6. Begin to debate the issues related to the role delineation and function of dental health care providers.

Rarely does a book begin with an exercise. This one does. The reason is that before a student or a clinician can recognize the importance of various issues confronting the delivery of dental care, he/she must take the time to sort out what his/her own beliefs and attitudes are and then listen to those of others who share an interest, and perhaps a devotion, to providing dental health care.

While there is a common culture surrounding dentistry and dental hygiene—and separate ones surrounding each of those—each individual professional has a variety of unique perceptions about the role, function, and future of dental care.

Most persons enter a career as a result of the perceptions they have acquired regarding its attractiveness. Men and women entering health professions may base their decision on how they perceived the profession as patients. Or they may have been influenced by family members who are in the profession. The attractiveness may be defined in terms of self-esteem, financial reward,

3

service to people, job security, independence, scope of responsibility, or pleasantness of the working environment.

Those perceptions are altered or reaffirmed as the persons enter educational preparation for the role and once again after having entered practice.

Depending on what an individual's total experiences are in relationship to the health career, the person develops a perception of the career People's perceptions therefore differ as greatly as their personal experiences. For a person in a health profession to acquire a better understanding of his/her career, there must be a sharing of perceptions among its members and with persons who stand outside the profession.

This may occur by accident as a health care provider overhears a conversation in which his/her career is being discussed. He/she may hear a rather inaccurate description of the activities or responsibilities that such a provider of care is supposed to perform or hear him/herself being cast into a stereotype. The humorous, albeit less than complimentary, ways in which the dental profession is often portrayed in films and on television programs are a hint of what the consumer may think about dental health care providers. An awakening may come from a conversation with another dental health care provider who has quite a different perception of the role of the profession. Each new experience as a patient, as a student, and as a practitioner will either alter or reaffirm certain aspects of a professional's view of his/her career.

To focus on the variations in people's perceptions, a planned group activity, referred to as values clarification, can point out clearly where the differences lie as well as provide insight into why certain people hold the views they identify as their own. Different solo or group methods can be used in values clarification.

The six exercises described at the end of this chapter can help a clinician clarify his/her own perceptions and those of others in the group. They also can introduce a variety of issues that currently are a center of debate in the professions. If the exercise rouses the interest of the group's participants, that is an ideal way to introduce the subsequent sections that provide information, opinions, alternatives, and new debate.

The main point is that being a health care clinician is more than learning how to diagnose, treat, and prevent disease. It is even more than working with people. It, by necessity, includes being aware of the internal and external forces and beliefs that will continually reshape the professions and the very way health care is delivered. Thus, a dental care curriculum includes more than clinical and basic sciences, and continuing education includes more than updated information regarding clinical procedures and new materials. The curriculum and continuing education programs should include seminars that focus on the delivery of dental care as a system that is part of social, economic, political, legal, and management systems that make or break what the individual clinician believes is right.

GROUP ACTIVITIES

1. Conduct a values clarification session in which foursomes identify the sources of the perceptions of their profession and explain the beliefs they hold and why. Other members in the foursome feed back what they heard the person say. Each person participates in both the sharing and the reflective feedback exercise.
2. Review editorials and presidential messages in the dental and dental auxiliary journals for excerpts that describe opposing views or cogent summaries of comtemporary issues. The point-counter-point material can be used to stimulate discussion by distributing copies of the excerpts to the students and asking them to take a stand and explain their rationale. Students may form groups to study the issues, ferret out addition information, and follow the development of trends.
3. Prepare a page of up to ten values statements. (See Appendix A for examples.) Obtain copies of the statements so that each student has a page. Students individually read the statements, circle the items with which they concur, and change the others so that they are acceptable. The students form groups of five to discuss their respective views and to draft a consensus statement for the group. A new group is then formed comprised of one member of each of the discussion groups. Its role is to share the various topics the students discussed in the respective groups and to identify

the areas with which they agree or disagree. One or two empty chairs should be included in the circle formed by the group. The rest of participants should gather around to hear the discussion and to move into one of the empty chairs in the group to add comments, vent frustration, or share opinions. As soon as his/her comments are completed, the person should return to the periphery of the group to enable discussion to continue. At the conclusion the facilitator should summarize the major areas of debate and discussion and indicate how they will receive attention later in the course.

4. Each participant is given six cards on which values statements are written (one statement per 3 × 5 card). See Appendix A for statements that can be used on the cards. Participants move around the room, trading cards with other participants until each person is satisfied with the six cards he/she holds. Satisfaction is described as holding cards that are acceptable as an expression of that person's beliefs or values. In other words, the person generally agrees with the statements on the six cards. There are no right or wrong cards. No one should have prejudged the appropriateness or truth of any of the cards. Each card should be considered neutral in terms of any external evaluation. The cards should be evaluated only in terms of the person's own particular beliefs.

When each person has six cards with which he/she feels reasonably comfortable, each participant should begin to form a partnership with one other person whose cards also seem to be reasonable reflections of his/her own values. To form the partnership, the dyad (twosome) may discard two or three cards on which they do not agree. The dyad should have between nine and twelve cards on which they both agree.

The dyad then sets out to form a foursome. A total of four more cards may be discarded if the formation of the foursome is blocked by them. A settled foursome should therefore have at least twenty cards and a maximum of twenty-four cards. Forming a group of four people may not be possible for all participants, in which case dyads may wish to remain unattached.

Once the foursomes are settled, each group should identify the four most important and four least important statements included in their values cards. The group should rank the four least important and then rank the four most important.

Depending on the size of the entire group of participants, the foursomes may need to write out their choices on sheets of newsprint with a felt-tip marker. This may assist the sharing process that follows, when each foursome or dyad explains its top and bottom four choices and the reasons why they were ranked as they were. Each person in the foursome should explain two of the eight choices.

During the discussion, noticeable similarities and disparities among the various groups will appear. On some points there may be general agreement in the entire group of participants; on other points polar opposites may be apparent between two or more groups.

It is important to achieve a thorough discussion of why people believe or value certain points. At the close of the session, each participant should be able to state the basis for six of his/her own personal convictions regarding dental health care providers and be able to state and explain the basis for six beliefs others have with which the person does not necessarily agree.

It is helpful to include faculty members and dental care providers currently in practice as long as these persons do not dominate the group discussions or become too influential in the decisions the students make about the values. If this exercise is conducted in a professional association as a beginning session of a study club, it may be helpful to invite several student members or consumers to participate. The shades of valuing should expand with the variety of persons involved in the process.

The entire process should take approximately 1½ hours, with 20 minutes allocated for initial trading of cards, 15 minutes for forming dyads, and 20 minutes for forming foursomes and ranking statements. Thirty minutes or more should be allowed for discussion.

The discussion can easily grow into a debate. In most instances it may be wise for the group facilitator to help participants focus on the open expression and sharing of beliefs and values and the reasons people hold them rather than allowing the group to begin condemning some and supporting others. This exercise should prepare people to be more interested in the differences and in the sources of their own beliefs, so that subsequent group activities can be opportunities for a more in-depth analysis of the issues that arose.

NOTE: This exercise was first described by the National Training Laboratory. It has been adapted for use in this context by the author.

5. If the group is a mixture of dental professionals, for instance dentists and dental hygienists, who feel they are in strong opposition on several issues, this group strategy may be used. There *must* be one independent person skilled in group process to serve as monitor to start and stop the activities and to lead the group discussion that follows.

The members of the groups split according to the factor that separates them (e.g., dentists in one group, hygienists in another). Each group lists all the things that are wrong with the other group's thinking and actions. Each group selects a representative to sit face-to-face in the center of the room with the other group's representative. They are given 30 seconds to ''hurl invectives'' at one another, citing all the things they find disagreeable and stating how tough each one's own group has it because of the other group's behavior. The ''crowd'' should cheer on their respective representatives.

After 30 seconds, new representatives should be sent in (quickly) to continue the shouting and fingerpointing. More cheering. Two more quick changes of representatives, with 30 seconds for each twosome, should be sufficient to elicit all the anger, disappointment, disagreement, fear, and disparagement that exists to separate the groups.

The groups each send in a new representative, who must now switch roles. The hygienist should play the part of the dentist and vice versa. The process begins again with the hygienist-playing-dentist hurling invectives against hygienists and the dentist-playing-hygienist hurling invectives against the dentists. The groups should be instructed to assist their respective representatives with ideas; the representatives should stay 30 seconds and be replaced by two new ones, who continue the role reversal. Allow a total of four rounds of representatives for 30 seconds at each round.

A calm usually comes over the group as the role-reversal takes over; the shouts become more thoughtful and considerate. The "cheering" becomes helpful ideas for understanding. Call the role reversal to an end.

Encourage a healthy 15 to 30 minute discussion of how the participants feel after the exercise and what they learned from it—about themselves and about the other group. Record their observations and new learning on newsprint. Encourage the group to specify new ways to help each other rather than fight each other.*

6. Prior to reading the chapters on ethics, ask each group member to list his/her reasons for deciding to become a health care professional. Also ask each person to list those factors that define *success* for the person. A list of the twelve most commonly cited reasons for entering the profession and the twelve most commonly listed success factors should be generated. The group should rank order them and discuss the differences among the perceptions of the group members. This list should be saved for further discussion in a later section.

---

*NOTE: This exercise is adapted from Jacob L. Moreno's sociodrama techniques as described in Shaffer, J.B.P., and Galinsky, M.D.: *Models of group therapy and sensitivity training,* Englewood Cliffs, N.J., 1974, Prentice-Hall, Inc.

CHAPTER 2

Origins of direct patient care dental auxiliaries

OBJECTIVES: The reader will be able to:

1. Briefly summarize the development of the profession of dental hygiene (as the first direct patient care dental auxiliary), including the following:
   a. The founder of the profession.
   b. The first dental hygienist of record.
   c. The date the practice of dental hygiene education was first defined.
   d. The first continuous dental hygiene education program.
   e. The function the educated dental hygienist was intended to serve in the provision of dental services.
2. Compare the purpose and function of the dental hygienist in the United States with the other operating dental auxiliaries that have been established as health care providers in other countries, including the following:
   a. Dental hygienists other than in the United States.
   b. The New Zealand School Dental Nurse.
   c. The New Cross Dental Auxiliary (later called a dental therapist).
   d. The Canadian dental nurse.
3. Summarize briefly the move to extend additional functions to dental auxiliaries (United States), including the following:
   a. Identification of the major experiments and demonstration projects that focused on expanded-function dental assistants.
   b. An explanation of dentistry's focus on dental assistants rather than on dental hygienists as auxiliaries to whom additional duties should be delegated.
   c. Primary experiments in the expansion of functions for dental hygienists.
   d. Overall results of the studies of the delegation of expanded functions to dental assistants and dental hygienists.
4. Describe the status of the second direct patient care dental auxiliary in the United States.
5. Compare the current scope of practice of the dental hygienist with that of the dental hygienist as defined by Fones and Newman.
6. Explain how the economic, political, and dental health changes of the past decade have affected dental hygiene and the movement toward expanded functions.

DEVELOPMENT OF DENTAL AUXILIARIES
Dental hygiene

The first direct patient care dental auxiliary in the United States that is acknowledged historically and that has continued to exist since the time of that profession's establishment is the dental hygienist. Dr. Alfred Civilion Fones, in 1906, established the profession by preparing Irene Newman to be a provider of care for his patients (Fones, 1927). There were earlier instances of women serving roles as preventive assistants as the concept of oral hygiene was periodically discussed as a proper role for nondentists. Fones was the person responsible for gaining widespread acceptance of the concept and for developing a lasting program of instruction for those persons. It was his expressed belief that there ought to be an auxiliary whose primary function was the prevention of dental disease. He believed that an auxiliary called the dental hygienist should be educated to remove calcareous deposits from teeth and to instruct patients in the care and maintenance of their teeth and supporting structures. The first educational program was long thought to be the Fones School of Dental Hygiene at the University of Bridgeport in Connecticut. However, recent findings indicate that the first program actually was at the Ohio College of Dental Surgery, from 1910 to 1911; it was closed down because of the opposition of area dentists (Motley, 1983).

Most activity in the development of the profession of dental hygiene occurred in the East, where dental hygienists were employed by school systems to provide dental health education and oral prophylaxis for children. The role was distinctly preventive and did not include restorative treatment (Motley, 1983).

In the profession's infancy, its members were not licensed. The first legal definition of dental hygiene was the Connecticut Dental Practice Act in 1915 (Motley, 1983). Licensure would be a trend the profession would both enjoy as strong support and later bemoan at times as a roadblock to its own evolution in the second 50 years of existence.

The period of greatest growth in dental hygiene was the 1960s and 1970s. Growth was in terms of numbers of dental hygienists (Malvitz and Mocniak, 1982) and in the scope of functions they could be delegated. The reason for this growth was the perceived need for a greater supply of health manpower that was to be available for the United States population once national health insurance was made law. Medicare and Medicaid were passed in 1965, providing financial access for the elderly and certain disadvantaged groups to health care (Albertini et al.,

1984). Congress considered numerous versions of proposed legislation that would have extended ''free'' health care to all residents, regardless of ability to pay. If this legislation had passed, the country would have immediately needed many more physicians, nurses, dentists, hygienists, and other allied health professionals to meet the expected demand for care.

While debate over national health insurance continued, federal funds were provided for health professions education, both to start new programs and to support increased enrollment in existing ones. Also, experimental programs were introduced to determine the extent to which routine care could be delegated. Dentistry emphasized streamlining the dental appointment and increasing productivity by delegating functions to dental auxiliaries.

Expanded function dental assistants

Dental assistants were considered first for expanded functions. Dental assistants originally did not provide direct intraoral care; they assisted dentists with office procedures and at the chairside. Since until the 1970s dental law did not restrict who could be hired as a dental assistant, many dental assistants were trained on the job.

There are, of course, educational programs to prepare trained dental assistants. The American Dental Assistants Association (ADAA) has a certification program to identify those persons who have demonstrated skill and knowledge in dental assisting through formal education, an examination program, and required continuing education (Hengl, 1984). Despite the educational programs and the certification credential, there is no mandate to hire these qualified persons. As a result, the association has had unique problems both in establishing its credibility as the voice of dental assisting and in establishing economic security for its members who continually compete with the on-the-job trained work force that staffs the majority of dental offices (Results, 1985).

However, what dental hygiene has in economic security in licensure, dental assisting has in flexibility of practice. Until the 1970s dental assistants were defined in few dental laws and therefore were not specifically restricted in practice, and they have always been available in large numbers (albeit not all educated or certified). These factors attracted many persons in the 1960s to begin experimentation in more productive patterns for the delivery of care with the focus on the dental assistant as the provider of the newly delegated services (Report, 1972).

The first documented experimentation was conducted in 1962 and 1963 by the United States Navy at Great Lakes Naval Training Station in Illinois. Setting the pattern for numerous experimental projects to follow, the U.S. Navy discovered that dental technicians with some didactic background could learn to place quality restorations in prepared teeth. Productivity was increased by up to 80% to 100% for the dental officers responsible for the care (Ludwig, 1964). The results in this study were reported to the American Dental Association in 1965 (Council, 1965).

The University of Alabama initiated a program in 1963 that eventually demonstrated that auxiliaries could successfully place rubber dams, matrices, temporary restorations, and amalgam and silicate restorations (Hammons, 1971). The Indian Health Service in 1963 demonstrated that appropriately trained auxiliaries could perform restorative procedures including placing and carving amalgam and silicate restorations (Abramowitz and Berg, 1973).

A landmark productivity study was conducted at Louisville, Kentucky, at the Division of Dental Health, U.S. Public Health Service (Latzkar et al., 1971). It demonstrated that assistants could perform the services as well as dentists and that with one dentist and four expanded function restorative assistants, productivity could be improved by up to 140%. Patient acceptance of auxiliaries performing such services was documented in this study, also. The University of the Pacific (Redig et al., 1974) and the University of North Carolina (Douglass, 1974) conducted studies also,

both utilizing specially trained dental assistants to perform restorative functions.

This trend toward delegating additional functions, particularly restorative functions, to assistants created a new breed of auxiliary, the expanded function (duty) dental auxiliary (EFDA or EDDA). This person was to be the second direct patient care dental auxiliary in the United States. The scope of responsibility of the EFDA varied with each experimental program and demonstration project that has been conducted and with the legal definition of each state (Council, 1976). It varied with the developer's perceptions of the relative importance of formal education, appropriate certification mechanisms, the autonomy of the employer-dentist, and the usefulness and availability of other dental auxiliaries.

This direct patient care auxiliary may be a completely new entity with some of the skills of the traditional chairside dental assistant and a full array of intraoral skills. Or he/she may be a dental hygienist with additional periodontal and restorative functions (Council, 1976). Regardless of the ambiguous definition, the EFDA emerged as a new operating auxiliary in the United States. The specific role of this provider of care has yet to be delineated or functionally integrated into the delivery of care in this country, more than a full decade after experimention.

EFDAs may not realize their potential in the delivery of dental care in the United States for many years, at least not as it was envisioned. Their role was invented to help meet the projected demand for dental care that was to follow the introduction of national health insurance. Such a program is highly unlikely given recent political and economic conditions and efforts to control government spending. Federal programs have been cut back, particularly social, educational, and health-related projects. Thus there has been no great increase in the number of patients seeking care. Actually, dental caries has reduced in prevalence, producing less need for restorative care (AAPHD, 1983; Ibikunle, 1985). Coupled with the marked increase in dentists (also as a result of projected demand for care), few practitioners feel compelled to delegate intraoral functions to an auxiliary. Dentists in many regions report partially filled schedules and can do the work themselves. If demand for restorative care increases, EFDAs may again be a focal point in accepting intraoral functions. For now, however, the movement is nearly dead.

Utilizing dental hygienists in expanded functions

The four primary experiments and training programs utilizing dental hygienists in restorative expanded functions were conducted at the University of Iowa (Sisty, 1975; Sisty et al., 1978, 1979), Howard University (Powell et al., 1974), the University of Kentucky (Spohn, 1975), and Forsyth Dental Center (Lobene, 1974). Experimentation included dental hygienists cutting tooth structure to prepare the tooth for a restoration as well as placing and carving the restoration. Dental nurses have had these functions, but U.S. dentists carefully avoided experimenting with dental assistants in restorative functions in the 1960s. The studies were conclusive in proving that cutting hard tooth structure and replacing it with amalgam or tooth-colored restorative materials could be delegated to specially educated dental hygienists without loss of quality. It was also demonstrated that dental hygienists could administer local anesthetic agents. The University of Iowa also assessed hygienists' abilities to accept expanded functions (cutting soft tissue) in periodontics. A similar study was conducted at the University of Pennsylvania (Cohen, 1976). Both demonstrated again that expanded functions could be delegated to dental hygienists without loss of quality and with patient acceptance.

On the basis of quality of care, patient acceptance, relative cost of educating auxiliaries rather than dentists, and the effect such personnel utilization could have on productivity in delivering dental care, the studies pointed directly toward delegating those functions to dental hygienists.

Supporters of that move cited the dental hygienist's substantial background in behavioral and clinical sciences as a solid basis on which to build expanded functions (Barish and Barish, 1971; Diefenbach, 1971; Lobene, 1974; Lobene et al., 1974). The fact that hygienists have an established national educational system and licensure mechanism was offered as further reason to consider the hygienist as a primary person to accept expanded functions in cutting hard and soft tissue and in administering local anesthesia. For persons concerned about a systematic program for preparing expanded functions personnel and then regulating their practice, these arguments were convincing.

There have been almost no opportunities, however, for implementation of these concepts in the health care system since few dental practice acts have been sufficiently altered to permit the delegation of restorative or advanced periodontal functions to licensed dental hygienists, regardless of their advanced educational preparation. In many licensing jurisdictions, the dental hygienist is still primarily described legally and in practice as the prevention-oriented person who may legally perform only the oral prophylaxis, preliminary oral examinations, fluoride applications, and patient education.

DENTAL AUXILIARIES IN OTHER COUNTRIES

Other countries have introduced various kinds of dental auxiliaries as direct providers of care, with many patterned after the scope of practice and the educational programs of those of the United States. Nigeria, Argentina, Brazil, Canada, Colombia, Mexico, Uruguay, Iran, Egypt, the Netherlands, Norway, Sweden, the United Kingdom, India, Thailand, Australia, Fiji, Japan, Saudi Arabia, Israel, Poland, and Korea have one or more educational programs to prepare dental hygienists (Curry et al., 1974; Myers, 1972). The first country to follow suit in developing the profession of dental hygiene was the United Kingdom, which introduced this auxiliary in 1944. In

1948 Japan introduced the dental hygienist and developed 63 programs to prepare persons for practice (Myers, 1972).

The United States may have established the model for dental hygiene, but it cannot claim the development of the dental nurse. New Zealand in 1921 introduced the dental nurse concept (Friedman, 1972; Gladstone, 1975). Dental nurses in New Zealand provide direct patient care to children in schools, but in addition to providing oral examinations, prophylaxes, fluoride applications, and patient education they are trained to prepare (cut) and restore deciduous and permanent teeth, to polish amalgam restorations, to perform pulp capping, to extract deciduous teeth, and to refer patients to private dentists for more complex services, including extraction of permanent teeth, restoration of fractured permanent incisors, and orthodontic care. They perform diagnosis and treatment planning. While the dental hygienist was developing in the United States in a preventive mode, the dental nurse was developing in New Zealand, providing both preventive and therapeutic services for children (Friedman, 1972; Gladstone, 1975; Roemer, 1975).

Just as a number of countries adopted the dental hygiene model in developing dental auxiliaries, many of the same countries and other countries opted for auxiliaries similar to the dental nurse model, permitting such direct patient care auxiliaries to provide, in varying ways, many basic restorative and therapeutic as well as preventive services to patients.

Dental nurses and therapists practice in Australia, Brunei, Burma, Canada, Ceylon, Colombia, Costa Rica, Cuba, Ghana, Haiti, Hong Kong, Indonesia, Italy, Jamaica, Kenya, New Zealand, Nigeria, Papua New Guinea, Paraguay, Senegal, Sierra Leone, Sudan, Singapore, South Vietnam, Taiwan, Thailand, Uganda, the United Kingdom, and Zambia (Roder, 1978).

The papers developed for the International Symposia on Dental Hygiene during the 1970s and 1980s provide a great deal of interesting information about the specific patterns of development and utilization that characterize many of the dental hygiene and other operating auxiliary concepts adopted by various countries.

In some countries there are distinctly separate roles for the dental hygienist and the restorative dental nurse. The United Kingdom provides a case in point. There are educational programs to prepare dental hygienists who perform the traditional functions related to prevention. And there was until recently an educational program to prepare dental therapists (called New Cross Dental Auxiliaries until 1979) who provide restorative and other expanded functions that are not in the realm of the dental hygienist. These two auxiliaries were not educated together nor did they usually function in the same practice setting after their education was completed. Dental hygienists mostly work in the private sector for individual practitioners, but the dental therapist is required to work within the dental hospital facilities or school health clinics (Holt and Murray, 1980; Millward, 1967).

Dental nurses have been functional in the northwest territories of Canada and in Saskatchewan for some years (Curry et al., 1974; Roemer, 1975). Countries with large underdeveloped areas such as Canada have found the dental nurse to be a primary means of extending care where dentists are not available. Also in Canada dental hygienists have been granted expanded functions in addition to their more traditional preventive role. In the mid-1960s prosthetic skills were delegated to licensed hygienists. Later operative functions were delegated to hygienists and prosthetic functions to dental technicians. The dental hygienist in the United States experienced some of this trend, largely through experimental programs that showed that restorative and periodontal functions can be delegated to dental hygienists.

The Federation Dentaire Internationale (FDI) laid out training requirements and career strata for dental auxiliaries that meet the majority of criteria established in countries that have auxiliary education programs (FDI, 1983). The four major strata are dental assisting, expanded functions dental auxiliary practice, dental hygiene, and dental therapy. Educational preparation expands for each strata. The strata have additional sublevels to account for length of training and experience.

The World Health Organization is considering strategies for controlling worldwide dental disease. One strategy presented (Songpaison, 1983) sees dentists providing leadership in planning, developing, monitoring, and evaluating programs, acting as specialists for complex care, and supervising auxiliaries. Auxiliaries will provide routine curative and restorative services. A midlevel group, "primary health care personnel," will be responsible for health education, provide preventive services and examine and refer those needing routine and complex care to auxiliaries and specialists. Thus, dental personnel other than the dentist are seen as critical components of a plan to help control the rise in dental caries in third-world countries and the continuing problem with periodontal disease.

ROLE SATISFACTION AND POSSIBLE GROWTH

Dental assisting and expanded function dental auxiliaries who emphasize restorative care are not currently experiencing a growth in demand. Demand for restorative care may rise in the future if large segments of the population seek care and need restorative services. Also, the "baby boomers" reaching middle age are doing so with teeth (with a much lower edentulous rate compared to previous generations); therefore there is a higher risk of caries activity for this age group (Douglass and Gammon, 1984). Whether they will experience caries or exhibit low levels of caries (typical of today's children) will determine the strength of demand for restorative care.

Population trends strongly indicate that there will be a demand for periodontal care in the coming decades. Adults with teeth are at even higher risk of periodontal disease than caries. Dental hygiene should be in demand for preventive and periodontal care.

In order to provide this care, hygienists will need the legal and practical feedom to provide the full range of services necessary for at least pre-surgical preparation, including root planing and curettage, periodontal pack placement and removal, and related pain control. A hygienist must be taught these functions, but some states limit what a hygienist can learn based upon current state law rather than upon the full scope of functions possible in other states (Legislative action, 1985). While 48 states permit root planing, only 34 permit curettage, only 13 permit administration of nitrous oxide-oxygen conscious sedation, and only 13 permit administration of local anesthesia (Legislative action, 1985), legally limiting the ability of hygienists to deliver complete pre-surgical care. In addition, there are practical limitations placed on the functions a hygienist can perform regardless of whether it is legally allowable. A hygienist working in a dental office or program is subject to the employer's decisions regarding scope of practice. Thus, a hygienist's variety of skills is limited by education, law, and the inclinations of the employer. This has an impact on the availability of care for the public and also upon hygienists' views of role satisfaction.

A survey of 16 graduating classes (1963-78) from Fones School of Dental Hygiene revealed that among the 316 respondents, job satisfaction is high. Although hygienists scored higher than technicians and paraprofessionals (purported to be comparable job classifications) on most dimensions, they scored lower than the other two groups in the areas of skill variety, task significance, experienced meaningfulness of work, and dealing with others. This supports the findings of several previous studies that show that hygienists are unhappy with the limitations placed upon their scope of work and upon career advancement (Sodano et al., 1984).

Another survey, this one of University of Michigan students and alumni, demonstrated that students expect a broader range of functions in daily practice than experienced by the alumni. It also concluded that hygienists who have a broad scope of functions in practice are more likely to report high job satisfaction (Farrugia, 1984). This study directly supports an earlier survey of practicing hygienists in California. Respondents in that investigation were more likely to report job satisfaction if they were practicing expanded functions and were not limited to traditional skills (Lawson and Martinoff, 1980).

A survey of a group of 111 hygienists attending a continuing education course found that the respondents generally were satisfied with dental hygiene, but that they had decreased feelings of accomplishment (Deckard and Rountree, 1984), a finding that fits with the other studies of hygienists' attitudes.

Generally speaking dental hygienists feel good about their work, but they need additional opportunities and the freedom to perform a variety of skills. In many ways, these factors may contribute toward the independent practice movement as much as the need for financial freedom and responsibility.

Independent practice

Independent practice is a controversial movement (Schwager, 1981). Some hygienists believe they can serve the public better and be unencumbered by the economic woes and the practice restrictions of an employer-dentist if they function in their own businesses, making referrals as necessary to dentists.

So far this is legal in only one licensing jurisdiction, Colorado (Colorado, 1986). However, hygienists have successfully established their own practices in several states, sometimes with a contractual agreement with a nearby dentist who serves as the legal ''supervisor.'' In one case, the hygienist has hired a dentist to work in the practice as an associate, thereby meeting the state's requirements for onsite supervision. Nonetheless, the hygienists are financially independent

and enjoy a greater sense of professional freedom and responsibility (O'Hehir, 1981; Schulz, 1981).

Other hygienists describe their financial situation as that of an independent contractor. It is often similar to the contractual arrangement made between a dentist who owns a practice and an associate dentist who works in the practice. The hygienist collects the fees for dental hygiene care and pays the dentist a certain portion for rent, utilities, and other specific expenses. The hygienist then pays taxes, social security obligations, and other professional expenses, and clears the remainder as net income (Woodall and Bentley, 1981).

As hygienists push for greater financial and professional freedom, the controversy will no doubt heighten. The majority of dental hygienists responding to a survey published in *RDH* favor having the legal option to practice independently from a dentist (Woodall, 1986). Organized dentistry continues to state its objections, claiming that the quality of care delivered to the public will suffer. Legislative activity began to focus on this issue in 1985; it will probably be the critical issue of the late 1980s.

Legislative change

There was a great deal of legislative activity in 1985. By April of that year, 17 states and the District of Columbia had legislation introduced to alter the legal practice of dental hygiene. Several of the states were considering laws that would give hygienists freedom to provide care with less supervision, in some cases the freedom to practice independently. Several states were seeking to add expanded functions to the hygienists' scope of practice, and others were seeking changes that would add a dental hygienist to the regulatory board (Legislation & Litigation 110: 605).

In 1985 the Hawaii Dental Practice Act was amended to permit dental hygienists to administer intraoral infiltration of local anesthetics under the direct supervision of a dentist. It also was amended to state that no dental hygienist may establish or operate any separate care facility that exclusively provides dental hygiene services (Legislation & Litigation 110:691).

The New Mexico dental law was amended also. Hygienists are permitted to perform all their traditional functions under general supervision; infiltration anesthesia under the indirect supervision of a dentist (must be present in the facility) was added to the scope of practice (Legislation & Litigation 111:375).

The Washington State dental practice act may undergo revision to permit independent practice. This move was recommended by the state's health coordinating council. The council also recommended that hygienists have their own examining committee (Legislation & Litigation 110:851).

The Federal Trade Commission (FTC) has studied the market restraints placed upon the dental hygienists by the state dental laws that prohibit independent practice. While the FTC has set aside the investigation until studies of the impact of independent practice upon consumer access and quality of care are conducted, it considers the topic open for discussion. The American Dental Hygienists' Association (ADHA) joined with other groups to influence the U.S. Congress to permit continued jurisdiction of the FTC over the professions, which makes it possible for hygienists to explore this avenue for change as they move toward financial and professional independence (FTC, 1984).

The issues relating to increased autonomy for dental hygiene will be a major topic of debate in the coming decade as the expanded functions movement waits for a more favorable time to re-emerge.

Hygienists can become involved in the issues and contribute financially to help support efforts to influence congressional decision making that affects health care in general and dental hygiene specifically. The ADHA HY-PAC is "a voluntary, nonprofit committee of dental hygienists, their spouses and citizens-at-large, who are interested in participating directly in our nation's political process by supporting specific candidates during their election campaigns for U.S. House and Senate seats" (Stanaland, 1985). While this political action committee may not be as large as the lobbying efforts made by dental organizations, it is one method for hygienists to feel their interests are transmitted to the legislators.

Changes in need and demand for health care

Changing patterns in oral health have been reported around the world. While there has been a sharp rise in caries in third-world countries, predictions are that caries can and will be brought under control through the use of fluorides and other preventive methods and to a lesser extent through the introduction of the auxiliary personnel to help restore diseased teeth, as was accomplished in New Zealand and Great Britain. In the meantime, developed countries are showing dramatically decreased caries rates. By 1985, two of the three schools for restorative dental nurses in New Zealand were closed, as was the school for dental therapists in London, England (Ibikunle, 1985).

In a survey of 36 dental schools from 22 countries, six respondents reported a decrease in periodontal disease, ten reported an increase, while the remainder reported no change. Dental caries was reported as decreasing in prevalence in 27 countries and rising in only 7 (Allen, 1985).

It is unlikely that there will be an increase in demand for restorative care among the U.S. population that currently regularly seeks dental care. Dental caries has decreased dramatically in prevalence among young people, with 37% of people under the age of 17 in 1982 having had no dental caries (Dental Statistics, 1984). Dentists can expect to provide less restorative care for that group and thus have less need for expanded-function auxiliaries performing restorative care.

A "more favorable time" could emerge if that portion of the population which does not currently seek dental care decides to knock at dentistry's door. There is still a substantial unmet need for dental caries treatment, especially among middle-aged and elderly adults. If a program were developed where those people could be attracted to dentistry, demand would be such that expanded function auxiliaries with skills in restorative care would be needed. As mentioned above, it is unlikely that any government program will fund such an effort. It is more likely that the untreated segment of the population will slowly trickle into dental practices. Demand for care will increase as dental insurance becomes available to those people through employee-benefit programs. It also will rise as the fear of pain and lack of care about one's teeth is outpaced by information regarding the relatively painless approaches to dental care and society's increased expectation that people will have healthy, clean mouths and teeth. Commercial advertising, totaling more than $90 million in 1985 (Freeman, 1986), for home oral care products that mention the importance of dental care may have an impact as well. However, since the increase is likely to be gradual, dentists who currently have open space in their appointment books may be able to handle patients' restorative needs with current staffing.

The greatest demand for auxiliaries in the coming years should be in the area of periodontics—diagnosis, treatment, and prevention. As the caries rate decreases, the need for periodontal care becomes more obvious. Currently such treatment comprises less than 1% of what a dentist does in daily practice (Kaplan et al., 1983). Unfortunately, most dental curriculums spend far greater time preparing dentists for a strong restorative demand than to identify and treat periodontal disease; typically dental hygiene students spend more clinical time working with periodontal patients than do dental students (Mescher, 1984). Meanwhile, more than half of the adult population has some form of the disease—from beginning gingivitis to advanced stages where teeth have lost most supporting bone (Dental Statistics, 1984).

Under continuing education programs sponsored by the Academy of General Dentistry and several dental schools and local groups, general practitioners are being reeducated to identify and treat the disease. This has been the focus of dentistry's efforts to respond to the decrease in dental caries. Likewise, commercial advertising has focused its messages on describing periodontal disease while promoting their products. The population should be learning that they need to see a dentist if their "gums bleed," and dentists should be better prepared to know what to do when those patients appear for care.

A general dentist just learning about periodontal disease, its treatment, and its prevention would do well to employ a dental hygienist to perform soft tissue assessments, perform scaling, root planing, curettage, and routine follow-up evaluations to determine whether further, perhaps surgical, care is needed to arrest the disease (Cohen, 1981; Ley et al., 1984; Schallhorn and Snider, 1981). The hygienist also can provide knowledgeable prevention-education for the patient so that health can be maintained. Few state laws need to be changed to permit this scope of function; these are recognized as traditional functions in most licensing jurisdictions, and hygienists are routinely skilled in these procedures. More often it is a matter of the dentist recognizing that a hygienist can and should perform these services and then taking steps to hire one. One study showed that fewer dentists employed a hygienist in 1984 than in 1983 (Anderson, 1985).

The trends in the population, most notably fluoride's impact on dental caries, and advances in periodontal diagnosis and treatment are driving the changes in dentistry today. Much of the experimentation with restorative functions from previous decades may become a historical footnote if these trends persist. The more traditional functions of the dental hygienist, with increased emphasis upon skilled periodontal scaling and prevention, may very well mark the growth for auxiliaries in the coming decade (Ley et al., 1984).

It will be dental hygiene's responsibility to carry that message to the public seeking periodon-

and to the dentists who currently supply jority of the employment sites for dental ..ygienists. Dental hygienists can become important assets to dentists who never before employed a hygienist or focused much attention on periodontal needs. Hygienists can meet the needs of those patients and pass them on to the dentists for treatment that requires their background and skill.

The development of dental auxiliaries in the coming decade will focus on how the current dental needs of the population are to be met. Development will focus on safe, effective delivery of care. It will also focus on the continued security of the professions.

Dental assistants and expanded function dental auxiliaries with skills in restorative care will continue to play a role in the delivery of those services. It is not expected that this area will grow given the population needs, although, as mentioned earlier, there will be a large adult population with teeth and thus the potential for caries.

Roles for dental hygienists will probably receive more attention, given the traditional role of hygienists as prevention specialists and as primary providers of periodontal care and given the profession's agitation for greater practice and financial autonomy.

Review questions

1. The founder of the profession of dental hygiene was _Dr. Alfred FONES 1906_.
2. The first hygienist was _IRENE NEWMAN_.
3. The original role of the dental hygienist can be briefly described as: _ORal disease prevention_
4. The functions of the New Zealand dental nurse differ from those of the dental hygienist in the United States because of the inclusion of: _prepare teeth for RestoRations, pulp capping, ExT deciduous teeth, Refer to private Drs._
5. What basic expanded functions have most often been included in experimentation with:
   a. Dental assistants? _placement of amal. + composite rest._
   b. Dental hygienists? _prep. teeth for rest, Local anes, perio therapy_
6. What major change in the oral health of the general public will affect how functions are delegated? _moRe perio. therapy than Restorative_
7. What major issue is replacing "expanded functions" as the topic of debate in dental hygiene? _the trend toward independent practice of R.D.H._

GROUP ACTIVITIES

1. Locate the original publications of data of the various experimental programs in extending restorative and periodontal functions to auxiliaries. Discuss the implications and findings of each study in terms of the dental health needs of the population of the United States.
2. Locate articles describing the various operating dental auxiliaries in other countries. Compare and contrast their function and their effectiveness with that of dental auxiliaries in the United States.
3. Poll local dentists or auxiliaries regarding the number of hours spent in providing periodontal treatment and restor-

ative treatment in a given period (week or month) in the practice, the number of procedures that involve dental auxiliaries for direct intraoral care, and which dental auxiliaries are assigned which components of care.
4. Invite local dentists and dental hygienists to discuss how dental hygienists are integrated into various dental practices. Include dentists who do not employ dental hygienists to discuss how periodontal and preventive care is delivered in the practice.
5. Scan the dental literature of the past year for articles that discuss changes in the demand for dental care, the caries and periodontal prevalence in the population, and changes in use of auxiliaries.

6. Read about the history of the American Dental Assistants' Association in the September/October 1984 issue of *The Dental Assistant*.

REFERENCES

Abramowitz, J., and Berg, L.E.: A four-year study of utilization of dental assistants with expanded functions, J. Am. Dent. Assoc. **87**:623, 1973.

Albertini, T.F., Hillsman, J.T., and Crawford, B.L.: Federal financing of dental services, J. Dent. Educ. **48**:606, 1984.

Allen, D.L.: The implications of changing patterns in oral health for dental education, Int. Dent. J. **35**:83, 1985.

American Association of Public Health Dentists, Subcommittee on Preventive Periodontics: Periodontal disease in America: a personal and national tragedy, J. Public Health Dent. **43**:106, 1983.

Anderson, P.E.: Staff salaries level or down for 1983, Dent. Econ. **75**(2):46, 1985.

Barish, A.M., and Barish, N.H.: Will dental hygiene become obsolete? J. Am. Dent. Hyg. Assoc. **45**:47, 1971.

Cohen, D.W.: University of Pennsylvania: Personal communication, 1976.

Cohen, D.W.: Dental education of the future, J. Dent. Educ. **45**:713, 1981.

Colorado passes unsupervised practice, ADA News, American Dental Assoc. **17**(10):5, 1986.

Council on Dental Education Annual Report, Chicago, 1965, American Dental Association.

Council on Dental Education Annual Report, Chicago, 1976, American Dental Association.

Curry, T.M., et al.: Saskatchewan studies with the British dental auxiliary model. In Lucaccini, L.F., and Handley, J., editors: Research in the use of expanded function auxiliaries, Bethesda, Md., 1974, U.S. Dept. of Health, Education, and Welfare, PHS-HRA, Bureau of Health Resources Development, Division of Dentistry.

Deckard, G.J., and Rountree, B.: Burnout in dental hygiene, Dent. Hyg. **59**(7):307, 1984.

Dental statistics handbook, Chicago, 1984, American Dental Association.

Diefenbach, V.: The 1970s: a new era for dental auxiliaries, J. Am. Dent. Hyg. Assoc. **45**:50, 1971.

Douglass, C.W.: Utilization of expanded duty dental assistants in a solo private practice. In Lucaccini, L.F., and Handley, J., editors: Research in the use of expanded function auxiliaries, Bethesda, Md., 1974, U.S. Dept. of Health, Education, and Welfare, PHS-HRA, Bureau of Health Resources Development, Division of Dentistry.

Douglass, C., and Gammon, M.D.: The epidemiology of dental caries and its impact on the operative dentistry curriculum, J. Dent. Educ. **48**:547, 1984.

Farrugia, N.S.: Traditional functions and job and career satisfaction, Dent. Hyg. **58**(7):300, 1984.

Federation Dentaire Internationale, Technical Report No. 19, Classification of dental auxiliary personnel based on strata training concepts, Int. Dent. J. **33**:308, 1983.

Fones, A.C.: The origin and history of the dental hygienist movement. In Fones, A.C., editor: Mouth hygiene, Philadelphia, 1927, Lea & Febiger.

Freeman, L.: Plaque fighters cool pursuit of ADA seal, Advertising Age **57**(5):36, 1986.

Friedman, J.W.: The New Zealand School Dental Service: lesson in radical conservatism. Presented at the Conference of Dental Examiners and Dental Educators, Chicago, February 11-12, 1972.

The FTC and the professions: an exclusive interview with FTC Commissioner Patricia P. Bailey, Dent. Hyg. **59**(9):394, 1984.

Gladstone, R.N.: International dental nurse programs, Dent. Hyg. **49**:169, 1975.

Hammons, P.E., Jamieson, H.C., and Wilson, L.L.: Quality of service provided by dental therapists in an experimental program at the University of Alabama, J. Am. Dent. Assoc. **82**:1060, 1971.

Hengl, R.D.: Certification: content and procedures, Dent. Assisting **3**(4):37, 1984.

Holt, R.D., and Murray, J.J.: An evaluation of the role of the New Cross Dental Auxiliaries and of their clinical contribution to the community dental services, Br. Dent. J. **149**:227, 1980.

Ibikunle, S.A.: The implications of changing patterns in oral health for the general practice of dentistry, Int. Dent. J. **35**:77, 1985.

Kaplan, A.L., Bader, J.D., Mullins, M.R., and Lange, K.W.: Measurement of effects of a state dental practice act on potential delegation and production in general dental private practice, J. Public Health Dent. **43**:161, 1983.

Latzkar, S.J., Johnson, D.W., and Thompson, M.B.: Experimental program in expanded functions for dental assistants: phase III experiment with dental teams, J. Am. Dent. Assoc. **82**:1067, 1971.

Lawson, E.S., and Martinoff, J.T.: Dental hygienists' perception of satisfaction in the private dental office, Dent. Hyg. **54**(2):74, 1980.

Legislation & Litigation, J. Am. Dent. Assoc. **110**:691, 1985; **110**:375, 1985; **110**:605, 1985; **110**:851, 1985.

Legislative action packet: A comparative overview of 51 practice acts, Chicago, 1985, American Dental Hygienists' Association.

Ley, E., Aker, D., and Mounts, C.: Maintenance of an adequate dental hygiene education system, J. Dent. Educ. **48**:556, 1984.

Lobene, R.R.: The Forsyth study of new duties for dental hygienists. In Lucaccini, L.F., and Handley, J., editors: Research in the use of expanded function auxiliaries, Bethesda, Md., 1974, U.S. Dept. of Health, Education and

Welfare, PHS-HRA, Bureau of Health Resources Development, Division of Dentistry.

Lobene. R.R.: Personal communication, January, 1986.

Lobene, R.R., et al.: The Forsyth experiment in training of advanced skill hygienists, J. Dent. Educ. **38**:369, 1974.

Ludwig, W.E., et al.: Report of clinical tests, Greater utilization of dental technicians, Dental Research facility, U.S. Navy Training Center, Great Lakes, Ill., May 1964.

Malvitz, D.M., and Mocniak, N.: Profile of dental hygienists licensed in the United States, J. Public Health Dent. **42**:54, 1982.

Mescher, K.D.: A new look at the educational preparation of dental hygienists: exploding the myths, Dent. Hyg. **58**(2):69, 1984.

Millward, E.: Dental auxiliaries: four years on, Dental Health (Brit.) **6**:15, 1967.

Motley, W.: Ethics, jurisprudence and history for the dental hygienist, ed. 3, Philadelphia, 1983, Lea & Febiger.

Myers, S.E.: Operating dental auxiliaries, WHO Chron. **26**:511, 1972.

O'Hehir, T.: Interview with Linda Krol, RDH, **1**(3):30, 1981.

Powell, W.O., et al.: Comparison of clinical performance of dental therapist trainees and dental students, J. Dent. Educ. **38**:268, 1974.

Redig, D., et al.: Expanded duty dental auxiliaries in four private dental offices: the first year's experience, J. Am. Dent. Assoc. **88**:969, 1974.

Report of the Inter-agency Committee on Dental Auxiliaries, J. Am. Dent. Assoc. **84**:1027, 1972.

Results of 1984 ADAA salary survey, Dent. Asst. **54**(1):7, 1985.

Roder, D.J.: The employment of dental nurses, J. Public Health Dent. **38**:159, 1978.

Roemer, R.: Credentialing dental auxiliary personnel in the United States and selected other countries. In Proceedings of the workshop on changing roles of dental auxiliaries, Bethesda, Md., 1975, U.S. Dept. of Health, Education and Welfare, PHS-HRA, Bureau of Health Manpower, Division of Dentistry.

Schallhorn, R.G., and Snider, L.E.: Periodontal maintenance therapy, J. Am. Dent. Assoc. **103**:227, 1981.

Schulz, D.: Out-on-a-limb and lovin' it, RDH **1**(3):14, 1981.

Schwager, M.: Hygiene independence: the dentists' reactions, RDH **1**(3):39, 1981.

Sisty, N.L.: Expanded-function dental hygiene student performance evaluations, Dent. Hyg. **49**:401, 1975.

Sisty, N.L., et al.: Evaluation of student performance in the four-year study of expanded functions for dental hygienists at the University of Iowa, J. Am. Dent. Assoc. **97**:613, 1978.

Sisty, N.L., et al.: Review of training and evaluation studies in expanded functions for dental auxiliaries, J. Am. Dent. Assoc. **98**:233, 1979.

Sodano, V.L., Javian, S., and Judd, B.B. Jr.: Job satisfaction in dental hygiene—fact or fiction? Dent. Hyg. **58**(8):346, 1984.

Songpaison, Y.: Manpower and the future role of dentistry in developing countries, Int. Dent. J. **33**:308, 1983.

Spohn, E.: Background and transition of the expanded duty program. In Agenda material for the meeting of the Educational Advisory Committee for the University of Kentucky expanded duty dental hygiene research program, June 1975.

Stanaland, J.: ADHA Hy-Pac letter, Chicago, 1985.

Woodall, I.: Survey of dental hygienists' values, RDH **6**(2):144, 1986.

Woodall, I., and Bentley, M.: Independent contracting as an alternative financial arrangement, RDH **1**(3):46, 1981.

CHAPTER 3

Health care delivery settings and systems and the concept of team health care

OBJECTIVES: The reader will be able to:

1. Describe briefly the traditional system of delivery of dental health care services, including the following:
   a. Practice settings.
   b. Payment mechanisms.
   c. Patient access to care.
   d. Utilization of health care providers in the system.
2. Summarize the movement toward the development of team dental health care.
3. Explain why a dentist might decide to join a health maintenance organization (HMO) or preferred provider organization (PPO).
4. Describe the major factors that have influenced recent changes in dentistry, including the following:
   a. Acceptance of professional advertising.
   b. Advent of retail and franchise practices.
   c. Increased competition among dentists.
   d. Increased emphasis upon cost containment.
   e. Decrease in caries prevalence.
5. Explain how the prevalence of periodontal disease may change how auxiliaries are utilized in dental practice.

PRESENT SYSTEM OF DENTAL CARE SERVICES

The present system for the delivery of dental care is quite different from what existed in the early 1960s. There have been, of course, major technological changes in how dentistry is practiced. Composite restorations have replaced the silicate restoration for anterior teeth, and silver alloy is far superior to its earlier versions. Methods for removing decay are much faster and less traumatic than earlier methods. Pain control is more effective. Advances in understanding dental disease have basically altered the way dentistry and dental hygiene are practiced.

Dental care delivery has changed in more ways than simply how specific treatment is provided. Attention is given to efficient, nonstressful, ergonomic approaches to how a given dental appointment is conducted. Dental auxiliaries are available to provide many of the functions previously reserved for the dentist. There are more dentists to provide care. Dental care is delivered in a greater variety of sites than it used to be, and the mechanisms for payment are quite different.

These changes have affected the availability of dental care to the population. The usual "access" issues in dental care remain intact; many people are still without adequate care. But there have been changes that make it possible for a larger percentage of the population to obtain care.

Dental care settings

For the most part, dentistry has functioned as a cottage industry. Traditional delivery of dental care occurs in isolated practice settings where individual providers of care (dentists) provide dental services to which the patient agrees. The dentist typically makes him/herself available for appointments during given hours in an office or clinic setting and attempts to meet the needs of the patients as they appear. There is no concerted, organized national or regional program to attract patients to dental care, and for the most part dental care is quite separate from any of the other health care experiences a patient may have.

The efficiency, pleasantness of care, and settings of the dental profession have been modified over the past 100 years as dental equipment became more functional, attractive, and more in keeping with minimal patient and operator discomfort. Practice settings have moved from Spartan environments to comfortable bungalow offices and medical arts buildings. Dental practices are more common in hospitals than they were, and they often are part of a larger ambulatory health care group. Dental care can also be obtained in retail stores, a phenomenon that was unheard of 20 years ago (Rovin and Nash, 1982).

Cost issues

Dental care, particularly regular, preventive dental care, has been more common among the middle and upper classes of the United States. This was partly a result of the community's view of the relative unimportance of dental care in overall health, but it was also caused by an economic factor. Dentistry until the mid-1960s was almost exclusively a fee-for-service enterprise (Rovin and Nash, 1982). Patients paid for each service from their private financial resources. There were almost no mechanisms for prepaid dentistry and very little dental insurance. Dental services therefore tended to be available only to those persons who were financially secure. Now, with health maintenance organizations and other forms of insurance, persons can subscribe to health care on an annual basis and be assured that needed care will be provided. The large labor unions have been able to negotiate for and obtain dental care benefits so that workers and their families are able to have dental care reimbursed through the company's insurance plan when it is needed or prepaid through a capitation plan. In addition, public funds are available in some states to pay for care for special beneficiary groups, such as the aged and children (Albertini et al., 1984).

Access issues

Improved access to health care implies more than providing the financial resources. Despite the fact that the patient may be able to have dental care paid for in its entirety, people still are not always able to receive the care they need (Colchamiro, 1976). Several reasons for this include the fact that the health care facility may be open on weekdays from 9 A.M. to 5 P.M., but the patient may not be able to come at those times because of conflicts with a work schedule. Perhaps transportation is not available to the site; the number of forms that need to be completed for each visit and the complexity of making an appointment may be more than the patient is able or willing to endure in obtaining health care. The more complex reasons include the possibility that patients covered by an insurance plan cannot locate a care facility willing to accept the plan. Or the plan itself may not provide realistic levels of payments for services provided, causing reimbursement to be insufficient for the requirements of various procedures, unless the patients supplement the plan's allotted amount with their own funds.

Attitudes affect access, also. People do not view dental disease as a life or death matter. Dental problems may cause a person great discomfort, but they rarely involve the life-threatening impact of many medical problems. As a result, the public often views dentistry as a luxury rather than a necessity, especially when financial resources are minimal.

Another major attitude barrier to receiving dental care is the population's fear of oral pain. Anesthesia by oral injection, the sound and vibration of the drill, the possibility of excruciating pain if anesthesia is not sufficient, and the dull pain that characterizes the aftereffects of having had several pieces of equipment and two pairs of hands in one's mouth all keep people away from the dentist. Even though dentistry is technologically miles ahead of its cumbersome and painful practice of previous decades, there are many skeptics who would rather suffer at home with painful teeth than suffer in a dental chair.

A broader issue related to access to health care is the problem of geographic distribution of health care providers. Certain segments of the population may not have access to care because the providers are not available in certain areas. This is often the case in rural areas and sometimes in the inner city. Very often the treatment facilities are clustered together in areas where care is already plentiful and accessible (Born, 1975).

The issues of access to and cost of care are problems common to both medicine and dentistry, but they may be compounded in dentistry since most providers are still operating largely independently of any larger system of health care planning to assess where care is most needed and how plans can be made to provide it.

Quality issues

Ensuring the *quality of care* is an issue related to past and current health care delivery systems. In the hospital or clinics in which a number of providers have frequent opportunities to review each other's performance in diagnosis and treatment, the elements of at least a rudimentary peer review mechanism exist. And in instances in which third-party payers, such as insurance carriers and public agencies, are paying for care, there may be more formal review mechanisms for individual providers and individual patient cases.

For these reasons, medicine has been involved on a more continuing basis with the issue of assessing the quality of care. In dentistry, especially in solo practices in which it is unlikely that another dentist may regularly see the work and in which third-party payers have been less common, the external constraints and reviews are less frequent. Only in the past 10 years has dentistry begun to formalize review mechanisms to assess the quality of care being rendered (Klyop, 1985; Milgrom, 1978).

Resource issues: dental auxiliaries

Another characteristic of the dental care delivery system is the proportionately fewer auxiliary personnel who are fully utilized in the provision of care. The dental hygienist, as noted earlier, is the only long-standing direct patient care auxiliary in dentistry. Dental assistants have been utilized as support personnel for many years, but they have been used to full advantage only since 1961, when attention was turned to the most efficient ways to provide care in dentistry. Recent literature indicates that many practitioners still use few auxiliaries and perhaps do not utilize the auxiliaries they do employ to their fullest potential.

One survey shows that 53.9% of all dentist respondents have only one assistant (Anderson, 1985), hardly enough to support a vigorous delegation of intraoral functions. Despite the growth in the number of hygienists, fewer than half of the dentists surveyed employ one. While the number of hygienists available for employment increased, the percentage of dentists employing hygienists actually decreased (Anderson, 1985). Furthermore, dentists have not generally delegated a substantial portion of delegable services to assistants and hygienists. In a study of 113 dental practices in Washington State, approximately 38% of what is delegable is delegated to auxiliaries (Chapko et al., 1985). A study of 14 Kentucky practices, found to be statistically representative of 76% of the practices in that state, showed that while 58.7% of all production was legally delegable to auxiliaries, practices varied greatly in what portion was actually delegated (Kaplan et al., 1983; Mullins et al., 1983).

The dental laboratory technician is viewed by organized dentistry as an auxiliary, along with the dental hygienist and the dental assistant. The dental laboratory technician fabricates appliances and prostheses according to the specifications of the dentist. The dental laboratory technician supports dental services in the laboratory rather than the operatory. Dental laboratory technicians, however, often choose to disavow themselves of the auxiliary concept and prefer to be acknowledged as free-enterprise business persons who contractually provide dentists with services they need performed by constructing intraoral appliances and prostheses. Those technicians who work directly with the dentist at the delivery site are more amenable to accepting the role or label of an auxiliary to the dentist.

Some laboratory technicians want authority to provide direct care to patients. This movement has been labeled *denturism*. The basic argument is whether a technician ought to be legally allowed to prepare dentures and removable partial dentures from start to finish for patients. Some technicians argue that their expertise ought to permit them to do this. In their testimony before various state legislatures in an attempt to modify the law to permit denturism, technicians cite the high cost of dentures prepared by dentists compared to the actual construction cost of the devices. Their primary argument is that they can provide dentures to patients at a lower cost than dentistry can—and that care may be more readily available if technicians are allowed to provide these services for patients (Hazelkorn and Christoffel, 1984).

Dentists complain that denturists would want to have the patient's teeth out and would not emphasize prevention of tooth loss; denturists counter that only dentists can remove teeth—the denturist has no say in the matter. Other dentists' concerns include the possibility that denturists would not use appropriate sterilization techniques; denturists

state that the same equipment and techniques available to dentists are available to them. One of dentistry's complaints, that fees for dentures would be just as high when delivered by denturists, has not been proven. After several decades of denturism in British Columbia, Canada, denturists fees remain half of what dentists typically charge (Hazelkorn and Christoffel, 1984). Further, a study conducted 6 years after the legalization of denturism in Oregon shows that the consumer price index (CPI) for all dental services was 14% above the expected value, but that denture prices were 15 to 20% below the expected value. Prices for dentures stabilized in that state (Rosenstein et al., 1985).

Despite the opposition of dentistry, the practice of denturism is legal in six states: Arizona, Colorado, Maine, Oregon, Idaho, and Montana. In Arizona, the state law requires that the patient see a dentist first for a thorough oral evaluation. Colorado and Maine state that the denturist must function under the general supervison of a dentist, and Oregon requires a dentists' examination and a statement of health. Idaho's law is one of the least restrictive, since denturists have their own licensing board (Hazelkorn, 1984). Montana approved an initiative in 1984 to establish a board of denturity and permit denturists to make and fit both full and partial dentures and to take radiographs of their denture patients. It was under challenge in 1985 by legislation brought by the dental association (Legislation & Litigation 110: 606).

Four other states, Michigan, Mississippi, North Dakota, and Washington, had legislation introduced during 1985 that would legalize denturists (Legislation & Litigation 110:606).

Hazelkorn describes the growth of the denturist movement as a sign that the political power and esteem of the profession are being tempered and that consumers are more likely to make decisions based on their own values than on those suggested by the professions. He also posits that if dentistry could achieve a cooperative relationship with denturists they might find a larger patient pool developing for general dentistry as people who have avoided the dentist seek advice from denturists.

A similar cooperative arrangement could develop between dental hygienists and dentists. Patients afraid of "needles and drills" might seek out care from dental hygienists, who can then wean them over to dentistry for restorative and other advanced care.

In summary, dental care delivery systems tend to be separated from other health care providers. Individual practitioners provide care as people present themselves for treatment, making payment through dental insurance or on a fee-for-service basis. Access to care varies with geographical location and financial resources. Practice sites may cluster in some areas and be totally inaccessible in others. There has been no formal widespread system of formalized peer review in dentistry, and auxiliary personnel remain underutilized and continue to function under the direct supervision of the dentist, with the exception of denturists and some dental hygienists who have made inroads into independent practice.

RECENT CHANGES IN THE SYSTEM
Advertising and competition

Until recently dental care delivery has been basically unchanged from the solo practitioner mode described earlier. Although there has been slow growth in the number of dentists who utilize dental auxiliaries, the system is not much different from what it was 20 or even 30 years ago. The changes that many dentists would consider major have occurred since 1976, when the U.S. Supreme Court made it illegal for professional associations to prevent their members from advertising. Business concerns began to market dentistry and to house services within shopping malls and retail department stores. Franchises were developed and sold to dentists to enable them to capitalize on their collective promotional strength (Rovin and Nash, 1982).

In the 1960s and 1970s many dentists were concerned that the federal government was trying to change the face of dentistry with its funding of experimental programs. It now appears that the most startling change ironically comes from the bastion of free enterprise. The retail dental clinics and franchises are using a free, competitive system to make dentistry more cost-effective and to meet the needs of the consumers who needed dental care but had not sought it. Their target was the large segment of the population that found dental care to be overpriced, inconvenient, and of unpredictable quality. In addition, corporate practices in which a company or corporation established an in-house dental practice to service the needs of its employees and their families have developed (Rovin and Nash, 1982).

The advertising retail or franchise practices and the corporate practices attract not only those patients who have not previously sought dental care but a percentage of those patients who are established with a practitioner. Regardless of the percentage of patients who are lost from independent dental practitioners, this movement is viewed by many dentists with caution and by some with alarm.

This new source of competition has encouraged some dental practices to form a network for purposes of pooling their resources to advertise. The network agrees on a common theme and then promotes its practices with a common advertisement. The advertisement lists all the practices or provides a telephone number interested consumers can call to locate the most convenient practice in the group. No doubt dentists who are interested in preserving their autonomy and also their livelihoods will be turning to this and other innovative strategies that make them more competitive with the larger practices that have greater financial backing and a more sophisticated understanding of marketing and management of systems (Bentley and Woodall, 1984).

New sites and organizations

There are other modes of dental care delivery that are not particularly new but are growing in importance and gaining attention as potentially effective and efficient systems of care for large numbers of consumers. They include health maintenance organizations (HMOs) and hospital dental services.

Health maintenance organizations were designed to promote the prevention of disease by enabling consumers to enroll for an annual fee and then to have access to nearly all health care that was necessary without having to pay additional fees. The theory behind the concept is that providers who receive capitation (a share of the enrollment fee) rather than a fee for each service will practice more conservative treatment and be more interested in maintaining the health of each person rather than treating disease as it occurs (Cowan, 1984). Opponents of the concept explain that it encourages providers to deliver minimal care even when more aggressive treatment is indicated.

A dentist can be an employee of the HMO or agree to treat patients on a capitation basis in his/her own practice. The latter form will probably continue to be more attractive to most established dentists since they can continue to treat other patients on a fee-for-service basis and because their mode of practice is basically unaltered. Two income sources exist: fees from independent patients and the capitation they receive for each organization enrollee. The latter source provides them with a more predictable income as long as the dentist has the resources to treat all the enrolled patients who request care.

Preferred provider organizations (PPOs) are increasing in number in medicine and dentistry. When a dentist joins a PPO, he agrees to provide dental care to patients enrolled in the PPO at discounted fees, which the PPO will pay upon delivery of the service under an insurance arrangement. In return the dentist is given access to a pool of patients who have dental coverage. The PPO directs its efforts at locating dentists who are willing to discount their fees and provide quality care; it then can sell its insurance program to employers and other groups looking for cost effec-

tive health benefits (Council, 1983; Cowan, 1984; Gabel and Ermann, 1985).

The emergence of HMOs, PPOs, and other programs that seek to limit the cost of dental care are signs of one of the major concerns of the 1980s—the delivery of health care in a system that contains costs. Individual dentists are looking for ways to economize while delivering quality care; insurance companies are looking for ways to put a ceiling on prices; and employers are looking for insurance packages that provide good health benefits to employees but that are not exorbitant in cost. This is accompanied by a growing number of people in the population who expect answers to their questions and an emphasis on prevention rather than expensive treatment.

Sites for the delivery of care have changed. Dental services are now available in approximately 50% of hospitals (Hospital Statistics, 1984). Many hospitals are expanding their primary and ambulatory care services in response to decreasing in-patient censuses and increasing difficulty in filling their beds. As a consequence, dental services will be offered as a part of comprehensive primary care programs if for no other reason than to offset losses from decreasing in-patient care (Rovin and Nash, 1982). These groups will no doubt also compete with the private practice of dentistry in providing services to a segment of the community that uses hospital services for most of its health needs.

Movement toward team health care

The efforts that initiated the first substantial changes in the way dentistry is practiced focused on ways to improve the efficiency with which specific intraoral services were performed (Cooper and DiBiaggio, 1979). The 1960s saw the era of time and motion studies, when the procedures performed by dentists were analyzed for the stress and strain they placed on the operator and for the amount of time they consumed. Systems analysts and efficiency experts analyzed the traditional stand-up dentistry approach that used few if any support personnel. They assessed the design of equipment and the manner in which storage was located in the dental operatory. The age of four-handed, sit-down dentistry resulted from these first efforts and established the "chairside dental assistant." This assistant became an active participant in the intraoral procedures provided by the dentist. The assistant passed instruments, aspirated fluids from the oral cavity, prepared materials at chairside for intraoral use, and generally facilitated the efficiency with which each procedure was performed.

In 1961 the federal government funded Dental Auxiliary Utilization programs at dental schools and supported the preparation of instructional materials and courses (Jones, 1977). Dental meetings almost always included lectures and seminars on how to implement four-handed dentistry. A good deal of effort was spent on designing dental equipment that would be compatible with these approaches to the delivery of care. The dental units of the 1940s and 1950s were immovable objects with little flexibility for accommodating dental assisting procedures. It was during this time that the ADA expressed its first significant interest in experimentation with the delegation of additional functions to auxiliaries. The success of four-handed dentistry in reducing chair time and in improving the ease with which various procedures could be performed prompted others to speculate how components of various clinical procedures could be delegated to auxiliaries. Increased efficiency could be achieved to an even greater extent by freeing the dentist to spend more time with the more demanding aspects of dental practice.

The first real focus on the low levels of health in the United States rather than on low productivity came with the publication of the Survey of Dentistry in 1961 (Hollinshead, 1961). The survey estimated that only 40% of Americans were obtaining at least satisfactory dental care and that 700 million cavities were unfilled in the population at that time. Since this report received the attention of the Great Society programs sponsored by the Johnson administration, dental health was in an ideal position to receive a boost from federal funding for programs for people otherwise unable to receive care. As federal money supported programs to provide health care and as national health insurance for all people became a recurring topic of debate in the legislature, the focus in health care became the human resources that would be necessary to deliver the care that would be financially supported.

The Carnegie Commission Report of 1970 projected that there would be a critical manpower shortage in the years to come unless more physicians and dentists were educated and unless additional functions could be delegated to allied health personnel.

The reports stimulated Congress to appropriate large amounts of money to assist dental and medical schools to improve their educational programs and to increase the number of students they were preparing (Schwager, 1981). Congress also funded a new grants program in 1971 called TEAM (Training in Expanded Auxiliary Management) (Jones, 1977; Redig, 1971), which extended beyond the four-handed dentistry concept and supported the learning of methods of delegating intraoral functions to dental auxiliaries. Federal legislation also supported the development of allied health education programs that would prepare personnel for assuming supportive roles in the provision of medical and dental services (USDHEW and USPHS, 1979). Dental hygiene and dental assisting were defined as a part of allied health for purposes of funding.

With federal support available, numerous community colleges and technical institutes started dental assisting and dental hygiene programs along with the myriad of other eligible allied health programs. The biggest growth period in dental hygiene programs occurred when the numbers of programs increased from 56 in 1965 to 183 in 1975. The emphasis was to increase the number of persons available to provide services and to extend various delegable services to auxiliaries.

In 1966 there were 3,072,000 health workers. In 1978 there were 5,412,000. The number of dental hygienists rose from 12,000 to 35,000 during those years, and dental assistants increased from 92,000 to 149,000 (USDHEW and USPHS, 1979).

As described in the previous chapter, dentistry turned first to dental assisting in designing experimental programs for delegating expanded functions. The reasons most frequently cited were (1) dental assistants were not governed by restrictive licensing laws that would inhibit the possibility of expanding their scope of function, (2) there were far more dental assistants (albeit many on-the-job trained) than there were dental hygienists, (3) dental hygienists were rendering an important service, the oral prophylaxis, and would find it difficult to add expanded functions to their responsibilities, (4) it would be difficult to logistically involve a dental hygienist in the provision of restorative care in a dental practice, whereas it would be relatively easy to involve the dental assistant, and (5) dental hygienists demand a higher salary than do dental assistants and therefore are an economic detriment to containing the cost of dental services. Another reason occasionally referred to in the literature is the dental hygienists' collective reticence with regard to expanding their scope of function.

A number of dental hygiene leaders, however, began to reexamine the role of the dental hygienist and to suggest ways in which new functions could be delegated. The broad educational base of the dental hygienist, the already existing curricula, the growing number of dental hygiene programs, and the fact that many dental hygienists believed that they were underutilized in terms of their education prompted a new perception on the part of the profession (Cavicchio, 1971; Gilman, 1977; Hayden, 1971; Mescher, 1972). Hygienists, with the support of interested dentists, began to pursue experimental programs within their own ranks. The Forsyth, Iowa, Kentucky, Howard, and Pennsylvania programs all went beyond the scope of study of the expanded duty dental assistant, since the experiments with dental hygienists involved the administration of local anesthesia, the cutting of preparations for the placement of restorations, and in two studies, gingival recontouring.*

An interesting historical note is that an experimental program to assess how well dental hygienists could learn to prepare children's teeth for the placement of restorations was proposed and funded in 1949 for the Forsyth Dental Center (Lobene et al., 1974; Lobene, 1979). Opposition from within both dentistry and dental hygiene caused the program to close, with the House of Representatives of Massachusetts passing legislation to end the program in 1950 (Hygienists, 1950; Legislation, 1950; Lobene, 1979; Maas, 1950). The Forsyth experiment was closed down again in 1974 as a result of political opposition among dentists in the state.

In 1985, Suffolk County Court turned down the Forsyth Dental Center's request that they be allowed the academic freedom to teach expanded functions to dental hygienists regardless of the provisions of the Massachesetts dental law (Lobene, 1986).

RESISTANCE TO CHANGE

In October 1975 after hearing testimony and reviewing the data available from the experimental programs, the ADA adopted a number of position statements that indicated their decision to pursue such experimental interests no further. A policy adopted in the early 1960s that supported experimentation with auxiliaries and that recommended extending every possible delegable function to auxiliaries was reversed. The House of Delegates of the ADA adopted a position statement that expressed its opposition to auxiliaries placing restorations in teeth that had been prepared by the dentist, thus disclaiming the numerous experimental

---

*References: Cohen, 1976; Lobene et al., 1974; Lobene, 1979; Powell, 1974; Sisty, 1974; Spohn, 1975.

studies performed with dental assistants as well as the more controversial studies utilizing dental hygienists. The association has continued to state its opposition to permitting auxiliaries to diagnose and prescribe, to administer anesthetics, or to cut hard and soft tissues (ADA, 24-1976-H).

Some critics cite these policy statements as denial of the evidence of experimental programs that demonstrate that properly trained hygienists and assistants can perform many of the functions previously reserved for the hands of the dentist. Organized dentistry contended that much of the research has been conducted in settings not reflective of the economic and logistical realities of most practice settings. They said that further research would be needed to determine the efficacy of how such procedures could be delegated. The discussions within the ADA, as described in reports of its continuing workshops regarding appropriate delegation of functions and as voiced in its reference committee hearings at its annual meetings, indicate that the dentists acknowledged that those functions *can* be delegated, but they were not convinced that they *should* be delegated.

Additional research was conducted to respond to these objections and to determine how delegation of functions could help dental practices.

Two studies supported by the American Fund for Dental Health and the Kellogg Foundation were conducted in the early 1980s to evaluate the use of auxiliaries in dental practice. Washington State was the site for one of the studies, where 126 practices employing expanded functions auxiliaries were studied every 6 months for 2 years. The study included extensive evaluation of dental hygienists functioning in expanded roles since they are the only auxiliary permitted by law to place restorations. The other study was conducted in Kentucky (which legally allows dental assistants and dental hygienists to place restorations), where 14 dental practices utilizing dental auxiliaries were studied in depth over a 2-year period (DeFriese et al., 1983).

The issues studied were (1) the reasons expanded functions were attractive to private practice dentists, (2) the characteristics that best predicted success with the scheme, (3) how productivity was influenced by expanded functions, (4) the impact of management training upon expanded functions productivity, (5) the levels of satisfaction of dentists and auxiliaries with expanded function practice, (6) the attitudes of patients toward this style of practice, and (7) differences in quality of care (DeFriese et al., 1983).

Results of the Washington State project suggest that while productivity rises significantly when expanded functions personnel are utilized, costs rise also, thereby resulting in no statistically significant increase in net income when all studied practices were evaluated. Net income did rise for practices having higher levels of delegation. Service mix did not change for the practices using expanded functions; the dentist did not perform increased numbers of complex or different activities. Job satisfaction was high for both dentists and auxiliaries, but dental assistants reported higher fatigue and stress levels when expanded functions were in place. Patients were satisfied with the care they received but were less satisfied with waiting times and with costs than under traditional systems. In general, delegation of services were "associated with more complete patient records, better preparation for emergencies, less use of cold sterilization, and better quality radiographs." In general, the study supported the hypothesis that productivity could rise substantially under this system and that providers and patients would be satisfied with it (Milgrom et al., 1983).

A second report describing the Washington State project found that high quality dental care was provided by most practices participating in the study. Those practices that delegated more tended to have higher quality overall in the structure, process, and outcome of care provided by the auxiliaries. The quality of restorations was highly correlated between expanded function hygienists and their dentists, with hygienists providing slightly lower quality composite restorations. In practices where the dentist attended to the evaluation of restorations placed by dental hygienists, the quality was correspondingly higher (Bergner et al., 1983).

The Kentucky project (Mullins et al., 1983) showed that using expanded function auxiliaries improves the productivity and income of the practice. The degree to which this occurred depended upon patient supply, the dentist's rate of production, number of operatories and staff, and scheduling intensity. There were no differences in quality of restorations placed by dentists and hygienists, and patient acceptance was high. The primary difference in the relative success of expanded functions in the practices was the individual's comfort level with delegation.

Both the Washington State and Kentucky projects supported the results of the previous studies that experimented with expanded functions in school or "nondental practice settings." The researchers concluded that there was no reason to rescind legal changes that extend expanded functions to auxiliaries and that there are numerous advantages to adopting this mode of practice.

Legal restrictions

The position of the ADA in the early 1960s was that dental practice acts would have to change to provide for the delegation of functions to auxiliaries. Many licensing jurisdictions moved rapidly to amend their laws to permit broader scopes of practice for at least the dental assistant, and often for the dental hygienist. Extension of expanded functions to dental auxiliaries rose from 9 states in 1968 to 49 in 1982 (Legislative action, 1985).

Programs preparing dentists to utilize dental auxiliaries in expanded function practice and programs preparing dental auxiliaries revised their curricula to provide the educational base for team practice involving expanded duties. Both the ADAA and ADHA continue their support of the delegation of expanded functions to dental auxiliaries, with their only conditions being that the

person be educated to perform the service and that a single minimum standard of quality of care be utilized to assess the services provided, regardless of who is providing the care (dentist, hygienist, assistant, or EFDA).

The educational programs expressed by means of a position statement from the American Association of Dental Schools (AADS) that they would not endorse pre-1960s utilization patterns in preparing their students for practice. This strong stand caused a separation between dental educators and organized dental practitioners (Jacobs, 1976). Much of the controversy was waged in the arena of academic freedom with individual programs claiming the right to teach whichever functions they chose, regardless of the particular dental law of the state in which the school was located (DiBiaggio, 1975; Robinson, 1976).

The ADA does not support schools teaching functions that cannot be legally performed in practice in that state. AADS policy (17-76-H) states that they ought to be free to do so since they have an obligation to prepare students to obtain licensure and practice in any licensing jurisdiction without requiring extensive additional education beyond traditional, basic preparation. The legal entanglements upheld the right of the state to enjoin those educational programs from teaching beyond that allowed in the letter of the law, thus limiting the opportunity for continued experimentation and precluding the preparation of large numbers of personnel for other states in which the laws are less constraining and health workers are needed (Eglit and Hauber, 1976).

The nuances of the law in each state caused basic dental hygiene education to offer a less generally understood, predictable curriculum. The basic courses may include one or more or none of the various expanded functions depending on the state in which the program is located. Although there is one title for all the persons graduating from those programs, the graduates are in actuality often drastically different from each other in terms of levels of knowledge, in terms of the services they are able to perform, and the competency levels at which they are able to perform them. This is a problem not only in the practice of the profession but in the identification of qualified teachers for educational programs.

Although federal and private funds continued to support experimental and educational programs for a time after the recision of the ADA policies, these funds have disappeared. Current policies espouse less governmental intervention and certainly less financial support of both business and education. Cuts in federal funding have been severe. Foundation funding has turned its attention to other projects. As educational programs accommodate increased financial needs and decreased sources of revenue, the curriculum takes on a back to basics theme from which experimental or nonessential programs are quickly expunged (Rovin and Nash, 1982).

For many auxiliaries it is difficult to understand why, despite the quality of care they learned to provide, dentistry chooses to oppose its being delegated to them. The hygienist who has learned to provide periodontal therapy may view the policy reversal and the subsequent stalling of progress in the delegation of functions as an unreasonable narrowing of his/her scope of function and as a step backward into a less challenging role in providing care. Dental assistants may see their opportunity for long-overdue, proper recognition of certification slipping away, along with the potential for a reasonable income level. And the EFDA trained specifically for restorative functions may feel and be totally obsolete.

The reversal is easily understood. It is frequently described as a reaction to a threat that dentists feel when they see the functions they have routinely performed—and which for some individual dentists actually comprise the operating definition of dentistry—being delegated to auxiliaries with 2 or less years of education. Dentists have described the phenomenon as a gradual eating away of their role in delivering dental services (Waldman, 1975).

Despite the theoretician's descriptions of the important, evolving role of the oral physician who engages in complex diagnosis, treatment planning, sophisticated therapy, and team management, the dentist who has been comfortable in a more simplified role may not be eager for the changes. The concept of team dentistry involving multiple personnel performing multifaceted services is not necessarily the goal of the contented solo practitioner. It may be that the results of the experimental programs and the accompanying legal and educational changes pointed too clearly toward radical change that would have a strong impact on the grass roots dentist. Some dentists prefer to support changes that are good for the practitioner, saying that what is good for dentistry will provide the best outcome for the population. The ADA has called for dentists to be utilized to fullest capacity before auxiliaries receive expanded functions (8-1976-H; 33-1976-H). Dentistry is quite understandably interested in utilizing the available manpower in dentistry before developing roles for auxiliaries.

This attitude was compounded in the early 1980s by the economic recession that kept patients away from their dentists. Workers with dental insurance did not seek dental care while they were unemployed. Thus, dentists reported that their appointment books were filled with white space, particularly in highly industrialized regions of the country. This temporary drop in business was accompanied by the decrease in dental caries prevalence in the population, particularly among children. One study showed that nearly 37% of children under 17 years of age had experienced no dental decay (Dental Statistics, 1984).

Periodontal disease is emerging as the oral malady that will replace dental caries. Therefore, the efforts to prepare auxiliaries with skills in restorative dentistry may now be an anachronism, as the dentist reserves those procedures for himself/herself.

In order to compete sucessfully for patients, dental practices will need to market the unique aspects of the care they provide. This will draw patients who are dissatisfied with the care they are receiving elsewhere. They also will need to attract

)le who have not routinely sought dental care, who are now willing and financially able to ~~ ~o. A dentist could still spend a major percentage of appointment time on restorative care if previously untreated patients are attracted to the practice. Otherwise, restorative care is likely to occupy an ever-decreasing part in clinical dentistry. As this occurs, auxiliaries will find their roles in restorative care diminished.

There may be a shift in delegated responsibilities as periodontal disease becomes a more central target in dental practice. Dental hygienists may be in greater demand; dental assistants, as well as hygienists, may spend more time educating patients about the prevention of periodontal disease and home care maintenance following treatment.

Dentistry has seen many changes in the past two decades. The treatment methods, efficiency strategies, practice sites, reimbursement mechanisms, attitudes toward competition and marketing, use of auxiliaries, and even the population's disease prevalence have changed markedly. These changes pose both opportunities and challenges to dentistry. To some, these changes are seen as signs of progress; to others they are seen as threats. The important point to most is that by and large the changes have made it possible for more people to seek care and for dentistry to see that it has conquered, mainly through the use of fluorides, the oral disease that preoccupied dentistry for centuries.

Review questions

1. Describe briefly the traditional system of delivery of dental health care services. *solo practices, fee-for-service, limited use of auxilliaries*

2. The primary stimulus for attempts to modify the delivery of dental care in the early 1960s was: *the prediction of ↑ demand for care in 1960's & 70's.*

3. The two early 1970s reports that shifted the reason for modifying dental care delivery are:

   a. *Carnegie Commission Report of 1970*

   b. *Survey of Dentistry, 1961*

4. Describe briefly the response of the ADA to results of experiments that demonstrate the degree to which auxiliaries can perform services traditionally defined as the practice of dentistry. *Dentists know that services can be delegated to aux. But question whether they should.*

5. List five major recent factors that have influenced how dentistry is practiced in the 1980s. *advertising → dental franchises, more dentists & change in dental disease, focus on cost containment, less caries seen today, more perio.*

6. Explain why a dentist might decide to join an HMO or a PPO. *to increase their income or patient load.*

REFERENCES

Albertini, T.F., Hillsman, J.T., and Crawford, B.L.: Federal financing of dental services, J. Dent. Educ. 48:606, 1984.

American Association of Dental Schools, 17-76-H, Amendment of 27-73-H.

American Dental Association, 8-1976-H.

American Dental Association, 33-1976-H.

American Dental Association, 24-1976-H.

Anderson, P.E.: Staff salaries level or down for 1983, Dent. Econ. 75(2):46, 1985.

Bentley, J.M., and Woodall, I.R.: Networking: the private practitioner's key to quality and marketing, J. Dent. Practice Admin. 1:3, 1984.

Bergner, M., Milgrom, P., Chapko, M.K., Beach, B., and Skalabrin, N.: The Washington State dental auxiliary project: quality of care in private practice, J. Am. Dent. Assoc. 107:781, 1983.

Born, D.O.: Factors affecting the distribution of dental auxiliaries. In Proceedings of the workshop on changing roles of dental auxiliaries, Bethesda, Md., 1975, U.S. Dept. of Health, Education and Welfare, PHS-HRA, Bureau of Health Manpower, Division of Dentistry.

Carnegie Commission on Higher Education: Higher education and the nation's health: policies of medical and dental education. Special report and recommendation, New York, 1970, McGraw-Hill Book Co.

Cavicchio, P.M.: An overview of dental hygiene expanded duties projects and consideration of relevant changes in state dental practice acts. In Hayden, H., editor: Training workshop on expanded functions for dental hygienists, Honolulu, 1971, District XI, American Dental Hygienists' Association.

Chapko, M.K., et al.: Delegation of expanded functions to dental assistants and hygienists, Am. J. Public Health. **75**:61, 1985.

Cohen, D.: University of Pennsylvania: Personal communication, 1976.

Colchamiro, S.: The challenge of dentistry in neighborhood health centers, J. Public Health Dent. **36**:254, 1976.

Cooper, T.M., and DiBiaggio, J.A.: Applied practice management: a strategy for stress control, St. Louis, 1979, The C.V. Mosby Co.

Council on Dental Care Programs.: Preferred provider organizations and dentistry, J. Am. Dent. Assoc. **107**:76, 1983.

Cowan, D.H.: Preferred provider organizations, Rockville, Md., 1984, Aspen Systems Corp.

DeFriese, G.H., O'Shea, R.M., Meskin, L., Pfister, J., and Barker, B.: The Kentucky and Washington State demonstrations: expanded-function dental auxiliary personnel in private general practice, J. Am. Dent. Assoc. **107**:773, 1983.

Dental statistics handbook, Chicago, 1984, American Dental Association.

DiBiaggio, J.A.: Academic freedom: a test case, Dent. Student News **5**:1, 1975.

Eglit, H.C., and Hauber, C.H.: The constitutionality of state restrictions imposed upon the dental hygiene education system, Educational Directions **1**:15, 1976.

Gabel, J., and Ermann, D.: Preferred provider organizations: performance, problems, and promise, Health Aff. **4**(1):24, 1985.

Gilman, C.W.: Comments on the inter-agency committee on dental auxiliaries, J. Am. Dent. Assoc. **95**:32, 1977.

Hayden, H., editor: Introduction, Training workshop on expanded functions for dental hygienists, Honolulu, 1971, District XI, American Dental Hygienists' Association.

Hazelkorn, H.M., and Christoffel, T.: Denturism's challenge to the licensure system, J. Public Health Policy **5**:104, 1984.

Hollinshead, B.S.: The survey of dentistry, Washington, D.C., 1961, American Council on Education.

Hospital statistics, Chicago, 1984, American Hospital Association.

Hygienists in Massachusetts to receive training in dentistry for children, J. Am. Dent. Assoc. **40**:77, 1950.

Jacobs, R.M.: Reflections on the controversy over expanded function dental auxiliaries, J. Dent. Educ. **40**:332, 1976.

Jones, P.F.: The changing role of the dental hygienist. In Boundy, S.S., and Reynolds, N.J., editors: Current concepts in dental hygiene, St. Louis, 1977, The C.V. Mosby Co.

Kaplan, A.L., Bader, J.D., Mullins, M.R., and Lange, K.W.: Measurement of effects of a state dental practice act on potential delegation and production in general dental private practice, J. Public Health Dent. **43**:161, 1983.

Klyop, J.S.: The dental profession's commitment to quality assurance, Dent. Clin. North Am. 239:521, 1985.

Legislation & Litigation, J. Am. Dent. Assoc. **110**:606, 1985.

Legislation: Massachusetts, J. Am. Dent. Assoc. **40**:115, 1950.

Legislative action packet: a comparative overview of 51 practice acts, Chicago, 1985, American Dental Hygienists' Association.

Lobene, R.R.: The Forsyth experiment: an alternative system for dental care, Cambridge, Mass., 1979, Harvard University Press.

Lobene, R.R.: Personal communication, 1986.

Lobene, R.R., et al.: The Forsyth experiment in training of advanced skills hygienists, J. Dent. Educ. **38**:369, 1974.

Maas, E.: President's corner, J. Am. Dent. Hyg. Assoc. **24**:37, 1950.

Mescher, K.: Summary of workshop discussions. In Mescher, K., editor: Training workshop on adaptation of dental hygiene practice to changing concepts in delivery of oral health services, Little Amana, Iowa, 1972, Iowa Dental Hygienists' Association.

Milgrom, P.: Regulation and the quality of dental care, Germantown, Md., 1978, Aspen Systems Corp.

Milgrom, P., Bergner, M., Chapko, M.K., Conrad, D., and Skalabrin, N.: The Washington State dental auxiliary project: delegating expanded functions in general practice, J. Am. Dent. Assoc. **107**:776, 1983.

Mullins, M.R., Kaplan, A.L., Bader, J.D., Lange, K.W., Murray, B. P., Armstrong, S.R., and Haney, C.A.: Summary results of the Kentucky dental practice demonstration: a cooperative project with practicing general dentists, J. Am. Dent. Assoc. **106**:817, 1983

Powell, W.O., et al.: Comparison of clinical performance of dental therapist trainees and dental students, J. Dent. Educ. **38**:268, 1974.

Redig, D.F.: The team program and its implications for expanded duties for dental hygienists. In Hayden, H., editor: Training workshop on expanded functions for dental hygienists, Honolulu, 1971, District XI, American Dental Hygienists Association.

Robinson, H.B.G.: Academic freedom and the issue of expanded-duty auxiliaries, Dent. Surv. **52**:12, 1976.

Rosenstein, D.I., Empey, G., Chiodo, G.T., and Phillips, D.: The effects of denturism on denture prices, Am. J. Public Health **75**:671, 1985.

Rovin, S., and Nash, J.: Traditional and emerging forms of

dental practice, with a commentary on cost, accessibility, and quality factors, Am. J. Public Health. **72:**336, 1982.

Schwager, M.: Expanded functions: RDH retrospective, RDH **1**(5):16, 1981.

Sisty, N.L.: Experimental program for dental hygienists at the University of Iowa. In Mescher, K., editor: Training workshop on adaptation of dental hygiene practice to changing concepts in delivery of oral health services, Little Amana, Iowa, 1972, Iowa Dental Hygienists' Association.

Spohn, E.: Background and transition of the expanded duty program. In Agenda material of the meeting of the Educational Advisory Committee for the University of Kentucky expanded duty dental hygiene research program, June 1975.

U.S. Department of Health, Education and Welfare, U.S. Public Health Service, Bureau of Health Manpower: A report on allied health personnel, Bethesda, Md., 1979, U.S. Department of Health, Education and Welfare.

Waldman, H.B.: Is dentistry's future threatened? Dent. Surv. **51:**50, 1975.

CHAPTER 4

Educational requirements and credentialing procedures

OBJECTIVES: The reader will be able to:

1. Briefly explain the purpose and role of educational standards and credentialing in the regulation of health care providers.
2. Define *accreditation*.
3. Given descriptions of credentialing processes for health care providers, identify whether the process is an example of the following:
   a. Licensure.
   b. Certification.
   c. Registration.
   d. Institutional licensure.
4. Explain the legal and economic constraints placed on employers that enforce the utilization of persons credentialed by licensure or certification.
5. Describe the advantages and disadvantages of licensure and certification.
6. Explain how supervision clauses in dental laws affect the opportunity for dental hygienists to deliver care and to grow financially.
7. State three mechanisms that could be used to change the supervision clauses.
8. Identify at least three major responsibilities that dental hygienists would assume if they were to become self-regulating.
9. Describe briefly the allied health movement.

The primary reason for standards of education and credentialing for health care providers is to ensure that the public receives quality care. Accreditation and credentialing by themselves cannot guarantee appropriate care, but they can influence programs to offer curricula that will adequately prepare persons for practice, and they can establish whether the candidate for practice possesses the knowledge and skill to deliver adequate care. Both accreditation and credentialing are focal points of control over the delivery of care and the maturation of the professional group of providers.

ACCREDITATION

Accreditation is a form of "regulation or control which is exercised over educational institutions and/or programs by external organizations or agencies." It is a "process whereby an association or agency grants public recognition to a school, institute, college, university, or specialized program of study having met certain established qualifications or standards as determined through initial and periodic evaluations." Institutions typically seek accreditation from a regional accrediting agency that evaluates the institution as a whole and from the individual specialty accred-

33

itation agencies for the specific programs offered that require accreditation for recognition (Pennell et al., 1972).

In addition to serving as a determinant of the quality of an educational program, accreditation has served as a means for establishing control over a specialty area of education by a special interest group (Proffitt, 1970). The accrediting body has great power in determining the future of a professional group or subspecialty by specifying which educational components and which educational structures are appropriate for that group. For instance, the profession of nursing has control of its own accreditation process (Kelly, 1974). The individual state boards of nursing accredit the programs established within their jurisdiction. The authority to accredit is granted to the boards of nursing and the National League for Nursing. The fact that nursing controls accreditation gives it far greater control over the growth and direction of its profession than dental hygiene and dental assisting, for instance, have in the control of their respective professions. Both dental hygiene and assisting programs are accredited by the ADA Commission on Dental Accreditation. In this case dentistry has control over the growth and direction possible in educational programs. The two auxiliaries rely on the input of their representatives (one dental hygienist and one dental assistant), on the commission, and on the wisdom of the dentists in control.

CREDENTIALING FOR HEALTH CARE PROVIDERS

Credentialing of individual health care providers is different from accreditation of an educational institution. It addresses itself to the capabilities of the person who has completed a formal education and wishes to enter the work force to provide care. It is similar to accreditation in that it is often administered by the same group that controls accreditation and because it is a force that shapes the nature of the profession for which the person is being credentialed. Both accredita-

tion and individual credentialing involve standards for approval and utilize measurement processes to determine whether standards are met.

Licensure and certification

Licensure and *certification* are utilized for credentialing allied health personnel. "Licensure is the credentialing mechanism or process by which an agency of the government (usually the state) grants permission to persons meeting the predetermined qualifications to engage in a given occupation and/or use a particular title, or grants permission to institutions (such as hospitals, nursing homes) to perform specified functions" (Study, 1971). Dental hygiene, dentistry, optometry, nursing, osteopathy, medicine, and pharmacy are examples of health professions that are licensed in all states and the District of Columbia. Legislation enacted by the state grants that licensing power to an agency such as a state board to protect the public from unqualified persons. The individual state dental practice acts are examples of such legislation. They empower the state boards of dentistry to regulate dentistry and dental hygiene by examining candidates for licensure and by ensuring that licensees remain within the law while providing care.

Certification refers to the "process by which a nongovernment agency or association grants recognition to an individual who has met certain predetermined qualifications specified by that agency or association. Such qualifications may include (1) graduation from an accredited or approved program of study, (2) acceptable performance on a qualifying examination or series of examinations, and/or (3) completion of a stated amount of work experience." The primary distinction between licensure and certification is that the former is granted by the state whereas the latter is granted by a nongovernmental agency, usually the professional association (Study, 1971).

Both licensure and certification imply a "restraint of trade" (Restrictive licensing, 1974). Credentialing does prohibit unqualified persons from entering the work force to perform services reserved for the licensed or certified person. In the case of licensure, the law specifies that an employer may not hire an unlicensed person to provide those services. The law also warns charlatans that to perform restricted services is a criminal offense. In the case of certification, the enforcement is economic rather than legal. For a health care facility such as a hospital to receive third-party reimbursement for services delivered at the facility, the facility must be accredited by the Joint Commission on Accreditation of Hospitals. To be accredited, the facility must employ only those persons who are qualified to provide care. The Joint Commission recognizes certification of the members of the professional association as an appropriate credential to designate persons as qualified (JCAH, 1984). Therefore to collect third-party payments, only certified persons can be employed in the key positions specified by the Joint Commission.

To enforce licensure restrictions, the state must send out investigators to scrutinize the credentials of persons providing care, an insurmountable task in a cottage industry such as dentistry. The enforcement of accreditation requirements to employ only certified persons occurs every few years for every hospital (JCAH, 1984).

The dental hygienist and dental assistant provide excellent examples of two allied health personnel who provide patient care but who are regulated under different mechanisms. The dental hygienist is licensed by the state according to the criteria stated in the law, after a minimum 2-year educational program.* The dental assistant is certified by the Dental Assistants' National Board after he/she graduates from an approved (accredited) dental assisting program, obtains certification in cardiopulmonary resuscitation, and successfully completes an examination. It is also necessary that 12 clock hours of continuing education be demonstrated each year to retain certifi-

---

*Alabama is the only state that licenses persons as dental hygienists without requiring formal education.

cation. Dental assistants with prescribed amounts of work experience but no formal dental assisting education can challenge the certifying examination.

Licensure has worked to the advantage of the hygienist more than certification has worked to the advantage of the dental assistant because of the nature of the health system in which dental care is delivered. It should be remembered that dentistry has been a fee-for-service enterprise, rarely located in a hospital facility. With no accreditation visits provided by the Joint Commission in individual dental offices and until recently little reason to be overly concerned about preferential status in the eyes of third-party payers, dentistry had no economic reason to employ only certified dental assistants. There was and is, however, a legal mandate to employ only licensed hygienists to perform dental hygiene care.

There are, however, disadvantages to licensure: restrictions on the scope of practice, difficulties in obtaining licensure in a different state when a person changes residence, and restrictions on where one may practice.

Restrictions on the *scope of practice* were discussed in detail in previous chapters. In summary, the differences in the various state laws make it difficult for educational programs to prepare their graduates for less restrictive practice acts; thus not all hygienists are qualified to practice in all states. Having duties defined in a state law makes it difficult for further experimentation with other duties and limits the freedom of dental hygienists to provide needed care that is within a hygienist's education and skill.

A major drawback of licensure that persists in several licensing jurisdictions is the difficulty involved in moving from one jurisdiction to another and *obtaining a new license.* In the 1950s, a dentist or hygienist had to complete a new clinical and a new written examination in whatever state he/she moved to in order to obtain a license. The National Board examinations (which were introduced in the early 1960s) in dental hygiene and dentistry are accepted by nearly all states, although many states require that the test be taken recently, within the past 5 to 10 years, depending upon each state's law.

Regional examinations were introduced in the 1970s which made it possible for a clinician to pass one clinical examination and be eligible for licensure in all the participating states. The applicant was still reviewed by each state in which a license was sought, but a candidate achieving a passing score on the national and regional boards was nearly always assured licensure. Therefore, the applicant experienced licensure delays only when moving from one region to another or when examinations were several years old. Some states review credentials obtained in other regions or in other individual states, sometimes issuing a license by credentials.

As of 1985, the states having provisions for licensure by credentials were: Alaska, Arkansas, Connecticut, Delaware, District of Columbia, Illinois, Indiana, Iowa, Kansas, Kentucky, Louisiana, Maine, Maryland, Michigan, Minnesota, Missouri, Montana, Nebraska, New Hampshire, New York, North Dakota, Oklahoma, Pennsylvania, Rhode Island, South Carolina, Tennessee, Virginia, Vermont, Washington, West Virginia, and Wisconsin (Legislative action, 1985). Dentists and hygienists moving from one licensing jurisdiction into one of these can apply for licensure by credentials, whereupon the regulatory board reviews their previous licensure and decides whether to issue a license to practice. States not listed require a licensure examination, including clinical testing by the state or the region of which it is a member and perhaps even written testing if it does not accept the National Board.

The third barrier posed by licensure is unique to dental hygiene—no other licensed profession has this particular limitation. As of 1986, every licensing jurisdiction in the United States, except Colorado, requires that a dental hygienist work under the supervision of a dentist. Therefore, the public is limited in its access to dental hygiene; it must occur through the office of a dentist or through a program supervised by a dentist. It also places a market limitation on dental hygienists. They must earn their living in settings where there is dental supervision. In most cases this means a dental practice, since the number of positions in public health or educational settings is limited. Therefore, if a dental hygienist cannot find a position where a dentist is willing to hire a hygienist, it is not legally possible to establish his/her own practice and succeed or fail.

Certainly not all hygienists have the inclination to take the business risk of establishing a dental hygiene practice. Such an endeavor requires capital and good business judgment as well as well-refined clinical skills and judgment. Independent practice can be an attractive alternative for a hygienist who has years of experience, financial resources, and no prospect for financial or professional growth as an employee.

The Federal Trade Commission may eventually issue an administrative ruling stating that such state laws are an unfair restraint of trade, or individual states may change the law through judicial overturn or legislative action when reviewed in this light (Restrictive licensing, 1974; Koopman, 1983).

An important point for the courts and the legislators to review is whether, in the case of required supervision for dental hygiene, the state board of dentistry and the dental association are acting in the interest of the public health or in the interest of professional security by minimizing competition. Whenever a profession regulates itself and others, it is possible to cross the line from a public interest body to a union or guild (Cohen, 1979).

Preparing for self-regulation

If an administrative ruling, judicial decision, or legislative change were to alter dental hygiene's practice restrictions, several results are possible. Included are:

1. A simple deletion in the phrase stating that a hygienist must work under the direct supervision of a dentist, with the remainder of the legal provisions remaining intact, and

2. The creation of a separate dental hygiene law and board that would permit dental hygienists to regulate themselves.

While the first alternative is the more likely of the two choices, the possibility remains that several jurisdictions will consider and establish separate regulatory provisions for dental hygienists. With such a change will come major responsibility.

Included will be the responsibility for interpreting and enforcing the dental hygiene practice act. Thus dental hygiene will do unto itself what dentistry has been doing for seven decades. The dental hygiene board will need to preserve those aspects of regulation that are helpful and essential for the public welfare; it also will need to carefully decide what it will do differently. The board will review candidates for licensure and consider punitive actions for hygienists who violate the principles of the law. It also will decide what criteria will be used for accreditation of dental hygiene education programs. The individual state boards will be responsible for deciding whether they will continue to accept the accreditation mechanisms of the Commission on Dental Accreditation of the American Dental Association or adopt a different set of criteria. For while it may appear that the ADA controls accreditation, each state law empowers the dental board to approve programs, and those boards accept the ADA criteria and then extend their own official approval and acceptance for licensure.

An important aspect of this change would involve whether special provisions need to be made for the education and licensure of hygienists who would be practicing independently. Issues presently on the table in discussions of independent practice relate to the need for a career-ladder approach where hygienists with more experience and education would be granted a special license to practice independently (Cameron and Olswang, 1984). This suggestion comes from the continuing charge from organized dentistry that a person with 2 years of education is not adequately prepared to practice without dental supervision.

Mescher (1984) presents interesting information about the length of preparation of the average dental hygienist. While many complain that most hygienists have only 2 years of college preparation, trends since the early 1980s show that approximately 74% of the students entering dental hygiene programs have 1 or more years of college before starting dental hygiene. Only 20.7% of the dental hygiene programs in the United States accept students with only a high school diploma, and of this group, half of the programs accepted classes where 50% had a year of college anyway.

Further, in 1981–1982, 70% of the programs required more than 2 years of college experience in order to graduate. Only 23 programs allowed completion in two years. Mescher summarizes by saying that the majority of graduating dental hygienists should not be thought of as 2-year graduates since the vast majority have sufficient credit hours to qualify for a bachelor's degree.

So while the debate around independent practice considers a realignment of minimum requirements for licensure and further education for an exemption from supervision, the actual preparation of dental hygienists may be only a few steps away from what people are suggesting or demanding. Articulation programs with 4-year degree granting institutions could make it possible for a much higher percentage of dental hygienists to be granted the degree they are so close to earning. It might also provide opportunities for hygienists to acquire management skills necessary for business success.

An extremely important development for dental hygiene would be the careful delineation of what dental hygiene constitutes, in contradistinction to dentistry. This delineation of the profession would help solidify the educational system for dental hygiene and help guide a research focus so that a scientific basis for dental hygiene is recognized.

This can be accomplished through a thorough statement of *dental hygiene diagnosis,* wherein all of the terms associated with dental hygiene assessment and treatment are identified and categorized into an array of related areas of expertise and responsibility.

Nurses began speaking publicly about the need for a classification of nursing diagnosis in 1973 when a national conference convened and developed a list of 30 tentative diagnoses. Nursing took this step in order to achieve greater clarity in role definition and to assist those nurses who had secured unsupervised positions where physical evaluation was their responsibility. A recent issue of *Nursing Clinics of North America* is devoted to the research carried on to validate those nursing categories (Dougherty, 1985).

Miller published an article on dental hygiene diagnosis in *RDH* in 1982 challenging dental hygienists to develop a taxonomy that defines the parameters of oral and general health evaluation. Preparation of such a taxonomy could help define dental hygiene, its education, and its licensure and continued evaluation. It also could establish guidelines for research emphasis. It would help establish how dental hygiene and dentistry interrelate in terms of patient evaluation and treatment. Such a step seems essential if independent practice and further advances in public health dental hygiene are to occur.

In 1985, the American Dental Association passed a series of policies stating clearly that dental hygienists are auxiliaries of the dental profession and that they are to work under the supervision of a licensed dentist (Legislation & Litigation 112:143). Thus it is unlikely that the change will occur without extended debate and a growing adversarial relationship between dental hygienists and the group of dentists who oppose greater practice freedom for hygienists.

Registration

The term *registration* is often used interchangeably with licensure and certification. Actually it is synonymous with neither. Registration is the process by which an individual is listed on an official roster maintained by the state or the nongovernmental agency offering certification. Registration is used to describe the entry of a name to the roster rather than credentialing.

Institutional licensure

Another distinct form of credentialing that has been discussed in medical fields is *institutional licensure* (Guy, 1973). Institutional licensure would grant to an institution such as a hospital or health maintenance organization the authority to define the role and responsibility of personnel on the basis of manpower needs in the facility and on the basis of the individual skills of the personnel employed. The institution would in effect control credentialing internally and be free to create staffing patterns based on its assessments. Few health care providers have voiced support for this alternative despite the flexibility it would provide. It removes credentialing control from the professions and places it in the hands of administrators of health care facilities.

The primary reason for suggesting the alternative is the need to sort out the vast array of certification requirements that the myriad of categories of allied health personnel have developed. Each category of worker has distinct criteria and a unique registration process, which again causes many headaches for employers attempting to create reasonable staffing patterns that meet accreditation standards (Mansfield, 1971). Even though the issue of multiple groups of personnel all requiring certification or licensure was addressed in detail in the early 1970s, it is still largely unsolved in the late 1980s.

DEVELOPMENT OF PROFESSIONAL REGULATION

Health professions began to adopt standards of professional competence before 1800 when the medical profession was concerned about the training and conduct of practitioners and had appealed to the individual states to establish and enforce controls. The most notable move toward the development of professional regulation occurred in the middle of the nineteenth century when professional associations were founded and licensure became more prevalent. The associations began to exert control over the educational institutions to improve and standardize educational programs. The American Medical Association was formed in 1847, the American Pharmaceutical Association in 1852, and the American Dental Association in 1859 (Pennell et al., 1972).

Those professions that were established to support medical and dental services were organized and regulated toward the late nineteenth and early twentieth centuries. The American Nurses Association was established in 1896, and the American Dental Hygienists' Association in 1923. Licensure was the primary mechanism for regulation during that period since there was no source for an economic mandate for employers to hire only those persons who held appropriate credentials. The legal constraint was the only mandate available.

The period for the development and delineation of health care providers as supporters of dentistry and (primarily) medicine occurred after World War II, with the greatest growth during the late 1960s. The allied health movement began when the necessities of war proved that persons could be prepared to perform various medical procedures without being physicians. Schools of allied medical professions were established and new categories of health workers developed to extend care to civilians in the postwar era. They were known at first as paraprofessionals or paramedical personnel. The terms *auxiliary* and *ancillary* were also used in the early years of development, but those terms were dropped as being nonreflective

of the scope of responsibility the providers h the delivery of health care.

The terms *allied health professional, physician extender,* and *midlevel practitioner* were used to describe the rapidly growing group of health workers who were established as the complexities of comprehensive health care demanded greater specialization among providers, particularly those who carry out the orders of the physician with specialized equipment and therapy. New advances in renal care, cardiology, medical technology, respiratory therapy, and nuclear medicine dictated that highly skilled technicians would be needed to operate the sophisticated equipment and to carry out the prescribed orders of the physician. With the health manpower scare of the early 1960s and the Allied Health Manpower Training Act of 1966, which funded new programs for such personnel and supported enrollment increases, new categories of health workers burgeoned. There was a specialist for every type of medical equipment and often an assistant for that person, each with a specified curriculum and specific standards to be met for association certification. No comprehensive plan was developed or followed.

CONCLUSION

This chapter has focused on the educational and credentialing requirements for health professions, citing their development, their strengths and limitations, and some of the issues and problems surrounding these forms of regulation.

The discussion leads naturally to an explication of the main issue, quality of care, which is found in the next chapter.

Review questions

1. Why are accreditation and credentialing important components of the health care delivery system? A method to ensure quality of care to the public. control over growth + direction of profession.

2. A state agency governed by a state practice act is empowered to license/certify (choose one) a health care provider.

3. A professional association sets up criteria for assessing candidates for licensure/certification (choose one) as health care providers.

4. Certification is not currently a strong mandate in dentistry for the employment of dental assistants because: *Insurance carriers usually didn't require all employees to be certified.*

5. Why is there such great variety in the methods of credentialing allied health personnel? *Rapidly growing allied health movement created many new jobs + each w/ its own certification process.*

6. How do clauses in dental laws that require that a dental hygienist be supervised by a dentist impact the practice of dental hygiene? *hygienists can't have their own office, compete w/ dentists, or have direct access w/ public to provide care*

7. How could the supervision clauses be removed from the dental law? *Administrative ruling by FTC, a judicial overturn if tested in courts, + a legislative change in laws.*

8. One possible outcome of the debate over supervision is the establishment of dental hygiene practice acts, with dental hygiene boards regulating the profession. Name three major responsibilities that would fall upon such a board. *Enforcing dental laws, Approving candidates for licensure, Approving D.H. programs w/in the state*

GROUP ACTIVITIES

1. Compare the specific credentialing requirements for the following:
   a. Respiratory therapists
   b. Dietitians
   c. Medical technologists
   d. Nurses
   e. Other health personnel of choice.
2. Read the Koopman article in the *Wayne Law Review* and summarize the major points made regarding the legality of the supervision clauses.
3. Review the Federal Trade Commission study of the control of dental hygiene by dentistry as a case of restraint of trade.
4. Debate whether dental hygiene ought to be allowed to practice independently. Include issues related to length of education, ability to make clinical judgments, the relationship between dentistry and dental hygiene in providing well-coordinated care, and the proposal for a two-tier system of dental hygiene licensure that would have stricter requirements for independent practice.
5. Review the editorials and interviews in *RDH* and in *Dental Hygiene* relating to independent practice and independent contracting.
6. Interview a nurse practitioner regarding the diagnoses and nursing judgments he/she makes in clinical practice. Inquire how nursing care, when conducted independently, is integrated with medical care.
7. List 20 terms that are integral to a dental hygienist's assessment of a patient's oral health; start with a brainstorming session and combine terms according to function (i.e., occlusion, home care routine) and according to structure (periodontium, enamel, soft tissue) until a comprehensive list of 20 is obtained. Discuss what diagnosis means and how dental hygiene diagnosis fits with dental diagnosis.

REFERENCES

Cameron, C.A., and Olswang, S.G.: Educating dental hygienists to be sole practitioners, Dent. Hyg. **58**:408, 1984.

Cohen, H.S.: Public versus private interest in assuring professional competence, Fam. Commun. Health **2**:79, 1979.

Dougherty, C.M.: Editor's foreword. In Dougherty, C.M., editor: Nursing diagnosis, Nurs. Clin. North Am. **20**:609, 1985.

Guy, J.S.: Institutional licensure: a dilemma for nurses, Nurs. Clin. North Am. **9**:497, 1973.

Joint Commission on the Accreditation of Hospitals: Accreditation manual for hospitals, Chicago, 1984, The Commission.

Kelly, L.Y.: Nursing practice acts, Am. J. Nurs. **74**:1310, 1974.

Koopman, E.L.: Are the supervision regulations which require a licensed dental hygienist to practice under the supervision of a dentist constitutional? Wayne Law Review **30**:127, 1983.

Legislation & Litigation, J. Am. Dent. Assoc. **112**:143, 1986.

Legislative action packet: a comparative overview of 51 practice actions, Chicago, 1985, American Dental Hygienists' Association.

Mansfield, E.O.: How the health care administrator looks at certification of allied health personnel in a changing health care system. An abstract in conference materials for an Invitational Conference on Certification in Allied Health Professions, College Park, Md., 1971, American Society of Allied Health Professions.

Mescher, K.D.: A new look at the educational preparation of dental hygienists: exploding the myths, Dent. Hyg. **58**:69, 1984.

Miller, S.S.: Dental hygiene diagnosis, RDH **2**(4):46, 1982.

Pennell, M.Y., Proffitt, J.R., and Hatch, T.D.: Accreditation and certification in relation to allied health manpower, Bethesda, Md., 1972, U.S. Dept. of Health, Education and Welfare, PHS-NIH, Bureau of Health Manpower Education.

Proffitt, J.R.: Accreditation as a stabilizing force in allied health professions, J. Am. Med. Assoc. **213**:604, 1970.

Restrictive licensing of dental paraprofessionals, Yale Law Journal, **83**:806, 1974.

Study of accreditation of selected health educational programs. In Conference materials for an Invitational Conference on Certification in Allied Professions, College Park, Md., 1971, American Society of Allied Health Professions.

The quality of care: the consumer interest, peer review, and continuing education

OBJECTIVES: The reader will be able to:

1. State the three issues on which consumers have focused primary concerns and complaints with regard to the delivery of health care services.
2. Explain three ways in which consumers have gained influence with regard to the way in which the health care system functions.
3. Identify the ways in which health care is monitored for its quality.
4. Differentiate *audit* and *clinical review* as two mechanisms for assessment.
5. Describe a mechanism for auditing patient records that can be instituted in a health care practice or local professional organization.
6. Explain two ways in which peer review mechanisms can function to assess the quality of health care in a health care practice or professional organization.
7. Explain how economic incentives can relate to a voluntary peer group of professionals.

THE CONSUMER MOVEMENT

The late 1960s marked a period when consumer awareness was awakened. Ralph Nader in his book *Unsafe at Any Speed* described how a major auto manufacturer had designed and was selling a product that was proved to be unsafe and a contributor to a number of accidents (Nader, 1965). Although many at first may have found such a book to be laughable in terms of its having any influence on big business, an auto described in that book was taken off the market a few years later. If the auto manufacturer did not respond immediately to the need to improve the design of the auto to improve its safety, it did eventually respond to the fact that people were no longer purchasing that product in sufficient numbers to warrant its continued production. The consumer had triumphed in a landmark confrontation, causing business to improve or retract faulty merchandise.

Nader has since continued investigating a number of industries, including the dental profession. He took the dental profession to task for what he believed was the unscrupulous use of x-radiation (Nader, 1968). The article resulted in practicing dental personnel needing to explain again and again to patients the rationale for the radiographs that needed to be exposed. There is no question that the article had a dramatic effect on the public's awareness of their right to question the services they receive, including health care services.

Nader sponsored summer programs for students to learn consumer advocacy, "Nader's Raiders," creating a team of people who could investigate corporate activities and consumer issues and publish their findings. While Nader believes the consumer movement would have started without him ("you could see it coming"), he attributes part of its growth to his leadership. He believes he was seen as legitimate and as knowledgeable of business and law (Dreifus, 1984).

Nader has reviewed the Congress as well, publishing fact sheets about the attendance records, voting records, responsiveness, and productivity of each of the representatives. The extent to which this investigative program has affected industry and government is not limited to what one man could perform.

With the advent of the Nader reports came a number of other consumer advocates who formed consumer organizations to inform buyers of unscrupulous business and professional persons and to provide advice to those seeking restitution when a product or service they purchased was shown to be inadequate or dangerous.

Dry cereals, long the staple of the American breakfast table, were examined for the nutrition they provided, resulting in part in legislation requiring food processors to include nutritive value amounts on their packages. Toy manufacturers were scrutinized for the quality and safety of the products they produce; consumer awareness announcements were carried on national television prior to the December holidays to inform shoppers of the dangers of some toys. Journalism turned increasingly to ferreting out those aspects of private enterprise that were suspect in their handling of the public, with newspaper columns devoted to assisting exasperated customers in achieving satisfaction and with television programming featuring several in-depth analyses of corruption in nursing homes, camps for children, hospitals, and any other endeavors, public or private, that squandered people's money or provided less than a fair return for the investment made.

In general, consumers are more informed, and they expect to obtain the necessary information to make purchaser decisions. This is true in the grocery store, at the used car lot, and in the dental office.

CONSUMERS AND THE HEALTH CARE SYSTEM

As noted previously, health care was not immune to this growing interest in what consumers were receiving in return for their money. Con-

sumers organized to form a strong lobbying force in the state and federal governments (Jones, 1977). Numerous pieces of legislation have been influenced by this interest group. As consumers they represent the American public as a whole, which is a force that is difficult to ignore in the legislature. Elected officials are eager to be viewed as consumer protectors and as responsive to the needs of the individual.

One of the forms of legislation consumer groups were active in shaping was the continuing stream of proposals for national health insurance. National health insurance is probably not going to be enacted because political and economic priorities have shifted. However, the public was and still is vocal in its displeasure with the health care system in this country. The high cost of care, the frequent inaccessibility of care, and the quality of care received have been and are matters of concern (Angevine, 1973; Jones, 1977; Tolpin, 1985).

While political lobbying has certainly been a strong force in the consumer movement to improve health care, consumers have made other inroads in affecting the health care system. Consumers objected to the way in which state boards controlling the practice of health care providers did not include consumer representation, or "public members." Their goal has been to ensure that the state boards are indeed protecting the public as they are mandated in the law and that they are not serving as a guild to control the numbers of practitioners or using questionable procedures in regulating the practice of dental personnel already licensed (Maurizi, 1975).

Consumers have been involved at least in the development of systems of peer review. Indirectly, they have affected private and public sector reviews of the quality of care through private insurance carriers and public assistance programs that cover dental care. These third-party payers conduct reviews of work to be performed and often evaluate the quality of the finished product before paying the health care provider (Bailit, Issues, 1980; Egdahl and Gertman, 1976).

In addition to the more overt impact of consumers on legislation and on state and private regulatory agencies, the consumer awareness era spawned a plethora of articles describing how good dental work can be found and how it can be evaluated by laypersons. These articles are written by inquiring consumers who have made it their business to investigate the health care industry (Quint, 1974), and by providers of care who feel a sense of responsibility for the well-being of the public (and who, perhaps, recognize the ready market for such publications) (McGuire, 1972).

The landmark consumer awareness text for dentistry is *Dentistry and Its Victims,* written by "Paul Revere," D.D.S. (1970). The book describes what to watch for in dental care and is less than complimentary in its evaluation of the kind of dentistry most patients receive. It stirred considerable wrath in the dental community since it marked a defection on the part of a dentist from the self-protective society of dentists. It had long been an unwritten ethical rule of associations to refrain from discrediting the profession.

The most significant impacts consumer awareness may have on the individual provider are patients' increased confidence in challenging treatment plans, in deciding to change providers when displeased, and in initiating litigation against dental care providers.

Consumers are interested in quality of dental care, supporting the idea of peer clinical review and continuing education as important avenues for ensuring quality treatment (Strauss et al., 1980).

ASSESSING THE QUALITY OF CARE
Grievance committees

Whether the move toward assessment of quality of performance in health care is a direct result of the consumer movement is questioned by some. There have been long-standing ethics committees of the state and local dental associations as evidence of dentistry's continuing interest in monitoring the quality of care its members provide the public. State boards of dentistry have had the power to revoke the license of any provider who did not meet the standards of the state practice act.

These review committees have existed for many years, but their impact in identifying and resolving weaknesses has been minimal because of the limited financial resources and the limited contingency controls they in actuality have over practicing dentists (Milgrom, 1978). The majority of complaints brought to them by patients may be resolved, but they have limited means to seek out or monitor the quality of care delivered by the individual practicing dentists to whom no disfavorable attention has been drawn. The committees usually do not have provisions for remediation for providers whose level of care is unacceptable (Milgrom, 1978).

State boards can revoke the licenses of practitioners they deem to be delivering substandard care. Often they need to prove their findings in a court of law, since they are often sued by the licensee for having taken capricious action. The state boards of dentistry review complaints and take official legal action, but there has been no claim that they have had a significant impact on improving the overall quality of care delivered by providers. They ensure that the very minimum of ethical and legal requirements are enforced but again only within the limited resources they are provided (Milgrom, 1978).

The audit

A more ambitious mechanism for reviewing dental care is the audit. One of the primary reasons for quality assessment, aside from greater consumer interest in the services they receive, was the need for third party payers to review whether care was being delivered and whether it fell within acceptable bounds of practice (Bailit, Issues, 1980). When care is delivered through a prepaid dental plan, the purchaser of the care, the patients who receive care, and the insurance company or HMO all are interested in the quality of care received. The patients certainly are interested in the way they are treated; those with a financial interest want to know the incidence of overtreatment or undertreatment, access to the providers of care, the technical quality of the work, and the amount of concern shown for the patient (Marcus, 1985). Thus, the movement toward third-party paid dental care has introduced momentum toward a workable system of quality assurance. The audit has great potential for monitoring the quality of care since it carries an economic contingency.

Insurance carriers use the audit process, which is a review by professionals and specially trained laypersons of a sample of patient records, radiographic surveys, data regarding appointment visits, sequence of treatment and fees, and study models (Egdahl and Gertman, 1976; Mayes, 1974). The basic goal is to assess the relevance of planned procedures to the needs of the patient, the emphasis on preserving teeth, and the appropriateness of the fees and filed claims. The economic contingency is that if the service is unnecessary or an obvious case of substandard care, or if the fees are unreasonable, the claim will not be paid.

This audit is apparently essential. When it was first instituted, discrepancies between reported and actual claims were numerous. Pennsylvania Blue Shield found 101 oral surgery offices with discrepancies for more than $500,000 in overcharges among the 152 offices they surveyed. A similar audit in New York revealed fraud in Medicaid claims. The audit, ferreting out practitioners who are cheating the system, is one step toward better quality (Milgrom, 1978).

A more global audit compares national norms with the frequency with which providers perform certain kinds of procedures. A provider who performs at a given number of standard deviations from the mean on certain key procedures is targeted by the reviewers for investigation. Again this procedure helps identify those who are outside the "usual and customary" practice of dentistry. It is another increment toward quality assurance.

An audit can be implemented in a group practice environment as an internal check on quality. It can be carried out by the providers or by a person employed to perform those procedures. An audit system could be developed for a local professional society review of care.

Audit systems do serve to reduce fraud and to identify providers who are outside the bounds of usual practice. However, like grievance committees, audit systems do not affect the process of dental care delivery. Records cannot speak to the gentleness and accuracy with which an injection is given. They cannot reflect the trauma induced during an oral prophylaxis or during the application of a rubber dam. The record does not reflect the quality of interpersonal communications with the patient. Moreover, record audits typically lead to punishment for improper behavior and offer no reward for above-average performance.

If quality assessment is intended to improve dental practice and encourage providers to learn new skills and sharpen old ones, it is doubtful that the audit alone will succeed. Both medical and dental quality assurance programs are looking at multiple measures of quality (LoGerfo and Brook, 1984; Morris, 1986).

Marcus, Koch, and Gershen (1979) described an audit (or records review system) that provides the practitioners with *quantitative information* about the care delivered and *qualitative information* that relates to the kind of care individual patients are receiving. One of his examples is that of a spur of calculus noticed radiographically at one of the reviews. If that same spur is detected on radiographs taken 1 year later, that is an indication that this one patient has not received adequate scaling. If this is a typical finding, where several patients are noticed to have residual calculus, the providers know they must take action to rectify the situation.

Also, it is important to look at the dentist-patient relationship to determine the extent to which the clinician's views of the patient affect treatment. The dentist's perceptions of the patient's manageability, treatability, and likability or attractiveness no doubt have an influence on how care is delivered. This could and perhaps should be incorporated into a system that looks at the process of care (Kerr, 1985).

These aspects of dental care, specifically the attention the clinician gives to patient comfort and to explaining treatment, are important to patients (Strauss et al., 1980).

Peer review: external committees

Complex process evaluations require more than a record audit. Direct observation and feedback from patients and co-workers round out the "hard data" from patient records.

A more sophisticated method of assessing quality of care is *peer review,* in which a group of colleague-providers audit records, evaluate the outcome of care, and actually assess the *process* used in the provision of care. The results of the group peer review can be measured against specific, predetermined criteria so that recommendations for improvement can be based on an objective definition of quality practice on which all can agree. With the refined behavioral descriptions of diagnostic, treatment planning, preventive, and therapeutic services that are available for nearly all phases of dental care, measuring provider performance is a logical step forward in measuring the quality of care.

Peer review committees have been used with success in California, Connecticut, and other states (Bailit, Quality, 1980; Demby et al., 1985). Special organized groups of dentists have used peer review and peer teaching as part of their program for clinical excellence. However, in most cases an external review committee defines the criteria and makes the judgments. Even if the criteria and evaluation procedures are reasonable and defensible, to many professionals the external review committee still smacks of policing. Positive behavior change (improved quality of care) is more likely to occur if the professionals are involved in setting the criteria and examining each other in a cooperative but noncollusive system and if there is an internal and external reward for participation rather than merely the threat of an external punishment.

According to dentists actively involved in peer review, participating as a reviewer and as a reviewee is one of the best ways to increase clinical competency (Harbo and Heaney, 1985).

Peer review: an extension of the voluntary study club

The framework for voluntary peer groups that can evaluate both the process and end product of dental care exists in the familiar study club. The study club traditionally has been a small group of interested dentists or auxiliaries who agree to work together to learn new information or a new skill. They may work together for a short time until the specific material is mastered. They may stay intact for years, moving from one point of interest to another. The study club is voluntary; the norm is learning together and from one another. It is unencumbered by association, governmental, or insurance carrier regulation. The move from a study club to a peer group involves agreeing not only to learn new skills but to identify the areas of practice that are most integral to quality care and to evaluate each other on how those aspects of practice are performed.

Study clubs are usually formed on the basis of common interest and values. Peer groups can be formed the same way—on the basis of common philosophies of practice or on other criteria that will maximize areas of agreement. Heterogeneous groupings may also be workable and desirable as long as there is sufficient time for the members to agree on the aspects of practice they wish to assess. A group trainer can meet with a local dental society and help the members explore the peer review concept and models that can be used in dentistry. The members are formed into groups on the basis of common philosophy or specialty or on the basis of location or availability. The individual peer group establishes which aspects of practice it wants to evaluate. It reviews samples of criteria and guidelines for the chosen areas and rewrites or creates guidelines on which the members agree. There can be more than one approved protocol for any given procedure. The only criterion is that all approved methods be documented in the literature and be in compliance with accepted standards of practice. This arriving at a consensus may require considerable time, but it is a keystone in creating a cohesive group.

Once the criteria are defined, the group is ready to observe and evaluate individual members' patient care. The group trainer prepares the members to conduct objective observations and to systematically compare observations with the guidelines of the group. By offering and soliciting constructive feedback and by active listening, the trainer helps the group sharpen its skills. The observations can be done in person with two peers observing a third. Immediately following the session the three peers review the notes for clarification. At the subsequent peer group meeting, all members hear the observed member relate the experience, including areas of strength and weakness. The peer group offers support, identifies areas in which the peer may need to improve or try an alternative approach, and praises work that is clearly within the parameters of good dentistry.

Clinical care also can be videotaped with relative ease, enabling the observed person to see him/herself and making it possible for the whole peer group to observe and comment on each other's performances.

Each peer receives two or three observations during a 6-month period. Progress in areas needing improvement can be charted. As the group is satisfied with the progress of members within the group, it can move on to other practice protocols or turn to learning new skills.

Members of voluntary peer groups similar to the one described above can accrue several benefits:

1. A sense of cooperation with other professionals in identifying strengths and needs
2. An affirmation of professional self-worth that is difficult to sustain when there is no source of external feedback from those who are best able to judge one's skills (Froebe and Bain, 1976)
3. A professional support group that can be relied on in times of professional or even personal crisis and with whom the professional can share triumphs and successes
4. An inexpensive, simple resource for improving the quality of dental care

There are, of course, some difficulties with the voluntary peer group model. One is the fact that it is a closed group that can become collusive. If all the members in the group tacitly agree not to criticize, few improvements in practice will follow. A related problem is competition among members (Waldman and Schlissel, 1977). The group trainer can assist in identifying these traps. If either appears in the early stages of the group, the trainer can play the role of consumer and point out the futility of having a peer group if candor is disallowed or if members are comparing each other's skills rather than using the guidelines of the group for evaluation. Third, few professionals may see the worth of joining the group. Those who need it the most will not be bothered; those who already have high standards of practice will be the first to join.

The incentives for joining a peer group include the desire for closer professional relationships and an opportunity for professional growth. This will be sufficient reason for a small percentage of practitioners. Other incentives, more attractive to the vast majority of professionals, can include exemption from audits by third-party payers. For instance, an insurance carrier may agree that dentists who participate in the voluntary peer groups in good faith will not need to submit treatment plans for preauthorization. Further, malpractice insurance carriers may offer lower premium rates to practitioners who demonstrate good faith participation in a voluntary peer group such as described here. Yet another incentive is the potential rise in income that can follow active participation in a practice network that uses a peer group system (Bentley and Woodall, 1984).

Networking: professional growth with economic incentives

A number of independent solo dental practices are experimenting with networking as a way to improve their patient pool and increase income. A group of dentists with similar practice philosophies agree to form a group (network) to pool funds. The marketing carries a common theme to the public. The theme may be prevention, quality care, low-cost conservative dentistry, flexible appointment hours, or some other message that they believe will attract new patients. For instance, an advertisement will mention a telephone number to call to locate the participating dental practice most convenient to the interested caller. Thus a solo practitioner can sacrifice minimal autonomy and relatively few resources to attract new patients.

As networks become more common and individual networks grow in size, one problem will undoubtedly emerge. Although each member agrees on the theme, some may not adhere to it. For instance, if the theme is prevention, there must be some standard of prevention that is met by all members of the network, or the advertising will be proven false, and in time the network will be ineffective in drawing patients seeking preventive dentistry. The peer group model can be used to enable a network to set a theme, establish the criteria for implementing it in all the practices, and monitor it to ensure that it is maintained. The peer group model can be extended to help participating dentists meet other standards that are critical for the economic and professional well-being of its members. The peer group can become the common link among networks of professionals (Bentley and Woodall, 1984).

PROJECTS, SUCCESSES, AND CONTINUING NEEDS

Quality assurance has been discussed and debated at great length in the last 20 years. However, it has yet to emerge as a viable mechanism for improving the quality of care. Many models are authoritarian or mechanistic. Others are impotent in changing the way providers deliver care. The profession needs a model that will draw members to it without threat. It needs a model that will meet the needs of the professionals as well as those of the consumers.

The insurance companies and other third-party payers are interested in establishing an acceptable, workable system that provides reliable, valid data and that encourages quality care. The

American Dental Association is also interested in developing a system that is acceptable to the members and that actually has an impact on maintaining quality standards.

In 1981 the American Dental Association gained membership on the Joint Commission on Accreditation of Hospitals (JCAH), helping establish the mandate that dental services provided in hospitals should be evaluated. With this move, dentistry moved closer to the "mainstream of medical quality assurance activities" (Gotowka and Bailit, 1981).

In addition to sharing responsibilities for quality assessment with medicine, the ADA has taken steps to support and coordinate efforts that focus on individual dental practices. In 1982 the American Dental Association Office of Quality Assurance was established to centralize and coordinate activities relating to quality assurance in dentistry. It interfaced with numerous projects. The most comprehensive project was the Development of Evaluation Methods and Computer Applications in Dentistry (DEMCAD), which developed practice assessment programs and computer analysis strategies over a 4½ year period (Klyop, 1985). A portion of this project brought together a group of dentists to define the criteria that are important in assessing a dental practice and then conducted field trials to establish the reliability and validity of the instrument (Morris, 1986).

An important distinction has arisen from this project and from the work of others. There are really two parts to the puzzle of quality: quality assessment and quality assurance. The assessment phase looks at what exists, describing the situation accurately and identifying improvements. Assurance implies taking steps to improve the situation and ensure that quality is maintained (Marcus et al., 1979).

The American Dental Hygienists' Association has also struggled with the idea of clinical competence and quality assurance. In 1979 the organization created the Commission for Assurance of Competence and subsequently the Task Force to Develop Standards of Practice. They have developed a detailed plan for the Competence Assurance Program (CAP), which addresses quality assessment, postgraduate education, study, and recognition of achievement (Standards, 1985). In the November 1985 issue of *Dental Hygiene,* the organization published the Standards of Applied Dental Hygiene Practice as a step toward a full program for competency assurance in dental hygiene.

The coming decade will see continued efforts at refining assessment methods, making it ble for reviewers and study clubs to feel more certain that what they are looking at are real indicators of the quality of practice in a dental practice. A more difficult challenge, the true bottom line of "quality," is implementing programs that actually help providers improve the skills, judgment, and attitudes that directly impact on a patient's well-being and, ultimately, the health of the practice.

Review questions

1. What two forces have brought dentistry to look at alternative ways of assessing quality of care? ① consumer movement ② third-party payers

2. What three issues have been the focus of consumer complaints regarding health care? Cost, Access, Quality

3. Briefly describe an *audit* system for assessing quality of care. External reviewers to match technique used for diagnosis + tx nec, ensures tx was actually done.

4. How is a small peer group *clinical review* different from an external audit? voluntary group of dentists to set the criteria used + observe ea other for techniques, discuss discrepancies + prescribe changes,

GROUP ACTIVITIES

1. Institute an audit system to review patient records, appointments, and the outcome of care.

2. Institute a peer review system of clinical performance that focuses on end product. Modify it to focus on *process of care,* using available task analyses to define the criteria. Introduce a public member and analyze how he/she affects intragroup competitiveness or reluctance to identify weaknesses.

3. Review articles reflective of consumer awareness of the problems in the health care system.

4. Review the Standards of Applied Dental Hygiene Practice for their ease of use in establishing a clinical competence (quality) assessment program among practitioners.

REFERENCES

Angevine, E.: The consumer's viewpoint of dental hygiene, Dent. Hyg. **47**:380, 1973.

Bailit, H.L.: Issues in regulating quality of care and containing costs within private sector policy, J. Dent. Educ. **44**:530, 1980.

Bailit, H.: Quality assurance in general dentistry, part 1, Compendium on Continuing Education **1**(1):49, 1980.

Bentley, J.M., and Woodall, I.R.: Networking: the private practitioner's key to quality and marketing, J. Dent. Practice Admin. **1**:3, 1984.

Demby, N.A., Rosenthal, M., Angello, M., and Calhoun, W.F.: A comprehensive quality assurance system for practicing dentists, Dent. Clin. North Am. **29**:545, 1985.

Dreifus, C.: The world according to Nader, The Progressive **48**(7):58, 1984.

Egdahl, R.H., and Gertman, P.M., editors: Quality assurance in health care, Germantown, Md., 1976, Aspen Systems Corp.

Froebe, D.J., and Bain, R.J.: Quality assurance programs and controls in nursing, St. Louis, 1976, The C.V. Mosby Co.

Gotowka, T., and Bailit, H.L.: Quality assurance systems for hospital outpatient dental programs: background, Spec. Care Dent. **1**:211, 1981.

Harbo, J.N., and Heaney, K.M.: Quality assurance: a reviewer's perspective, Dent. Clin. North Am. **29**:589, 1985.

Jones, P.F.: The changing role of the dental hygienist. In Boundy, S.S., and Reynolds, N.J., editors: Current concepts in dental hygiene, St. Louis, 1977, The C.V. Mosby Co.

Kerr, I.L.: Quality assurance and the dentist-patient relationship, Dent. Clin. North Am. **29**:581, 1985.

Klyop, J.S: The dental profession's commitment to quality assurance, Dent. Clin. North Am. **29**:521, 1985.

LoGerfo, J.P., and Brook, R.H.: The quality of care. In Williams, S.J., and Torrens, P.R., editors: Introduction to health services, ed. 2, New York, 1984, John Wiley & Sons.

McGuire, T.: The tooth trip, New York, 1972, Random House, Inc., and Berkeley, Calif., 1972, The Bookworks.

Marcus, M.: Quality assurance and prepaid programs, Dent. Clin. North Am. **29:**497, 1985.

Marcus, M., Koch, A.L., and Gershen, J.A.: A record review model for assessing dental practices. Calif. Dent. Assoc. J. **7**(10):51–54, 1979.

Maurizi, A.R.: Public policy and the dental care market, Washington, D.C., 1975, American Enterprise Institute for Public Policy Research.

Mayes, D.S.: Blue Shield's quality assurance program, J. Public Health Dent. **34:**215, 1974.

Milgrom, P.: Regulation and the quality of dental care, Rockville, Md., 1978, Aspen Systems Corp.

Morris, A.: Personal communication, 1986.

Nader, R.: Unsafe at any speed: the designed-in dangers of the American automobile, New York, 1965, Grossman Publishers.

Nader, R.: Wake-up America: unsafe x-rays, Ladies Home Journal **85:**126, May 1968.

Quint, B.: A closemouthed look at bad dentistry, Money **3:**11, 1974.

"Revere, Paul," DDS: Dentistry and its victims, New York, 1970, St. Martin's Press, Inc.

Standards of applied dental hygiene practice, Dent. Hyg. **59:**510, 1985.

Strauss, R.P., Claris, S.M., Lindahl, R.L., and Parker, P.G.: Patients' attitudes toward quality assurance in dentistry, J. Am. Coll. Dent. **47:**101, 1980.

Tolpin, B.B.: The role of the consumer in quality assurance, Dent. Clin. North Am. **29:**595, 1985.

Waldman, H.B., and Schlissel, E.: Honor codes and peer review: Is peer review really possible? J. Dent. Educ. **41:**126, 1977.

PART TWO

Legal considerations

The way in which a health care provider relates to patients to obtain and sustain health has often been regarded as both a matter of common sense and an ethical mandate. To a large extent the "proper" way to relate to a patient can indeed be understood in terms of everyday courtesy and sensitivity to the patient's wants, needs, and expectations. With the addition of the sobering realization that the care to be provided does affect the health and well-being of a person, most health care providers demonstrate an ability to establish a professional, caring relationship with patients.

The law has something to add to the common sense and ethical mandate of relationships between patients and providers. The law has defined over the years some specific rights and duties that the patient and health care provider have. Failure to fulfill a duty can mean unhappy days in the courtroom, financial loss, and a tarnished reputation.

These chapters provide an overview of those rights and duties, along with important guidelines for avoiding legal entanglements that could arise from ignorance of the law, a failure to understand the consequences of acts, or omissions that violate patients' rights. The chapters also give the health care provider some working definitions of terms. These definitions should make it easier to communicate with legal counsel about preventive measures to follow and to discuss possible legal actions against oneself or against another.

An important overlay on these chapters is the need to consider the patient's perspective—the trusting, but more fully aware person who seeks only necessary care and who expects appropriate information, attention, compassion, and careful, competent treatment. Basic principles of communication—listening, providing full information, anticipating needs, and responding to questions—are important adjunctive skills which help to prevent legal action and to ensure that patients maintain trust in the work the clinician provides.

CHAPTER 6

Rights and duties in the patient–health care provider relationship

OBJECTIVES: The reader will be able to:

1. Describe the nature of the legal relationship between the health care provider and the patient.
2. Recognize those circumstances under which a health care provider is legally obligated to render care to a patient.
3. Define *duty.*
4. List the legal duties required of a health care provider.
5. Given a set of circumstances
   a. Indicate if a duty has been breached.
   b. Identify the duty that has been breached.
   c. Specify the possible result of that breach.
6. List the duties that a patient owes a health care provider as a result of the contractual relationship.
7. Define *reasonable care* in terms of the duties the law expects the health care provider to fulfill in a contractual relationship with a patient.
8. Given a set of circumstances in which a patient is claiming that a health care provider did not exercise reasonable care, analyze whether the claim is supportable in terms of the duties the patient and the health care provider owe to one another as a result of the contractual relationship.
9. Define
   a. *Negligence.*
   b. The legal standard of the *reasonably prudent man.*
10. Define *privileged communication.*
11. Recognize that there is an *agency* relationship between dental auxiliary personnel and employers.
12. Provide examples of how the principle of *respondeat superior* affects an employer-dentist as well as the accused employee should he/she be charged with an alleged tort committed against the employer's patient.
13. Project the probable impact of expanded functions delegation on the legal definition of standards of skill and care for dental auxiliary personnel.
14. Assess personal rules of conduct in dealing with patients to determine if rights and duties are being respected and alter conduct when necessary.

ESTABLISHING THE LEGAL RELATIONSHIP

When a patient requests that a health care provider perform some service for the assessment, maintenance, or improvement of the patient's health, the health care provider legally has a choice. He/she can agree to provide the service or can refuse. Although there is an ethical mandate to provide care when it is needed, health personnel are not required by *law* to accept a patient. One exception to the rule is government-funded programs in which regulations may stipulate that any and all persons meeting eligibility criteria be accepted as patients by the health care staff (Miller, 1970). Another is when the patient is enrolled in a prepaid program, such as a health maintenance organization or a preferred provider organization (PPO), and the provider has contracted to provide care for enrolled persons.

Once the patient is accepted for care by the provider of care (or once the patient is enrolled in a prepaid program), a contract is established (Morris and Moritz, 1971). It may be *implied* by the actions of the provider and the patient, or it may be an *express* contract in which the terms of the agreement are discussed by the two parties or formalized in a written agreement. There are many advantages and disadvantages to be considered in deciding what kind of contract is "best," which will be discussed in the chapter concerning contracts. What is important to consider now is what this consensual, *contractual* relationship means in terms of basic rights and duties shared by the persons in the contract (Miller, 1970).

Rights and duties

A health care provider owes certain duties to the patient, just as the patient owes certain duties to the provider. A *duty* is "that which a person owes to another. An obligation to do a thing" (Black, 1979). The patient has certain specific rights by virtue of the contractual relationship, and the health care provider is obligated to respect those contractually defined rights. Conversely, the patient has certain duties that correlate to the rights of the heath care provider.

The duties of the health care provider include: (1) protecting and respecting the personal and property rights of the patient, (2) providing only that care that is necessary and that the patient has agreed to have provided, (3) completing care within a reasonable amount of time, and (4) achieving reasonably satisfactory results if satisfaction was guaranteed (Morris and Moritz, 1971). These four duties are integral to the legal, contractual relationship. Two others, implied by law, are that the provider exercise "reasonable care"

in performing health care services and that the charge for the services provided be a "reasonable fee" (Miller, 1970).

If any of the duties is unmet, the patient has grounds for a civil action against the health care provider. If the patient proves by a *preponderance of evidence* that a duty was unmet, the patient may be awarded damages (financial restitution) for the wrong-doing (Black, 1979; Prosser, 1971).

It should be remembered that the patient has duties to pay the reasonable fee and to cooperate in treatment (Miller, 1970; Sarner, 1963). The patient may lose a case against a health professional or even find him/herself the object of a civil suit if either of these duties is unmet.

It should be obvious that the contractual nature of the relationship provides a built-in set of checks and balances established by the law that helps ensure equitable and "reasonable" business, as well as professional procedures.

What is most crucial, however, in daily clinical practice is a full understanding of what those duties mean. The description provided here, after all, is really quite vague. What does it mean to protect the personal and property rights of a patient? How should that be interpreted?

Does it mean that the dental hygienist must refrain from asking prying questions of the patient's personal life that have no relevance to dental health? Does it mean that the physician should ensure that the walkways in the office are free of obstacles that could harm a patient? Does it mean that the dentist must respect the patient's right to ownership of dentures and in some instances x-rays? The answer to these questions is yes. And the law offers additional practical interpretations.

The patient has a right to confidentiality regarding his/her condition and the care received. Displays, presentations, and publication of photographs of patients are a breach of the right of privacy of each patient.* Written permission to use patient records, photographs, and the patient's

---

*Radiographic surveys that do not readily identify the person are an exception to this rule.

name in any public manner is absolutely necessary (Morris and Moritz, 1971). The patient may understandably not want his/her ailments or cures to be known to others, and the health provider has the duty to ensure confidentiality. This includes permitting only personnel contributing to the performance of health care services to be present in the treatment room. Specific permission must be obtained from the patient before nonessential persons may be admitted.

This right to privacy includes not only the particulars of the health care procedures but also any information about the patient acquired in the course of treatment. The law considers such information to be *privileged communication,* and the health care provider is bound by the law not to reveal the information even in a court of law (Black, 1979; Kessler, 1978). This right is personal to the patient and can be waived by him/her, for example, when the patient asks the provider of care to testify regarding his/her condition. The only exceptions relate to information regarding child abuse and communicable disease. Some states expect such information will be revealed in a court of law, and most further require that such information be promptly reported to the appropriate authorities (Miller, 1970; Morris and Moritz, 1971).

The second duty mentioned in defining the obligations of the health care provider to the patient relates to the requirement that the provider complete the agreed-on care and not abandon the patient (Morris and Moritz, 1971). The explicit condition of entering a contract is that the agreed-on treatment be completed—and within a reasonable period of time. Long waiting periods to commence or complete treatment violate this duty. If treatment is going to exceed one year, it is best to secure the patient's agreement in writing.

It is *not* the provider's right to terminate treatment before it is completed. There are appropriate ways to withdraw from the contract to perform health care services, including a written notice of intent to withdraw, a statement of what care remains to be performed, and suggestions for obtaining the described care. But under no circumstances may the provider purposely extend treatment over an unreasonable amount of time or simply stop making appointments for a patient. To do the latter is to abandon the patient in the eyes of the law (Miller, 1970).

For a patient to prove abandonment, he/she would have to show that the prescribed series of treatments was left incomplete and that it was unreasonable to expect the patient to resume treatment under the care of another provider. In the case of temporary or extended absence on the part of the provider, the patient will need to show harm as a result of not having had access to another provider of care. In any case the provider does have an obligation to see treatment to its completion and to make some provisions for access to care during periods of absence.

An example from a 1982 case provides a description of abandonment. A patient was continuing to have discomfort in her teeth and gums after root canal treatment and fixed bridgework was placed on her anterior teeth. Despite the fact that the bridgework continually loosened and even fell out on several occasions, the dentist "reassured her at all times that she was 'progressing nicely.' " The abandonment occurred when the dentist's receptionist told the patient that the dentist wanted her "to go elsewhere for treatment as he could no longer help. . . [the plaintiff] inasmuch as [she] complained too much." The main thrust of this suit was the poor standard of care exercised in preparing the root canal and the bridgework, but the abandonment of the patient contributed to the finding that the dentist breached the patient's rights (Jobson, 1982).

Experimental or nonstandard drugs, equipment, and procedures should not be used in the care of any patient (Miller, 1970). The patient has the right to expect that commonly accepted, standard care that would be provided by at least a "respectable minority" of practitioners will be provided. Even knowledgeable consent documented by written permission does not provide immunity from liability if the innovation fails and harm is caused to the patient.

A closely related duty requires that the provider perform *only* those services to which the patient has agreed (Miller, 1970). Performing a procedure that the patient has not agreed to constitutes technical battery. The patient can recover damages if he/she can prove that something was performed that was not in the treatment plan to which the patient agreed.

There are, of course, instances in which the law presumes consent, such as when a patient is unconscious and is in need of oxygen, cardiopulmonary resuscitation, or medication to reverse the medical emergency.

It is the health care provider's duty to ensure the safety and well-being of patients by making certain that there are no hazards present on the premises. All equipment used should be safe, and the patient should have a clear pathway to and from treatment rooms.

Other duties included in the concept of providing reasonable care include keeping the patient informed of the progress of treatment and his/her condition, arranging for care of the patient during periods of temporary absence, and referring the patient to a specialist if necessary (Miller, 1970). If the scope of care required to meet a patient's needs is beyond the skill and/or knowledge of the provider, the patient should be referred promptly to another provider or specialist who will be able to meet those needs.

Two suits reported in the recent appellate literature relate to the requirement that the patient be kept informed. One of the suits involved a dentist leaving a fractured root tip behind when attempting extractions and not telling the patient what had occurred. The failure to inform was worsened by his subseqent failure to take proper steps to remedy the situation. It is important to note that the fracturing of the root tip is, in itself, not necessarily negligence; a reasonably prudent dentist using ordinary skill and care can fracture a root tip. The malpractice enters the picture when the dentist does not disclose the accident to the patient and, further, takes no action to have the tip removed (Dailey, 1983).

The second case involved a dentist who did not inform a patient of the extensive nature of caries in her child's teeth. Parents or guardians have the right to be fully informed about their children's health and the treatment suggested and carried out (Lee, 1982).

Standards of care

With the introduction of the word *reasonable* in describing duties, the concept of legal standards or guidelines to ascertain whether a duty has been breached is likewise introduced. What does *reasonable* mean—especially as it relates to the law?

The dictionary definition of reasonable care is care that is "just; proper. Ordinary or usual. Fit and appropriate to the end in view." And the measure the law uses in determining whether a provider has exercised reasonable care is known as the standard of what would be exercised by the *reasonably prudent practitioner* (Black 1979; Murchison and Nichols, 1970). The law has gone even further, saying in a 1974 court case that what is typically practiced may not be sufficient to meet the standard of reasonable care (Helling, 1974).

This measure of conduct applies to all persons in society in their daily activities with other human beings. When a person does not measure up to the reasonably prudent person and harm results to another, *negligence* may be charged. When the charge specifically relates to a professional person's lack of reasonable care in serving a patient or client, the charge of negligence is referred to as *malpractice* (Willig, 1970).

Malpractice is the "failure of one rendering professional services to exercise that degree of skill and learning commonly applied under all the circumstances in the community by the average prudent reputable member of the profession with the result of injury, loss or damage to the recipient of those services or to those entitled to rely upon them" (Black, 1979).

In *Costa v. Storm* (1984) a judgment was affirmed against a general dentist who did not refer

*EXception
is CPR*

his patient to a specialist despite the patient's persistent "gum infection." An expert witness (another dentist) testified, in addition, that a tooth the defendant extracted would normally be saved by other treatment and that "the ordinary reasonably prudent dentist" would try to save it. The evidence supported claims that the patient was left in a "dentally unstable condition" for "extended periods" (Costa, 1984). This case highlights three of the major judicial points made in this chapter: failure to refer, failure to meet a reasonable standard of care, and failure to complete treatment in a reasonable amount of time. In this case, more than one duty was breached; it is possible to file a suit citing one breach of duty or several.

There are three main classifications of charges that a patient may bring against a health care provider as a consequence of the explicit and implicit duties the provider owes the patient as a result of the consensual, contractual nature of the relationship. The patient may charge *breach of contract* if his/her property and privacy rights have been violated, if the services agreed to are not performed, or if they are delayed for an extended period of time. The patient may charge *technical battery* if the provider performs some service to which the patient has not agreed (Miller, 1970; Prosser, 1971). Or the patient may charge *negligence* if the care provided does not satisfy the duty of reasonable prudence *and* causes harm to the patient, or if a hazard is allowed to exist in the office that harms the patient.

All of the previous charges are covered by civil law since they relate to disagreement between two individuals and do not connote any wrong against society (the basis for criminal law). Only in the case of gross, wanton negligence may criminal proceedings also be appropriate actions against the defendant. Civil law has two branches relevant to this discussion: contracts and torts. Breach of contract is considered under contract law, whereas charges of negligence and technical battery are parts of tort law (Black, 1979). Later chapters will discuss the distinctions between these branches of the law.

LEGAL ASPECTS OF EVOLVING ROLES

The implications of the basic issues of contracts and torts have a special meaning for health care providers whose roles in delivery of health services are evolving. The increased scope of the role of the dental auxiliary in providing care is quite obvious in some states in which it is legal for dental hygienists to administer block and infiltration anesthesia and in which other services previously performed only by the dentist may now be delegated to the dental hygienist or dental assistant.

Just as every right has a correlative duty, an expansion in the role brings an accompanying increase in responsibility. The auxiliary with the legal right to provide direct patient care has the duty to provide that care with the caution, foresight, and skill expected of the "reasonably prudent person." For instance, in 1984 the District Court of Appeals of Florida confirmed that a dental hygienist "when cleaning teeth, is a provider of health care within the meaning of [that state's] statute of limitations for actions for medical malpractice." The courts see dental hygienists as responsible for their professional activities, which, while limited to the oral prophylaxis in this particular case, can be extended to all clinical dental hygiene functions (Estes, 1984).

The contemporary issue that becomes obvious is whether the auxiliary performing a service is properly held to the standard of other auxiliaries or to the standard of the dentist, whose function it also is to perform those services (Murchison and Nichols, 1970). The law has historically said that the auxiliary will be measured against other auxiliaries and that the dentist will be measured against other dentists (Murchison and Nichols, 1970). But this may imply a dual standard of quality for the patient.

With each step toward greater responsibility in providing health care, the health care provider is held against a greater measure in terms of the law. This fact has been confronted by nursing, which has an ever-expanding definition of practice and which often includes practice without any direct supervision. Irene Murchison described the parallel situation in nursing this way:

Although there has been no change of legal doctrine, the advances of medical science have been accompanied by radically new developments in nursing practice which require careful legal evaluation. As the nurse assumes increased responsibility for complex acts requiring greater skill, she should be aware that the boundaries of reasonable conduct are shifting. Indeed, were a nurse to harm a patient today, she could well be held to a level of knowledge of medical science and medical practice unknown a generation ago (Murchison and Nichols, 1970).

The proper caution of the evolving health care provider certainly includes adequate preparation to knowledgeably perform new functions before accepting them as part of the scope of practice. No new function should casually be added to that scope, even as a response to urgent health care needs. Educational preparation and a careful assessment of the legal implications of such an additional function should precede its acceptance. In addition, health care providers who delegate certain functions to dental auxiliaries must be certain that (1) the person designated to perform a given procedure is competent, and (2) the dental statutes of the licensing jurisdiction in which the practice is located permits such delegation. To do otherwise can result in a malpractice action against the primary health care provider as well as against the auxiliary *and* the state board can revoke the privilege to practice (Addiego, 1978; Kunkle, 1978; Little, 1983).

Rise in malpractice actions

Malpractice actions are common in an age of consumerism when the public is becoming aware of its rights and is learning how to assert those rights (Morganstern, 1973). The increase in civil actions against physicians and dentists is a sign of that new awareness. Higher premiums for professional liability insurance, the growing difficulty of obtaining such insurance at any price, and the significant increase in the incidence of claims and suits along with larger damage awards should be strong indicators that the public will not tolerate lack of reasonable care and should warn the health professions that reasonable care had better be provided.

In the past this threat of malpractice or breach of contract action was felt primarily by the physician and to a lesser extent by the dentist. Dentists incurred an increase in the number and severity of malpractice claims during the 1970s. In 1985 the malpractice claims against dentists, and the concomitant rise in malpractice insurance premiums, were still rising. The incidence of malpractice claims in 1978 was 6.85%; it jumped to 8.27% in 1982 and was continuing to rise. In 1978 the average damages payment was $6,600; in 1982 it was nearly $20,000. The rises in frequency and severity of such suits cause insurers to raise their premiums. While the reality of escalating costs poses a serious problem, the greater threat comes from the possibility of lack of availability of insurance as carriers become more selective in whom they will insure (Council, 1985).

The factors cited as probable causes of the growth of malpractice claims and their severity were:

growth in the number and complexity of medical treatments; proplaintiff trends in common law in general, and in particular the demise of traditional malpractice defenses such as charitable immunity and the locality rule; an increase in the number of lawyers and passage of no-fault automobile legislation in some states; and such intangible factors as the erosion of physician-patient relationships (Danzon, 1984).

A 1983 study, using multiple regression analysis (a statistical technique that determines the extent to which each of a variety of variables explains an outcome variable), concluded that the legal reform laws of the late 1970s have been shown to successfully curb the severity and frequency of legal claims against physicians. It also concluded that urban living, regardless of the density of physicians and lawyers, was a major contributing factor in the number and severity of malpractice suits. The researcher did not have an explanation for this phenomenon; pursuing the issue further would most likely lead researchers to examine sociological conditions such as alienation, limited resources including space and privacy, and impersonal delivery of care by multiple providers, which may occur more often in dense-population areas than in other areas (Danzon, 1984).

Health care providers who are employed by a dentist, clinic, or institution should be aware of the need for malpractice insurance. Health professionals, such as nurses and dental auxiliaries, whose scope of practice usually finds them employed by physicians and dentists, have suffered from the delusion that all liability for their own negligence would be absorbed by the employer. However, the law relating to the *agency relationship* between the employer-physician and the employee-nurse is clear on the fact that even though the employer may be vicariously liable, the employee *is* personally responsible and liable for his/her actions while furthering the objectives of the practice (Black, 1979; Creighton, 1970; Murchison and Nichols, 1970; Seavey, 1964).

Therefore it is necessary that the employed health care provider (including the dental hygienist) conduct his/her professional affairs with the same respect for the patient's rights as that of the wise physician or dentist.

It is true that the employer is often named in a suit in which the employee caused some harm to a patient. This is legally allowable under the concept of *respondeat superior*, which means literally, "let the master answer" for the wrongful acts of his servants or agents. The attraction of suing the master is a practical, economic one (Seavey, 1964). "It is in the interest of every plaintiff to have as many financially responsible persons as defendants as he can legitimately find" (Murchison and Nichols, 1970). However, this does not mean that a dental hygienist, dietitian, nurse, respiratory therapist, or other allied health professional does not need personal malpractice insurance. Despite the person's position as an employee, a suit brought solely against him/her for a tort or one brought jointly against him/her and the employer may result in devastating financial losses to the individual if no personal malpractice coverage is in effect. Even if the employee is covered under the employer's "umbrella" policy, it is possible for the employer's insurance carrier to sue the employee if the employee lost a malpractice suit for which the carrier paid damages. *It is essential to carry one's own insurance protection* (Peterson, 1985).

It should be apparent that the legal ramifications of health care practice can have a profound impact on the individual health care provider. A good reputation, as well as financial assets, requires the application of these basic legal principles in daily practice to ensure that the duties owed the patient are fulfilled.

Review questions

Case 1

A 25-year-old man arrives for the first time at a dental office for an oral examination and necessary treatment.
1. Is the dentist legally obligated to provide dental care? ~~Not necessarily~~
2. Under what conditions is the dentist obligated to provide care? ~~If dentist is employed by federal clinic, if dentist has already started tx, if the pt is enrolled to a pre-paid dental plan that the Dr. has a contractual arrangement~~

Case 2

A patient has been accepted for dental treatment. The dentist provides a treatment plan and fee schedule to which the patient agrees, in writing. The dentist indicates that the patient will be called for his first treatment appointment. Given that the dentist has indicated that he will call the patient for the first appointment, what duty must the dentist be especially careful in fulfilling?

the duty to do the tx in a reasonable time frame.

Case 3

A patient trips over the rheostat in a dental operatory and fractures her arm in the fall. The rheostat had been left directly in the path of the patient.

1. Has a duty been breached? *yes*
2. If so, what duty has been breached? *to protect pt from hazards in the office*
3. What could be the likely legal consequences of the harm the patient suffered?
   pt may sue for negligence, the provider could claim contributory negligence on the part of the pt,

Case 4

A patient has been highly offensive in his mannerisms and language while receiving care from a dental hygienist. The dental hygienist tells the patient that she will call him for his next appointment. She never does, despite the fact that the treatment plan is incomplete.

1. Has a breach of duty occurred? *yes*
2. If so, which one? *to complete tx cotarted, pt has been abandoned.*
   In this case the dental hygienist is employed by a hospital in the outpatient clinic.
3. Legally, the hygienist is an ___*AGENT*___ of the hospital.
4. Because of this relationship of the hygienist to the hospital, liability for any breach of duty on the part of the hygienist is charged to *the R.D.H. & the hospital.*

Case 5

A dental hygienist is doing clinical research in the area of myofunctional therapy. "Before-and-after" study models and photographs are prepared for all patients included in the program. The models and photographs are displayed at a professional meeting as a part of a presentation of the clinical results.

secure written permission from pts

1. What procedures must the clinician follow to display legally those articles?
2. What duty if any would be breached if the procedure was not followed? *invasion of privacy*

Breach of contract

3. What legal action could be taken against the dental hygienist, if any?
   In this case, the dental hygienist often invites dental hygiene students to observe

Breach of contract or invasion of privacy

therapy sessions. The hygienist always asks the patient's permission to allow these "nonessential" persons into the therapy room.

4. Is this a necessary procedure? _yes_

5. Why or why not? _the hygienist must protect the pts right to privacy_

Case 6

A patient has had full-mouth reconstruction completed by his dentist. The oral contract between the dentist and patient called for six separate, equal payments of $300. The last payment was due at the final visit. The first four payments were made on schedule, but at the last visit the patient left without paying, explaining that he had forgotten his checkbook. Six months and a collection agency later, the patient still owed the last two payments.

1. Has a duty been breached? _yes_

2. If so, which one? _duty to pay a reasonable fee_

3. What legal action, if any, can be taken as a result? _Dr. can sue for breach of contract_

4. Is there any countercharge the patient could make?
   pt may attempt proceedings charging negligence

Case 7

A patient is under general anesthesia for the extraction of two impacted molars. The dentist notices that there is a badly decayed tooth next to the first extraction site and decides to remove it also. When the patient regains consciousness, the dentist tells the patient that three teeth were removed rather than just the two agreed upon.

1. Has a duty been breached? _yes_

2. If so, which one? _duty to perform only services agreed to_

3. What legal action may result?
   pt can charge technical assault or battery but recovery will be minimal unless pt can show significant harm.

Case 8

A dental hygienist is scheduled to perform a root planing and curettage for a reluctant patient. The patient clearly needs the services to be performed, so in his zeal to have the patient consent and cooperate the hygienist promises that the patient's mouth will feel much better within a week after treatment. As luck would have it, the patient's teeth develop sensitivity and remain sensitive even after 2 weeks.

1. Has a breach of duty occurred? _yes_

2. If so, which one? _that of satisfaction promised, informed consent about poss. outcomes_

3. Why? _we shouldn't guarantee our results but are liable if we do, we should inform pt of outcomes before tx is given,_

4. What legal action can the patient take against the dental hygienist? _Breach of contract_

5. Assuming that the patient wins the case, what harm will the dental hygienist suffer?
   time + anguish in court, tarnished reputation, financial loss

Case 9

A dentist fractures a root tip during an extraction. He does not tell the patient about it and decides he will retrieve it at a later date. The patient develops severe pain, fever, and malaise and is hospitalized. An oral surgeon removes the root tip in the hospital, and the patient recovers.

1. Did the first dentist breach a duty? *yes*
2. Is the fracturing of the root tip *in itself* a breach of duty? *No*
3. If there was a breach of duty in the case, what was it? *didn't inform pt*
4. Could it have been avoided? *yes. Tell pt about it + suggest waiting to remove it.*
5. What charge may the patient bring against the dentist, if any?
Breach of contract since the duty to keep pt informed is a contractual matter, Also charge of negligence since pt suffered harm as a result of professional duty.

Case 10

A woman has developed periodontal disease after 20 years of regular prophylaxis and oral examinations. She needs $1200 worth of periodontal surgery. Curious about how this could develop "over the last 6 months," she visits the local library and learns that it is a process that can usually be controlled by thorough daily control of plaque and microorganisms in addition to regular prophylaxis. She is appalled that the hygienist casually mentioned brushing and flossing but never emphasized the need for plaque control and the real consequences of allowing accumulation of those soft deposits on a daily basis. The woman sues the dental hygienist and the dentist for negligence, claiming that she was given substandard care over a long period of time.

1. Does the patient have a legitimate suit?
2. Explain how the legal standard of care can be applied to this case.

yes, if she can prove she wasn't given reasonable care by not having the benefits of plaque control info.

see p. 272

Case 11

A dental assistant who has had no formal training is responsible for instrument sterilization. Because of his lack of knowledge, instruments that are autoclaved are stored in the open air or loose in drawers, allowing air contamination before they are used. A patient proves that an oral infection she developed was directly linked to the contaminated instruments.

1. Has a breach of duty occurred? *yes*
2. If so, which one? *duty to protect safety of the pt.*
3. Whom will the patient probably sue? *Both dentist & dental assistant*
4. How will the legal "standard of care" be applied in this case?

see p. 273

GROUP ACTIVITIES

1. Research law review articles to determine the typical size of financial damages awarded to patients winning civil cases against health care providers.

2. Survey local dental hygienists to determine how many carry malpractice insurance, what type, coverage limits, etc.

3. Visit a courtroom during malpractice proceedings. Report

to the class on how the legal principles of rights and duties, negligence, breach of contract, standard of care, and *respondeat superior* were applied.
4. Conduct a seminar discussion involving graduating dental hygienists and licensed hygienists at the local society meeting regarding the application of these principles in clinical practice.
5. Recall any incidents in clinical practice that should have been handled differently to protect the patient's rights.
6. Review the typical steps followed in completing an initial assessment appointment for a patient. Identify all the points at which a deviation from the acceptable protocol could result in harm to the patient and possible legal action (e.g., clear the pathway to the chair to protect the patient from accidental injury, update medical history to avoid clinical procedures or medications that could aggravate a medical condition, etc.).

REFERENCES

Addiego v. State of New Jersey and New Jersey State Board of Dentistry, 394 A.2d 179 (1978).

Black, H.C.: Black's law dictionary, ed. 5, St. Paul, Minn., 1979, West Publishing Co.

Costa v. Storm, 682 S.W.2d 599 (Tex. App. 1 Dist. 1984)

Council on Insurance, American Dental Association: The outlook for dental malpractice insurance. J. Am. Dent. Assoc. **110:**395, 1985.

Creighton, H.: Law every nurse should know, ed. 2, Philadelphia, 1970, W.B. Saunders Co.

Dailey v. North Carolina State Board of Dental Examiners, 309 S.E.2d 219 (N.C. 1983).

Danzon, P.: The frequency and severity of medical malpractice claims. J. Law Econ. **27:**115, 1984.

Estes v. Rockinson, 461 So.2d 989 (Fla. App. 1 Dist. 1984).

Helling v. Carey, 83 Wash. 2d 514, 519, P.2d 981–985, 1974.

Jobson v. Dooley, 296 S.E.2d 388 (Ga. App. 1982).

Kessler v. Trom, 392 A.2d 662 (N.J. 1978). The defendant dentist was found to be entitled to assert physican-patient privilege and thus was not required to reveal details of other patients' conditions and treatment results as requested by the plaintiff.

Kunkle v. Commonwealth of Pennsylvania State Dental Council and Examining Board, 392 A.2d 357 (1978).

Lee v. State Board of Dental Examiners of the State of Colorado, 654 P.2d 388 (1983).

Little v. North Carolina State Board of Dental Examiners, 306 S.E.2d 534 (N.C. App. 1983).

Miller, S.L.: Legal aspects of dentistry, New York, 1970, G.P. Putnam's Sons.

Morganstern, S.: Legal protection for the consumer, Dobbs Ferry, N.Y., 1973, Oceana Publications, Inc.

Morris, R.C., and Moritz, A.R.: Doctor and patient and the law, ed. 5, St. Louis, 1971, The C.V. Mosby Co.

Murchison, I.A., and Nichols, T.S.: Legal foundations of nursing practice, New York, 1970, Macmillan, Inc.

Peterson, R.G.: Malpractice liability of allied health professionals: developments in an area of critical concern, J. Allied Health **14:**363, 1985.

Prosser, W.L.: Handbook of the law of torts, ed. 4, St. Paul, Minn., 1971, West Publishing Co.

Seavey, W.A.: Handbook of the law of agency, St. Paul, Minn., 1964, West Publishing Co.

Willig, S.H.: The nurse's guide to the law, New York, 1970, McGraw-Hill, Inc.

CHAPTER 7

The contract relationship

OBJECTIVES: The reader will be able to:

1. Describe the health care provider–patient relationship as both contractual and consensual.
2. Differentiate express and implied contracts.
3. Given hypothetical situations, identify whether the health care provider may be subject to a breach of contract suit.
4. Given hypothetical situations, identify when the health care provider has taken reasonable precautions to prevent a breach of contract suit.
5. Given hypothetical situations, identify when the contributory action or lack of action on the part of the patient may negate a charge of breach of contract against the health care provider.
6. List the criteria for *informed consent*.
7. Prepare case presentations that meet the criteria for informed consent.

As mentioned in the previous chapter, when a person seeks the care of a health professional and the professional agrees to provide a service, a legal contract exists between the person and the professional. The professional has the *legal* right to accept or reject a patient (unless the professional is employed in a federally funded health care program or the patient is enrolled in a prepaid plan, such as a health maintenance organization, with which the provider has a contract). The patient has the right to agree to or reject the proposed care. Therefore the patient–health care provider relationship is both consensual and contractual. Once both parties *consensually* agree to the service, they have contractual obligations to each other (Black, 1979; Miller, 1970).

This contractual relationship may be *express* (stated orally or in writing), or it may be *implied* (agreed to by the actions of the two persons) (Black, 1979). The former is readily identifiable when a treatment plan is presented to the patient, and the patient agrees orally to the plan or actually signs the treatment plan. The latter type is

more difficult to identify since it is implied by the actions of the health care provider and the patient (Miller, 1970). A typical example of an implied contract to permit an oral examination is: The patient opens his mouth for the dentist, and the dentist looks in. The patient has implied a request for professional assessment of his oral health and the dentist has, by action, agreed to provide that service. Another is: A patient offers his arm for an injection, and the nurse injects a prescribed medication. No words or signed statements may have been exchanged between the patient and the professional. Yet another type of implied contract is the *quasi contract,* which the law recognizes when, for example, a provider of care renders necessary emergency treatment to an unconscious person. Implied contracts are viewed as valid in a court of law as long as there is compensation for the service.

In the years that preceded the consumer movement the vast majority of health care providers relied heavily on the implied contract. It seemed logical that a person behaving in a manner that said, "Provide me with health care," really wanted it, and the implied contract requires no special series of forms nor a lengthy discussion of procedures and alternatives.

However, in the current age of consumer awareness of rights and privileges, the implied contract is a less tenable approach to health care. If nothing is said or written about what care is to be provided or what cooperation is needed on the part of the patient, the nature of the contract is open to wide interpretation. What *was* the patient agreeing to in his silent submission? What *was* the health care provider expecting of the patient? Simply stated, a charge of breach of contract is difficult to defend when the contract was never specifically stated. Conversely, the charge of breach is difficult to prove, and the plaintiff bears the burden of proof. A written express contract offers greater protection to both parties than does an oral express contract, which relies on good expressive and listening skills and which fades with the memory (Miller, 1970). However, a written contract provides firm grounds for proof of breach of contract if it is not fulfilled by one or more parties to the contract.

Breach of this contractual relationship is one of the two most frequently filed charges against health care providers. A breach of contract suit may be initiated whenever a partner in the contract does not perform as agreed. So in the contractual relationship with a patient the provider is liable for breach of contract if he/she fails to attend to the agreed-to needs of the patient until care is completed. For instance, unreasonable delays in providing care may trigger a breach of contract suit. If the health care provider *promised* satisfactory results, and reasonable satisfaction is not obtained, the charge of breach may result. (NOTE: Promising satisfaction is an extremely unwise practice in an inexact field such as health care (Miller, 1970)).

There are several defenses against a charge of breach of contract. A health care provider faced with such a suit may be able to demonstrate that the patient did not cooperate in the contractual re-lationship. If the patient missed appointments, did not adhere to the prescribed pretreatment and posttreatment procedures, or refused certain integral phases of the proposed care, the health care provider may be able to prove that there was no opportunity for the agreed-to procedures to be performed or to be successful. If it can be demonstrated that ample opportunity for successful care was not possible as a result of the patient's lack of cooperation and that the provider made every effort to perform the agreed-on services, the health care provider will likely be able to turn aside a charge of breach of contract (Miller, 1970).

The best avoidance of breach of contract is the explicit statement of proposed treatment, in writing, which provides the patient with the following information: (1) a description of the condition the patient has, (2) the treatment proposed, (3) the possibilities that that treatment will or will not be successful, (4) the probable results of not treating the condition, (5) the risks involved, and (6) other possible ways to approach treatment of the condition. Providing the patient with this information will permit the patient to provide an *informed consent,* either orally or in writing (Bailey, 1985; Miller, 1970).

Informed consent is based on our society's belief that every adult person has "a right to decide what should be done to his or her own body, and that consent in the absence of adequate information is equivalent to no consent at all" (Bailey, 1985).

In general, courts require that the dentist fully discuss all information that is relevant to the patient's decision to proceed, even if it is not customary within the profession to disclose such information. An example could be discussing possible toxic reactions to a fluoride treatment. Even though most dental hygienists may not discuss this with patients or with a minor's parent, a plaintiff may be able to win a suit on the basis that if the toxic reaction had been explained, he/she would not have agreed to the treatment.

Consent is typically implied for routine procedures such as oral examinations, but informed consent is required for complex procedures and for those involving risk (Bailey, 1985).

In a study of behaviors that patients prefer in their dentists, it is clear that full explanation of treatment and truthfulness about pain and discomfort are important communication elements. Patients want to be fully informed (Rankin and Harris, 1985).

A California case concluded that if a dentist does not provide a patient with enough information to enable the patient "to intelligently decide whether to undergo [the] dental procedure," the dentist is "liable for injuries sustained by the patient during the course of dental treatment, *whether treatment was negligent or not*" [emphasis added] (Willard, 1981). Thus, if risks are known, give the patient the opportunity to avoid or choose risks associated with the procedure.

In addition, estimates of cost and the number and length of appointments should be included in the treatment plan. If payments are expected during the course of treatment, the patient should be informed of this expectation. Otherwise, the patient is not legally obligated to pay until treatment is completed. The patient should have an accurate appraisal of how much time will be necessary to complete all phases of the treatment. If the time is to exceed 1 year, a written contract is necessary (Miller, 1970).

The best precaution is to put *all* this information in writing and to share a copy signed by both parties with the patient. A format or checklist should be obtained from an attorney.

An interesting point can be drawn from a 1982 case against a Pennsylvania dentist. The dentist claimed he gave the patient three alternative treatment approaches aimed at replacing a large number of mandibular missing teeth (only three teeth remained, all in the anterior sextant). The alternative selected was a 10-unit cantilever bridge, which ultimately failed and cost the patient great discomfort and money. The dentist contended that the patient was "fully informed" and selected the alternative freely. The patient contended in her suit that she relied upon the dentist's recommen-

dation, which was for the extensive bridgework. Expert opinion concluded that this particular treatment recommendation was folly; the number of teeth and the amount of supporting bone were inadequate to support the prosthesis (Kundrat, 1982). Thus, despite meeting the mechanical requirements of informed consent, the dentist was not immune from civil action *and* punitive action by the state board. The dentist was shown to be incompetent in selecting and suggesting a treatment alternative.

Just as a clinician can be held liable for recommending a poor alternative while meeting all informed consent criteria, he/she can also be excused from liability in a few instances when a procedure *to which there is no alternative* fails or causes harm, even when the risk was not fully stated. An Illinois appellate court determined, based on expert testimony, that a badly involved molar *required* extraction; to leave it in place would cause systemic infection and other serious side effects. Even though the patient stated she would have refused treatment if she had been informed of the possibility of the loss of feeling that followed the extraction, the court stated that since there was no viable alternative, the patient had no justifiable action against the dentist (St. Gemme, 1983). This point might, however, be decided differently in another court or jurisdiction. The clinician should follow informed consent procedures completely so that if a legal question is raised, the clinician is standing upon solid legal precedent and good clinical practice.

In the State of Washington a case was won against a dentist because he had not taken a medical history or taken blood pressure measurements prior to commencing dental treatment. The patient had high blood pressure, but the dentist gave no notice of the risks of proceeding since he had taken no steps to learn about the patient's existing medical condition. The patient suffered a stroke. The plaintiff won the case because the dentist did not use standard skill and care (negligence) and did not fully inform the patient of the risks she would undertake if treated (breach of contract) (Le Beauf, 1980). Often cases are based on more than one legal principle; lack of informed consent frequently is cited in cases where negligence is also at issue.

A Louisiana case brought against a dentist was turned aside, despite the fact that the patient had not been warned of a possible specific negative outcome—breaking off an endodontic reamer that became lodged during an attempted root canal treatment. The dentist told the patient that the reamer had broken off and was lodged and then gave her alternative treatment steps and a recommended action. The patient did not return for care. The patient's claim of lack of informed consent was denied because "a physician or dentist is not required to inform a patient of a remote or rare possibility, or an event which can not be reasonably anticipated" (Wiley, 1982). Thus, as supported in this case, it is not necessary to recite a litany of rare, possible outcomes. However, known negative results sometimes or often associated with a given procedure should be addressed in a case presentation to a patient.

There are times when a health care provider may file a breach of contract suit against a patient—usually when the services have been satisfactorily performed and the patient has not paid. The patient, being on the defensive in this case, may contend that the services either were not completed or that they were unsatisfactory, and therefore nonpayment is justified. The breach of contract suit may stimulate the patient toward even further defensive legal actions (Miller, 1970). A patient charged with a breach of contract for nonpayment of fee may choose to countersue, charging negligence or malpractice, particularly if he/she is displeased with the outcome of treatment.

Logically enough, negligence or malpractice suits constitute the other most frequent charge made against health care providers. The unique considerations surrounding the "standard of care" issue related to charges of negligence will be discussed in the next chapter.

Review questions

1. The relationship between a patient and health care provider is both _CONSENSUAL_ and _CONTRACTUAL_.

2. What are the two forms of an express contract?
   a. _ORAL_
   b. _WRITTEN_

3. How is an implied contract different from an express contract? _relies on the CONSENTING actions of pt & DR, w/ NO oral OR written agreement._

4. True or false:
   a. Having a written contract is a "two-edged sword"; it defines those responsibilities for which the patient is responsible, but it also specifies the requirements expected of the clinician. It can protect the clinician in a legal action, but it also holds the clinician to a firm agreement. _true_
   b. If a health care provider stops to assist a person in distress, the law considers a *quasi contract* to exist between the two parties. _true_
   c. If a clinician *promises* satisfaction, a court will hold the clinician to that promise or expect compensatory damages be paid to the patient if the dissatisfied patient files suit. _true_
   d. One risk in filing a suit against a patient for nonpayment is that the patient may countersue, charging malpractice. _true_

GROUP ACTIVITIES

1. Using hypothetical treatment plans, prepare case presentations for the patients that include the six necessary components for consent to be legally considered informed.
2. Consult with an attorney regarding the likelihood of a countersuit, if the health care provider sues the patient for payment of a fee.
3. Review clinical services provided for patients by a dental hygienist or a dentist listing possible negative outcomes (e.g., root planing—sensitive roots, extraction—fractured root) that can result from a dental procedure even when due care is used by the clinician.
4. Discuss how a court would/could rule on the following cases involving dental hygiene care. Base your conclusions on the legal principles discussed in this chapter:
   a. A dental hygienist fractures the tip of a curette deep in a periodontal pocket. The patient had not been informed prior to treatment that such an event could occur. The patient sues for lack of informed consent.
   b. A dental hygienist fails to tell a parent that his child could feel nauseated following a fluoride treatment. The child becomes quite ill; the physician attributes the illness to fluoride toxicity. The parent sues for lack of informed consent and negligence.
   c. Sealants placed on a child's first molars have required replacement at 6-month and 1-year inspections. The parent complains that she had no idea she would be required to spend money at each dental visit to replace sealants; she sues for lack of informed consent and for negligence, hoping to prove that the reasonably prudent dental hygienist would be able to place a sealant that would last longer than 6 months.

REFERENCES

Bailey, B.L.: Informed consent in dentistry. J. Am. Dent. Assoc. **110:**709, 1985.

Black, H.C.: Black's law dictionary, ed. 5, St. Paul, Minn., 1979, West Publishing Co.

Kundrat v. Commonwealth of Pennsylvania State Dental Council and Examining Board, 477 A.2d 355, 1982.

LeBeauf v. Atkins, 621 P.2d 787 (Wash. App. 1980).

Miller, S.L.: Legal aspects of dentistry, New York, 1970, G.P. Putnam's Sons.

Ranking, J.A., and Harris, M.B.: Patients' preferences for dentists' behaviors, J. Am. Dent. Assoc. **110:**323, 1985.

St. Gemme v. Tomlin, 455 N.E.2d 294 (Ill. App. 4 Dist. 1983).

Wiley v. Karam, 421 So.2d 294 (La. App. 1982).

Willard v. Hagemeister, App., 175 Cal./Rptr. 365, 1981.

CHAPTER 8

The "standard of skill and care" in providing health care

OBJECTIVES: The reader will be able to:

1. Define *negligence* and *malpractice*.
2. Describe the condition under which a health care provider may be liable for malpractice.
3. Define *proximate cause* and explain how it is a key factor in charges of malpractice.
4. Explain the use of the "prudent-man rule" in litigating charges of negligence.
5. Define *contributory negligence* and explain how it may constitute a defense against malpractice.
6. Explain the importance of informing the patient of any accident or wrong judgment and ensuring that any damage that may have resulted has been rectified.
7. List at least ten errors in dental practice that could be grounds for a malpractice suit.
8. Define "Good Samaritan Law."

In the area of patient–health care provider rights and responsibilities, the most basic considerations are that the patient has the right to expect at least "reasonable" care and the provider has the responsibility to ensure that each patient receives it. When the level of care is not reasonable, the provider may face a tort liability for negligence or malpractice. A *tort* is a civil wrong, such as an injury to another's person, property, or reputation (Black, 1979; Pollack, 1985). In discussing levels of quality of care provided by health professionals, *negligence* and *malpractice* are synonymous, referring to the omission of an act that the reasonably prudent health care provider would include in treatment or the commission of an act that the reasonable provider would not perform (or would perform differently) (Miller, 1970).

Basically, there are four factors that must be apparent before a person may be liable for negligence. First of all, the provider must have undertaken to care for the patient. Second, the provider must have breached a duty of care owed to the patient. Third, there must be damage or harm to the patient; fourth, this harm must be causally related to the breach of duty. If any of the four factors is missing, the ruling will be in favor of the health care provider and not the plantiff (Miller, 1970).

The "reasonably prudent man" rule is applied as the measure of the appropriateness of the action, the basis of the required standard of care. The rule requires only that the practitioner possess and exercise that standard of skill and care that the reasonably prudent practitioner in the same or similar locality would possess and exercise under the same or similar circumstances (Black, 1979). An example is: A hygienist agrees to provide an oral inspection and radiographic series for a patient (acceptance of the patient). The patient contracts subacute bacterial endocarditis (harm done) as a result of (causal relationship) the probing for

69

spontaneous gingival hemorrhage points that occurred as an integral part of the oral examination, despite the fact (breach of duty of care) that the patient has a history of rheumatic fever, as indicated in her medical history.

With all four factors evident, the plaintiff has only to show that reasonably prudent dental hygienists, given the same circumstances, would have the patient premedicated before proceeding with probing for hemorrhage (Miller, 1970). If the plaintiff can show that dental hygienists are expected to exercise this higher level of care according to stated standards, the plaintiff will probably win a judgment against the dental hygienist in question.

The reasonably prudent man or woman is not perfect, and the law does not expect any person to be perfect. But the prudent person "has average courage and average caution" (Murchison and Nichols, 1970), exercises professional foresight, and is careful to prevent injury to fellow human beings.

Even complete failure of a dental case is not sufficient evidence of negligence. In a 1985 case, an orthodontist whose treatment was unsuccessful was able to turn aside a malpractice case. The point to prove was that the orthodontist did not meet the standard of care exercised by other reasonably prudent orthodonists; apparently the plaintiff was unsuccessful in establishing this proof (Gurdin, 1985).

Negligence does not necessarily imply lack of competence "since the competent may be negligent." Negligence implies carelessness, lack of caution or discretion, without the positive intention of harming the person (Black, 1979). However, lack of competence may in many instances be the cause of the harm done. The law does expect that a health care practitioner will constantly be seeking to improve his/her level of competence, and a provider is not excused from liability on the grounds of ignorance of proper procedure.

Based on these legal principles, the dental hygienist who probed without premedicating may find him/herself in some difficulty. However, one or two other considerations might spare the dental hygienist from a judgment of malpractice (Miller, 1970). If the dental hygienist can identify more than one *proximate cause* (the cause directly linked to the harm) of the subacute bacterial endocarditis, the judgment of malpractice will be turned aside. For instance, could the patient have contracted the disease from having brushed her own teeth the day on which the gingiva hemorrhaged? Or what if the patient had seen another dental health care provider that day or one day earlier or later and bleeding occurred and no premedication was provided? Proximate cause is "that which is nearest in the order of responsible action" or that which "produces the injury and without which the accident could not have happened" (Black, 1979).

Nerve damage associated with an injection of anesthesia is not necessarily negligence. Expert testimony could cite a chemical reaction that the reasonably prudent dentist or hygienist would not be expected to predict. With more than one proximate cause established, the clinician could turn aside a malpractice action. Such was the decision in a 1983 case (Myers, 1983). If more than one likely cause can be shown and the provider is not the source of all the identified likely causes, the court may decide that the provider is not liable for the damage. If the court recognizes that the cause, by a preponderance of proof, more than likely *is* attributable to the provider, it will find for the plaintiff.

The second consideration that might spare the dental hygienist from judgment would be proof that the patient contributed to the negligence (Miller, 1970). For instance, if the patient had a prescription but did not take the medication or if the patient when specifically questioned did not inform the hygienist of the history of rheumatic fever, the patient could be proved to have contributed her own negligence in creating the harm. Failure to follow instructions or disclose pertinent information may be evidence of *contributory negligence* (that is, the patient contributed her own poor judgment to the ultimate harm).

It is essential to understand that accidents or instances of poor judgment are not in themselves proof of negligence (Miller, 1970). The malpractice suit is more likely to focus on how the accident or poor judgment is or is not rectified. Was the patient informed? Did the health care provider take all possible measures to correct the problem? If the provider chooses to hide the error, a judgment against the provider is probable, since not only the duty of reasonable care was breached but so was the provider's duty to inform the patient. Whenever accidental harm occurs to the patient, it is best to calmly inform the patient and then take steps to correct the error.

In dental practice there are several errors that account for the majority of dental malpractice claims. They include errors in judgment causing harm to a patient by means of slipping with an instrument, extracting too many teeth at one appointment, delivering improperly fitting dentures, using drugs and anesthetics improperly, and allowing a foreign body to be aspirated into the respiratory tract, failure to refer the patient to a specialist when necessary, failure to keep the patient informed, and failure to sterilize instruments or to prepare adequate x-rays are other frequent errors that may prompt a malpractice suit. If the patient was accepted by the provider and one of these errors can be proved to be the proximate cause of some harm to the patient, the provider of dental care will in all likelihood find him/herself in court. He/she will be compared to the mythical peer, "the reasonably prudent dentist" or "dental hygienist," and if found to have conducted him/herself short of that standard, he/she will probably lose the case (Miller, 1970).

In many instances, the plaintiff does not need to call on expert witnesses or create a substantial base of evidence to prove negligence. The doctrine of *res ipsa loquitur* (the matter speaks for itself) may be invoked, when injury is obviously directly related to some clear instance of negligence (Black, 1979). An example might be harm caused by not recording a medical history or by providing services while intoxicated. Once it is

proved that there was no medical history or the provider was indeed intoxicated, the court needs no further proof of fault.

In a Colorado case, a patient tried to invoke *res ipsa loquitur* in an action against a dentist who extracted all the patient's teeth without having taken a complete radiographic series. The court ruled that expert testimony would be required in hearing this case, and that the dentist's failure to act was not sufficiently apparent to be negligence (Smith, 1982). Decisions in such matters vary greatly among states and courts within states.

There may be some comfort in the realization that the criteria historically used to determine the appropriate standard of care for health care providers were dependent on the practice of other health care providers in the profession in the same locale. The plaintiff would then need to call on professional peers to testify regarding how they would perform under the same circumstances. This is no longer the case, however. The courts now turn to stated professional standards of practice for the criteria rather than to individual peers (Medicolegal, 1976; Murchison and Nichols, 1970), and to regional or national practice norms rather than to local custom (Dailey, 1983; Guide, 1984).

The "locality rule" was developed when standards of practice varied greatly from one community to another and when there were wide differences in opportunities for continued education for the professions. Thus a professional practicing in a large city with numerous, high quality opportunities for updates might be held to a stiffer standard than one practicing in a remote community with few continuing education courses. Greater uniformity in the health professions nationwide has led to regional or even national standards of skill and care (Guide, 1984).

During the 1970s and early 1980s malpractice suits have increased in frequency. Hygienists are not free from the threat of suit. An awareness of this fact alone may prompt dental hygienists to assume greater responsibility for the quality of care they are delivering.

s the growth in number of malpractice ac- ... it caused malpractice insurance premiums ...cket. Exorbitant premiums, especially for anesthesiologists, surgeons, and other high-risk specialties, drove some insurance companies out of the medical malpractice business and caused some physicians to consider leaving practice. Annual premiums of $30,000 per practitioner are not uncommon in some specialties. A health care provider who is sued and loses the case may find it difficult thereafter to obtain insurance coverage, which literally may force him/her from practice. State legislatures and medical societies worked to resolve this problem by placing ceilings on malpractice awards and ensuring by various state measures that physicians will have coverage available. (See Chapter 6.)

Ironically, the advent of consumer awareness and the resultant increase in litigation regarding quality of health care resulted in a decrease of certain kinds of care, especially on-the-spot, voluntary emergency care. Physicians may well fear litigation if some harm came to the patient that might be attributed to the inadequacies of first aid efforts.

All states have enacted special legislation to protect health personnel from litigation in the event they stop to render emergency care. Such legislative provisions are known as Good Smaritan Laws or clauses (Black, 1979; Guide, 1984; Mancini and Gale, 1981; Morganstern, 1973). They specifically protect the provider by turning aside litigation charging negligence except when harm is the direct result of wanton or gross negligence. The attempt to help cannot be recklessly or rashly made, or the doctrine provides no safety. Also, if the volunteer worsens the condition of the person in distress, liability can be imposed if it can be shown that the volunteer was negligent (Black, 1979).

Many Good Samaritan Laws address themselves only to physicians and nurses, making no mention of other persons (such as dentists or dental hygienists) who could provide emergency care. The laws are therefore unclear in the possible protection they could offer such a provider who, for instance, ''almost'' saves a person's life.

The general rule is that the reasonably prudent man or woman measure is applied to assessing whether the provider of first aid was negligent. Dentists are ''measured'' against dentists, physicians against physicians, nurses against nurses, and dental hygienists against dental hygienists. Despite the minimal protection provided by such laws, knowledge of state provisions and just what safeguards they contain is wise for any health care provider. In the meantime, it is imperative that one develop a constant awareness of the quality of care being provided and the duties owed the patient. Negligence or a violation of a patient's rights can be very costly—in time, money, and reputation.

Review questions

1. Define *negligence*. *doing an act NOT NEC. OR omitting an act that IS NEC.*
2. What is the measure of whether a person is guilty of negligence or not?
3. What four factors must be present for a suit of negligence to be successful against a person?
   a. *duty is owed to a person (contract exists)*
   b. *there's a breach of that duty*
   c. *the person has been injured or harmed*
   d. *breach of duty is the proximate cause of the harm.*

4. What is *contributory negligence?* pt contributed his own ignorance or action to the situation

5. What is *proximate cause?* factor that can be related to the harm

True or false:

6. A Good Samaritan Law protects any health care provider against all related negligence suits if the provider renders first aid care to an injured person. _false, or unlikely (P state LAW)_

7. The recently established criteria for determining what is reasonably prudent are to determine the average person's quality of activities. _false_

8. Hygienists are safe from malpractice suits. _false_

GROUP ACTIVITIES

1. Review current literature to identify what suits have been brought against dental auxiliaries, whether the suit was successful, and the amount of damages awarded the plaintiff.

2. Review the Good Samaritan Law of your state. Analyze it for the actual protection it provides and whom it protects.

3. Discuss or debate these issues:
   a. Dental hygienists performing curettage should be held to the standard held for dentists who perform curettage.
   b. Dental hygienists who are required by state law to be supervised by dentists should be immune from liability for the services they provide.
   c. One national standard should be used when measuring the "reasonably prudent hygienist."

REFERENCES

Black, H.C.: Black's law dictionary, ed. 5, St. Paul, Minn., 1979, West Publishing Co.

Dailey v. North Carolina State Board of Examiners, 309 S.E.2d 219 (N.C. 1983).

The guide to American law, vol. 7, St. Paul, Minn., 1984, West Publishing Co.

Gurdin v. Dongieux, 468 So.2d 1241 (La. App. 4 Cir. 1985).

Mancini, M.R., and Gale, A.T.: Emergency care and the law, Rockville, Md., 1981, Aspen Systems Corp.

Medicolegal Rounds: *Shier v. Freedman,* J. Am. Med. Assoc. **235:**1614, 1976.

Miller, S.L.: Legal aspects of dentistry, New York, 1970, G.P. Putnam's Sons.

Morganstern, S.: Legal protection for the consumer, Dobbs Ferry, N.Y., 1973, Oceana Publications, Inc.

Murchison, I.A., and Nichols, T.S.: Legal foundations of nursing practice, New York, 1970, Macmillan, Inc.

Myers v. Dunscombe, 669 P.2d 388 (Oreg. App. 1983).

Pollack, B.R.: Risk management in the dental office. Dent. Clin. North Am. **29:**557, 1985.

Smith v. Hoffman, 656 P.2d 1327 (Colo. App. 1982).

CHAPTER 9

Technical battery

OBJECTIVES: The reader will be able to:

1. Define *technical battery*.
2. Differentiate between technical battery and breach of contract.
3. Given hypothetical cases, identify instances in which health care professionals commit technical battery or take appropriate precautions to protect themselves from claims of technical battery.
4. Compare express and implied contracts with regard to the protection they provide against charges of technical battery.

The previous chapter explained that when a patient seeks and accepts care from a health care provider, the patient enters a contractual relationship with the health care professional, and the health care professional is obligated to provide the care agreed to, according to the accepted standard of skill and care. The patient is expected to cooperate in the provision of care and to pay a reasonable fee for the services received.

If the health care provider does not provide the care or if the patient does not pay the fee, one may sue the other for breach of contract. If an appropriate standard of care is not met, resulting in some damage to the patient, the patient may under tort law sue for *negligence*. The patient will not be successful in the suit if *contributory negligence* (lack of agreed-on cooperation or other act or omission of the patient significantly contributing to the patient's injury) can be proved.

But what happens if the health care provider performs some service over and above that which is agreed to? Is this some special bonus for the patient? The health care provider may think so. However, if some service other than those specifically agreed to is performed, the patient may sue, charging *technical battery*.*

Negligence and technical battery are the two components of tort law. The former is applicable when some damage can be proved to be causally related to an act omitted or committed by another person and that is judged to be a dereliction of duty when compared to the action performed by the "reasonably prudent" person. The latter refers to those instances in which a "touching" to which the patient has not agreed has occurred (Bailey, 1985; Black, 1979; Pollack, 1985; Prosser, 1971). It is different from breach of contract because it generally refers to some procedure *not* included in the contract that *has* been performed rather than to some procedure *not* performed that is included in the contract.

A 1983 Michigan case provides an instance where technical battery applies. The patient consented to have two small marks removed from her maxillary central incisors. The dentist, however, went on to file her teeth down so that they were to points and did not match the teeth on the other

---

*Unlawful touching is referred to as *battery*. In some cases, *assault* is used to describe the actions of health care providers performing services to which the patient did not consent (Black, 1979).

side. Even if the result had not been so obviously deleterious, the patient could have charged a battery since she did not consent to having the procedure performed. Since the procedure did result in harm (poor appearance and sensitivity to temperature changes), she could also claim negligence (Sullivan, 1983).

The difficulty for health care providers arises when the provider assumes that because the patient has sought his/her care, the patient is agreeable to anything that appears necessary. Many health care providers believe that the trusting patient is providing them with blanket authorization.

Legally, it is not possible for a patient to give up his/her right to be informed by signing any statement that says the provider may do "whatever appears necessary"(Miller, 1970). Nor does a blanket verbal release provide health care personnel with the right to proceed with whatever procedures they choose. Each procedure or combination of procedures must be specifically agreed to by the patient if the provider is to be protected against battery. However, the law clearly recognizes an "extension doctrine," which allows the provider to do related things not specifically agreed to that sound professional judgment requires be done as part of the same procedure and circumstances preclude consulting the patient.

For instance, using a rubber dam may be considered an integral part of performing a root canal treatment and would not require separate consent. Polishing the teeth or using an antiseptic during scaling could be considered integral to an oral prophylaxis. Applying a plaque disclosant could be argued to be a normal part of giving oral hygiene instructions.

In contrast, a child whose parent specifies "oral prophylaxis and fluoride treatment" as the procedures to be provided should not have a radiographic series prepared unless the parent is asked and agrees. A man expecting that one tooth needs to be prepared and restored should not have two teeth receive that treatment unless he is asked and agrees. A woman who agrees to have a biopsy of a lesion should not awaken to realize she has had more extensive surgery, unless before the biopsy she has agreed that if surgery is necessary it may be performed.

Persons who participate in express and implied contracts have the legal right to be apprised of intended procedures, and they have the right to agree or to decline (Miller, 1970; Morris and Moritz, 1971). It should be apparent that the concept of the implied contract leaves the health care professional in a precarious position: the open mouth may legally, contractually imply "You may look in," but it does not provide much protection when the patient claims that it did not imply permission was granted to do what was performed after the provider looked in.

The "sole element of an assault and battery or trespass action is an unconsented touching." In early cases, patients did not have to demonstrate that any harm occurred. While patients can still win suits that show only unwanted touching, if actual benefit came to the patient as a result of the unwanted action, the damages awarded the plaintiff will be very small. In general, the courts now require that the plaintiff show he/she suffered some harm; but cases still appear that award damages even when no injury came from the incident (Bailey, 1985; Black, 1979).

Once again, the requirements for obtaining informed consent apply. The patient should be fully informed of the condition he/she has, the proposed treatment, the possibilities of successful or unsuccessful outcome, the probable result of leaving the condition untreated, the risk and cost involved, the expected duration of treatment, and other possible ways to approach treatment of the condition. (See Chapter 7 for further discussion on obtaining informed consent.)

The express contract, in which the procedures and conditions are agreed on either verbally or in writing, provides greater protection (Bailey, 1985; Miller, 1970), assuming of course that the provider does not deviate from the original written agreement. By discussing the proposed procedures with the patient or by presenting a written treatment plan, the provider allows the patient the opportunity to agree or disagree with what is planned. The patient has the opportunity to say "yes," and "proceed," which is all that is necessary in most instances to protect the patient from battery and to protect the health care provider from the charge that technical battery was committed (Prosser, 1971).

In most instances the simple request, "Should we proceed?" following a discussion of the need for and nature of the procedure is adequate. However, a complex treatment or series of treatments would best be agreed to in writing. This may be appropriate especially when a complex treatment plan could result in a less than perfect result because of the difficulty or tenuous nature of the procedures. The patient should be aware of the likelihood of an "imperfect" result from agreeing to treatment; a written, signed statement may make it a good deal easier to prove knowledge as well as the agreement.

As mentioned earlier, often the procedures provided in health care involve more than one "component" of care, depending on how they are defined (Miller, 1970). For instance, an oral prophylaxis may include some root planing. Some root planing procedures include soft tissue curettage. It is possible that a patient could successfully sue, charging technical battery, if he were to learn that his roots were planed when all he wanted was to have his teeth cleaned. The suit would be successful if the definitions of the two procedures were proved to be distinctly different. However, the suit would probably be turned aside if it could be proved that the root planing was an integral part of the oral prophylaxis and necessary for the prophylaxis to be considered complete. Because many treatments are actually composites of more than one distinct procedure, it is probably wise for the health care provider to distinguish components in any treatment when discussing the treatment plan with the patient.

For instance, a routine oral prophylaxis might be identified as scaling and polishing. A complete radiographic survey might be described as a series of fourteen periapical and four bitewing or caries-detection radiographs so that the patient is aware of the scope of the procedure.

Regardless of the scope of the procedure, the best way to avoid technical battery is to explain fully the procedures planned and *ask* for permission to proceed. This relatively simple practice may prove to be invaluable in an era when patients are more aware of their legal rights. Aside from legality, the explanation and permission-seeking may greatly improve patients' cooperation in the delivery of care, since they may have a greater feeling of participation and may more fully understand the nature of procedures.

There is another responsibility owed to patients that is related to performing only those procedures agreed to by the patient. The health care provider may be charged with technical battery if he/she touches the patient in places or in manners that have no direct relationship to the provision of health care (Miller, 1970; Prosser, 1971). Using a patient's chest as a prop for one's arm is one example. Just because the patient agrees to some intraoral procedure does not mean that the patient has agreed to being used as a shelf.

A second easily understood example is the "bear hug" some dental clinicians give their patients' heads when performing some procedures from behind the patient. If the patient is positioned too high in relation to the operator, it may be convenient for the operator to provide an extra source of support for the patient's head with his/her chest. The patient has not agreed to this extra contact, and if he/she reacts strongly enough to the touching, he/she may sue in tort law, claiming technical battery. The obvious conclusion is that all health care providers ought to be more aware of the liberties they take in touching the patient incidental to providing care.

A second conclusion worthy of some discussion is the possible liability for technical battery a health care provider may have if specific permission is not asked before commencing palpation examinations. For instance, the oral examination procedure performed for a patient includes extraoral palpation as an integral component. But what if the oral examination the patient thought he/she agreed to did not include the palpation? What reaction may the patient have to having his/her neck "massaged" when he/she thought he/she was having his/her mouth looked at? The patient may immediately react to the palpation procedure as an assault. The patient may sue if his/her reaction is strong enough. This example may appear to be extreme, but it could occur, and as a practical matter it provides one more reason to describe intended services to patients an their agreement.

A simple precaution is to inform that the oral exam is visual, but that it also includes feeling the face and neck for lumps, texture deviations, and other indicators of normal and abnormal conditions and then to ask for permission to proceed.

Explanation and a request for permission to go ahead with the procedures are the two keys to preventing a charge of technical battery.

Review questions

1. The act of "touching" or performing some procedure for a patient that was not agreed to is known as: technical battery
2. Breach of contract occurs when: person in contract doesn't perform as agreed to.
3. Breach of contract and technical battery differ because: performing procedure not agreed to.
4. *Review:* Tort law is comprised of:
   a. negligence
   b. technical battery
5. An implied/express (choose one) contract is the better safeguard against technical battery.
6. Identify, for each of the hypothetical cases, whether a charge of technical battery by the patient could be upheld:
   a. A dental hygienist performs a fluoride treatment for a child patient whose mother specified teeth cleaning and x-rays. could be upheld
   b. A dentist extracts three teeth from a patient while the patient is under general anesthesia. The patient agreed to having only two extracted. could be upheld
   c. A dental hygienist explains that the oral prophylaxis to be performed will include smoothing roughened roots. He performs an oral prophylaxis and root planes fifteen surfaces. Not likely to be upheld
7. Current case law supports the health care provider because in cases where no actual harm has resulted from the battery, the court will: provide minimal damages award

GROUP ACTIVITIES

1. Outline case presentation formats that are most likely to prevent technical battery.
2. Consult "consumer awareness" handbooks to determine what guidelines patients should have to protect themselves against technical battery.
3. Record or observe various case presentations to assess whether the express contract is sufficiently comprehensive to prevent technical battery from occurring during the actual provision of treatment.
4. Describe personal experiences as a patient and as a care provider in which technical battery occurred.
5. Attend a trial in civil court in which technical battery is the charge.

REFERENCES

Bailey, B.L.: Informed consent in dentistry. J. Am. Dent. Assoc. **110:**709, 1985.

Black, H.C.: Black's law dictionary, ed. 5, St. Paul, Minn., 1979, West Publishing Co.

Miller, S.L.: Legal aspects of dentistry, New York, 1970, G.P. Putnam's Sons.

Morris, R.C., and Moritz, A.R.: Doctor and patient and the law, ed. 5, St. Louis, 1971, The C.V. Mosby Co.

Pollack, B.R.: Risk management in the dental office. Dent. Clin. North Am. **29:**557, 1985.

Prosser, W.L.: Handbook of the law of torts, ed. 4, St. Paul, Minn., 1971, West Publishing Co.

Sullivan v. Russell, 338 N.W.2d 181 (Mich. 1983).

CHAPTER 10

Fees, forms, and good judgment

OBJECTIVES: The reader will be able to:

1. Define *fee* and identify it as an integral part of the contract agreement.
2. Compare the two types of fees with the two types of contracts.
3. Explain how a reasonable fee is determined.
4. Explain a patient's likely response to an unexpectedly high fee.
5. Describe the advantages and disadvantages of the following:
   a. Quoting a fee
   b. Estimating a fee
   c. Not discussing fees at all
6. Given a partial payment accompanied by a statement marked "paid in full," identify what consequences may occur if payment and statement are accepted without comment.
7. Identify the courses of action available to a provider of services whose client or patient does not pay as agreed.
8. Recognize the characteristics of a well-kept patient record.
9. Relate the importance of a well-kept record to its use as evidence in a court of law.
10. Define *admission against interest* and *res gestae* and identify how these concepts apply to use of evidence in a court of law.
11. List the steps a person should follow when (a) confronted with a lawsuit and (b) an incident occurs that could lead to a suit.
12. Describe how the "patient as partner in care" concept can prevent legal action.
13. Explain the concept of consumer advocacy and how it relates to the ethical duties owed to patients.

The contractual relationship between a health care provider and a patient has been described as one in which some service is provided for the patient for which the patient pays a *fee*. A fee is a consideration, usually in money, for services. It is an essential part of a contract between two competent parties (Black, 1979; Creighton, 1970; Miller, 1970; Stetler and Mortiz, 1962).

Just as a contract may be express or implied, so may a fee. A fee may be stated either orally or in writing, or a fee may be implied by the actions of the parties—an assumed component of the fact that the patient requests care and the health care provider performs the services (Miller, 1970; Morris and Moritz, 1971). Few patients would honestly expect care for free. So the issue of debate then centers on the question, "How much?"

Most court actions regarding fees relate to the patient's contention that the fee was unreasonably high. So how is a fee determined to be reasonable or unreasonable? The simplest answer is that it ought to be in keeping with the complexity of the services provided and comparable to the "going rate" for services of similar complexity.

A more specific determination of what is reasonable is based on four considerations: (1) what is customary in the geographic area for the particular procedure, (2) the cost of materials and other overhead considerations (such as time) to provide the services, (3) the complexity of services and the skill and expertise of the operator, and (4) (some have contended) the ability of the patient to pay (Miller, 1970).

Professional organizations may actually publish a list of suggested fees to which they hope their members will adhere. However, the U.S. Supreme Court in a case involving lawyer's fees has declared this practice to be price-fixing and therefore an illegal restraint of trade in violation of the federal antitrust laws (Goldfarb, 1975). But even without published, suggested fees, a community of professionals is often aware of the ''going rate'' and may not deviate from it too drastically. Despite the fact that most professionals do not advertise their services and fees, patients often are aware of what various procedures cost. And if a fee greatly exceeds their idea of ''reasonable,'' they may choose not to pay part or all of it. An unexpectedly high fee may be countered by more than just nonpayment. It may trigger a malpractice suit, particularly if there is some measure of dissatisfaction with the procedure (Miller, 1970). Such a suit can present problems to the practitioner even when there is little doubt that the patient's case ultimately will fail.

Once again, the danger of an implied contract or fee is apparent. If the fee has not been discussed, there is a significant possibility that it will be an unpleasant surprise to the patient. Many health care providers may view the discussion of the fee as an unprofessional or embarrassing occurrence. The fact is that patients do expect some sort of a fee, and the health care provider may be able to allay their concerns if it is simply discussed in an open manner at the time of case presentation.

Since not discussing the fee is risky, there are two remaining approaches worthy of consideration. One approach is quoting the fee; the other is estimating the fee. Quoting the fee gives the patient an exact indication of what dollar investment will be needed to receive care. There are no surprises, and the fee is either paid in a series of partial payments during or after care is completed or paid in full on completion. Although surprise to the patient is eliminated, a surprise may be in store for the health care provider. A quoted fee does not usually allow for unexpected materials costs or for treatments not anticipated to be necessary at the time of the treatment plan. If the case involves more time, effort, or other cost, the fee legally remains unchanged when it is quoted exactly (Miller, 1970).

A health care provider who has been stung by the quoted fee may decide to take the second approach, the estimated fee. In this instance, the case presentation includes an estimated fee, which is subject to costs incurred in providing the outlined care. If more effort is needed, this can be explained to the patient and the fee adjusted upward. Likewise, if the procedures progress more easily than anticipated, the fee can be adjusted downward. The estimated fee provides the patient with a reasonably accurate idea of what the cost will be, but it also ensures a measure of flexibility to cover the unexpected. Even though the estimated fee allows the provider legal flexibility, it is wise for him/her to advise the patient when unexpected circumstances necessitate a substantial deviation from the estimated figure.

In most instances a policy of expressing the fee either orally or in writing will prevent legal encounters over fees. However, even in cases when a fee is stated and agreed to, some patients will refuse to pay. One tactic patients may take is to make a partial payment by check and label it ''paid in full.'' In a few states, accepting the partial payment without comment may be interpreted as meaning that the balance due is not expected. So it is important to compare payments labeled ''paid in full'' with the actual balance due. Any discrepancy should be resolved before the partial payment is accepted by depositing the payment (Miller, 1970). It is advised that the provider ask an attorney whether the state still follows the old rule allowing for discharge of the obligation by acceptance of an ''in full payment'' check.

When the patient simply refuses to pay, the health care provider does have some recourse.

The provider can issue warning letters in increasingly persistent language. If the letters are not successful, the account can be turned over to a collection agency, which continues the dunning process and which can alter the patient's credit rating (Miller, 1970). The agency charges a percentage of the fee ultimately paid by the patient in return for its efforts. It is doubtful whether this collection fee can legally be passed on to the delinquent patient unless this practice was made known to him/her prior to the rendering of the services in question.

If the letters and the efforts of the collection agency prove to be futile, the health care provider can bring a suit for breach of contract against the patient. However, it is important to recall that litigation is costly in time, money, and aggravation, and legal fees are not recoverable from a losing defendant. Furthermore, given the possibility of a countersuit, legal action for fee collection should be viewed as a last resort and be used only when the unpaid balance is substantial.

It should be clear that express contracts and agreed fees are good preventive measures. Can the provider, then, go a step further and get the patient to sign an agreement not to bring legal action against the provider? Such a statement would be a blanket waiver.

A dentist or hygienist cannot relieve him/herself of the responsibility to provide due care by having the patient sign a blanket waiver of his/her right to pursue legal action if the care provided is believed to be negligent. A 1981 court decision nullified a dental school's blanket waiver that would have released it from responsibility for providing a reasonable standard of care (Emory University, 1981). Such a decision would probably also be reached in instances where a practicing professional attempted to use such a contract to prevent malpractice actions.

One legal safeguard that can be used effectively is a clear, concise, accurate patient record. The patient record is probably the most important piece of evidence in court. If it is easily understood, meticulously recorded, and focuses on the needs of the patient and the care provided to meet those needs, the rationale and quality of care will be much easier to defend. Sadly enough, the best of care may be indefensible in court if it is indiscernible in the record. Poor radiographs, pencil entries, undated entries, or missing or incomplete entries do not present a picture of quality care. The patient record should include radiographs of diagnostic quality; the entries should be made *in ink* and be dated with the month, day, and year. All patient visits and procedures should be described. The progress of health should be discernible. A medical history, kept up to date, should be present in the chart. Before and after intraoral photographs can be invaluable when the practitioner is confronted with a malpractice suit. A well-kept record can have a very positive impact on the judge and jury. The fact that the patient knows the records are accurate may dissuade him/her from filing suit.

In contrast, the scribbled, incoherent, misspelled chart may smack of lack of due concern or even incompetence. By tolerating inaccurate charts, the health care provider is stacking evidence against him/herself.

There are other ways in which the health care provider can create evidence that is harmful in a court of law. One such way is for the health care provider to make some spontaneous statement during treatment that is self-incriminating. For instance, if during an oral prophylaxis, an instrument slips and cuts the tissue and the operator exclaims, "Oh, I should have had a better fulcrum," the operator has made a comment that can be used against him/her. This self-incriminating spontaneous utterance constitutes *res gestae*, which means "a part of the action," since the statement occurred simultaneous to the action in question (Black, 1979). Evidence that might otherwise be barred from court by the rule against hearsay may be admitted under the *res gestae* exception.

If a person makes an out-of-court statement, either spoken or in writing, which proves the opposite of what he/she is contending in court, the statement is an *admission against interest* and is admissible as evidence against the person (Black,

1979; Miller, 1970), again in exception to the general rule barring hearsay evidence. For example, a nurse may write a letter to a friend describing an error she made in administering a medication and explaining that she is fighting a charge of malpractice. The letter may end up as evidence against the nurse, since it may contradict what she is contending in court. An admission against interest differs from *res gestae* because it is a statement made at any time, which goes against the pecuniary or other legal interest of that person. A patient-plaintiff, of course, could make an admission against interest just as the provider could.

The use of *res gestae* and admission against interest as evidence should provide an indication of an important rule to follow if the health care provider finds him/herself in a potential legal tangle: He/she should discuss it with no one except his/her attorney and the malpractice insurance carrier (Miller, 1970). Direct communication with the patient may prove disastrous. When an injury occurs, the patient should be informed of the injury and appropriate steps should be taken to correct it. However, no incriminating explanations should be offered about the reason for the error. It is important to avoid estranging the patient while one is protecting him/herself from legal difficulties. The problem should not be discussed with colleagues or friends, except as advised by the attorney. Any injury that could be viewed as a stimulus for a lawsuit should immediately be reported to the insurance carrier.

In addition, it is a good practice for dental professionals to have at least a rudimentary awareness of the legal principles that guide good practice. For instance, knowing the difference between negligence, breach of contract, technical battery, and civil and criminal charges can result in more intelligent procedures in daily clinical practice. Such knowledge can also result in a more informed discussion with one's attorney if a legal action is pending. Even attorneys make mistakes in filing or defending actions (Steinmetz, 1984); a dentist or hygienist should know enough to ask informed questions and to supply important information to assist legal counsel in preparing a defense or in initiating an action.

Express contracts and fees, accurate records, and careful responses to potential lawsuits are all useful preventive measures. But they imply a defensive approach to the legal aspects of health care delivery. While it is appropriate to be protective of one's own well-being, it is more in keeping with a service-oriented profession to conduct oneself with the well-being of the patient as the primary consideration.

The very philosophy that a health care provider provides services *for* a patient rather than *to* a patient can create a "partnership" approach to health care. Including the patient as a responsible codeterminer of the nature of health care services is probably the most significant step in preventing lawsuits and in ensuring success of treatment. Patients who feel a commitment to the care they receive by virtue of understanding their needs will cooperate more fully in obtaining and maintaining the successful treatment.

It is of utmost importance that the clinician and the patient maintain clear communication about the care that is being delivered and about the responsibilities of both parties. It is possible to end up in court debating an issue that is clearly due to a failure to communicate rather than to any specific negligent act on the part of the dental professional or the patient (Lazar, 1980). Informed consent procedures carry the clinician a long way toward ensuring good understanding, but throughout the course of treatment the patient should be kept well-informed and statements of concern or possible misunderstanding should be pursued and rectified.

Consumer awareness of rights dictates involving the patient as a partner in health care. If care is indeed patient centered rather than procedure centered, the health care provider might look beyond the matter of care to be provided to issues relating to the dignity of the patient, the procedures to which the patient is subjected (including the red tape of forms and multiple visits), and the quality of overall care the patient is receiving.

If a health professional or a group of professionals adopts the role of consumer advocate, patients whose rights are violated might be assisted in obtaining restitution. Patients can be informed of their rights, be provided with guidelines for determining the quality of care delivered, and be directed to legal aid, if necessary. Poor quality health care, fraud in charging for procedures not performed, and the unhelping, elitist attitudes of some health care personnel cost the public a deal in terms of time, money, discomfort, dignity. A commitment to changing these negative aspects of health care may in itself change the negative reputation that some believe health care has acquired in recent years.

Review questions

1. How do the two types of fees relate to the two types of contracts? *implied & expressed*
2. How is a reasonable fee determined? *customary locally, scope of procedure, skill of DR, overhead costs, ability of pt to pay*
3. A patient pays only 60% of the fee due. The physician files a breach of contract suit for nonpayment. What is a possible legal response from the patient? *countersuit of malpractice*
4. Identify four characteristics of a well-kept patient record:
   a. *accurate, coherent, quality x-rays*
   b. *med hx*
   c. *care is related to need*
   d. *progress of health is discernible (to detect w/ eyes)*
5. A spontaneous statement accompanying some injury or error is referred to as *res gestae*.
6. A statement made by a person which conflicts with the position taken by that person in court is known as *admission against interest*
7. True or false: A patient can sign away his/her right to file a malpractice suit.

GROUP ACTIVITIES

1. Have a panel discussion to debate whether fee determination ought to be based in part on the patient's ability to pay.
2. Poll professional associations to see if recommended fees are published for members.
3. Assess sample patient records for their usefulness as evidence. Design a set of records that clearly depicts care needed and provided and the progress of health.
4. Conduct two mock trials in which the patient record offered in defense is (1) unhelpful, even detrimental and (2) helpful.
5. Role play instances of *res gestae* and admission against interest.
6. Read and critique one or more books written to serve as a guide for consumers of dental care.

REFERENCES

Black, H.C.: Black's law dictionary, ed. 5, St. Paul, Minn., 1979, West Publishing Co.

Creighton, H.: Law every nurse should know, Philadelphia, ed. 2, 1970, W.B. Saunders Co.

Emory University v. Porubiansky, Ga., 282 S.E.2d 803, 1981.

Goldfarb v. Virginia Bar Association, 96 Sup. Ct. 2004 (1975).

Lazar v. Federal Insurance Company, 380 So.2d 719 (La. App. 1980).

Miller, S.L.: Legal aspects of dentistry, New York, 1970, G.P. Putnam's Sons.

Steinmetz v. Lowry, 477 N.E.2d 671 (Ohio App. 1984).

Morris, R.C., and Moritz, A.R.: Doctor and patient and the law, ed. 5, St. Louis, 1971, The C.V. Mosby Co.

CHAPTER 11

Civil — to a person
Criminal — to society

Criminal charges

OBJECTIVES: The reader will be able to:

1. Differentiate between civil law and criminal law.
2. State the purpose of a state practice act, governing the practice of health care professionals.
3. Explain how the health care practitioner's actions are governed by the two branches of law: civil and criminal.
4. Given a series of hypothetical situations, identify whether each situation is covered by civil law or criminal law.
5. Describe the role of the state board in enforcing the practice act.
6. Differentiate open practice acts and closed practice acts.
7. Describe briefly how the trend toward greater scope of practice for auxiliaries is affected by the practice act.

So far the legal considerations for health care providers have been within the realm of the patient-provider relationship, described as consensual and contractual and in which certain rights and duties are reciprocal between the parties involved. Difficulties encountered in this contractual relationship are dealt with through one of the two branches of the civil law: contract law or tort law. In civil law, the individual who believes a wrong has occurred files against the offender through a private attorney. The previous chapters have identified rights and duties owed in the patient-provider relationship. The chapters offered suggestions for preventing such difficulties.

The health care provider is also obligated to observe the limits defined in *criminal law*.

A 'crime' [is] punishable upon conviction by:
1. Death; or
2. Imprisonment; or,
3. Fine; or,
4. Removal from office; or,
5. Disqualification to hold any position of trust, honor or profit under the state.
6. Other penal discipline (Hall and Mueller, 1965).

Criminal law involves actions that constitute a wrong against society. Civil law is related to actions causing harm to an individual. In criminal law, the state takes action against the wrongdoer, whereas in civil law, the plaintiff (wronged individual) files suit through a private attorney. Statutory law (enacted by the legislature) forms the basis of most criminal law, with case law (which is based on precedents established by the courts) comprising a smaller portion. Case law and statutory law are of equal importance in civil law.

It may not be obvious at first how a health care provider may commit a criminal act in the normal course of a day's professional activities. The ''crime'' that a provider commits is rarely the kind dramatized on television. It is usually an infraction of the state practice act (statute) covering the scope of activity of the particular provider in question.

Many health care professions are covered directly by a state practice act, which defines the practice of the particular profession and stipulates the means by which a person may be granted a license to practice as a member of that particular

84

profession. All licensed health care provider groups are regulated by state statute.

In all states or licensing jurisdictions, there is a state board to administer the written word of the practice act. The state board is an agency of the state; its members are usually appointed by the governor. The primary purpose of the practice act is to protect the public from incompetent would-be practitioners of the profession. The practice act prohibits persons from practicing unless they have specific, proven qualifications and competencies. The practice act empowers the state board to review the qualifications and competencies of applicants and to issue or deny a *license* to practice. The act also empowers the state board to suspend or revoke a license, if the practitioner violates the regulatory provisions of the act (Miller, 1970; Sarner, 1963; Woodall, 1972).

Any act committed by a person in violation of the applicable state practice act is a crime against society and subject to prosecution. If convicted, the individual is subject to punishment. The action is brought against the offender by "the people" in the person of the attorney general at the request of the state board (Miller, 1970; Sarner, 1963).

An illegal act need not result in actual bodily injury or property damage to be a criminal offense. The "harm" is considered to be the violation of the principles set down by the people through the action of the legislature (Black, 1979; Hall, 1960; Hall and Mueller, 1965; Miller, 1970; Sarner, 1963).

For instance, if a state dental practice act stipulates that dental hygienists or dentists are the only persons recognized to perform the oral prophylaxis, any other person who performs that procedure has committed a crime—even though no actual harm to the patient may have resulted. If a graduate hygienist begins to practice before he/she is issued a license, that hygienist has committed a crime. If a dental practice act empowers a dentist to delegate specific functions to an auxiliary in the office and a dentist delegates more procedures than those permitted, the dentist has com-

mitted a crime, but the person who performed the procedure has also committed a crime by engaging in unauthorized practice. Violation of the state practice act is regarded as a criminal offense. The seriousness of the violation determines what the punishment will be if prosecution results in a conviction (Black, 1979; Hall, 1960; Hall and Mueller, 1965). The state board may levy a fine or revoke the person's license or at least suspend it for a specified time. If court action is involved, the practitioner may be heavily fined or even imprisoned, depending on the severity of the infraction.

Examples of infractions beyond those cited previously that could result in a criminal conviction are: (1) the illegal prescribing or dispensing of narcotics by a licensed professional, (2) fraud (for instance, in making insurance claims), (3) income tax evasion, (4) sex offenses against patients or employees, or (5) gross negligence that results in wrongful death. Criminal activities not directly associated with practice of dentistry can also be grounds for license revocation. Thus, the state board may conduct its investigation of professionally related misconduct and recommend license revocation; then the attorney general may bring criminal charges against the licensee and succeed in exacting additional punishment. Likewise, if a dentist or hygienist is found guilty in criminal court of some offense, the state board may take action to revoke that person's license on the grounds that only ethical, trustworthy individuals of sound character may be considered worthy of state licensure to practice a profession.

Criminal acts committed by persons governed by one of the practice acts may be reported to the state board by a patient, another practitioner, or any other person who recognizes the infraction. The state board then sends out an investigator to gather evidence necessary to determine whether an infraction has occurred. If sufficient evidence is gathered, the board conducts a hearing. In extreme cases the attorney general may be asked to begin criminal proceedings. It should be obvious from the list of possible punishments that charges of violation of the state practice act can be substantial for the person found guilty.

In some instances, the board may decide to suspend or revoke a practitioner's license on the grounds of incompetence or negligence, even if no patient has sued the practitioner in a civil court. If complaints are brought to the state board rather than to the civil court or are brought concurrently with a patient's civil action and board investigation shows that the licensee is not fit for practice, the board's police powers enable it to withdraw the privilege to practice. The case may still end up in civil court, but usually with the licensee suing the board for wrongfully withdrawing the license.

In 1980 a dentist successfully sued the Oregon State Board for having wrongfully revoked his license for "unprofessional conduct." The statutes, rules, and regulations in Oregon did not define unprofessional conduct, and thus despite the distasteful nature of the dentist's activities the court ruled that the board had no power to revoke the license (Megdal, 1980).

However, a year later the Supreme Court of Wisconsin ruled the contrary in a similar case, where 14 patients were shown to have had negligent dentistry (Strigenz, 1981). The dental board claimed "conduct unbecoming a professional," which the supreme court supported, stating that a specific definition of the term was not required.

In a judgment rendered by the Supreme Judicial Court of Maine, an orthodontist who was shown to be incompetent in his care of orthodontic patients was not permitted to retain his license to practice general dentistry. Thus, in this case, incompetence in a specialty area did not permit the dentist to resume general practice (Board of Dental Examiners, 1982).

Going one step further, a Texas dentist who was determined to be practicing medicine without a license "under color" of practicing dentistry was not only prohibited from continuing his medical practice activities, but also was prohibited from practicing dentistry (Kelly, 1975).

A 1982 case in New Hampshire against a dentist was based in part on the dentist's failure to inform the patient and her parents of the risks associated with the placement of an implant. When the implant damaged the roots of the adjacent teeth, the patient's parents filed a complaint with the dental society, with the state dental board, and then in civil court. The New Hampshire Supreme Court upheld the board's action to suspend the dentist's license (Appeal of Beyer, 1982).

An additional wrinkle in the state board's enforcement of the dental law involves the legality of having public members (consumers) and dental hygienists on the board and making decisions regarding dental licensure. The Supreme Court of New Hampshire affirmed the appropriateness of the composition of the board, which did include a public member and hygienist (Appeal of Beyer, 1982). Similar affirmation was obtained in a Pennsylvania case (State Dental Council, 1974).

The responsibility of the health care provider in recent years is complicated by the status of most practice acts. In the 1930s, when many dental practice acts were enacted, frequently all provisions for practice were stated in the law (a *closed* practice act). The state dental boards were empowered to enforce what was clearly stated in the act. However, with the trend toward utilizing auxiliary personnel to support dental practice, the states' acts went through a period of change. This trend and period of change reached a peak in the late 1960s and early 1970s (Woodall, 1972). The changes that were enacted often provided the state dental practice act with only general descriptions of the scope of functions of dental personnel. A few functions were listed in the act as allowed and a few functions were listed as disallowed to provide a semblance of a definition of the health care provider being described. In addition to the skeleton listings, many revised acts added a phrase such as, "This person may perform any other functions which the state board of dentistry determines to be appropriate," resulting in an *open* practice act. This catchall phrase and others similar to it give power to the state boards to decide what activities are appropriate for each covered health care provider (*Manual, 1973*). Many states' laws include statements permitting the supervising dentist in the practice to delegate a wide variety of functions, according to his/her judgment.

There are many advantages to the open practice act, the most important of which is the fact that the entire state legislature need not reconsider the practice act to allow delegation of certain additional functions to personnel. As the times change and the need for support services changes, the state board through an official ruling can alter what is allowed to be delegated. The most liberal or open act reads, "The health care provider may perform those procedures which he/she has mastered through formal education." The state board must then identify a limit on what procedures are allowable, which it includes in its rules and regulations relating to the practice act.

The difficulty with this trend in the structure of practice acts belongs primarily to the health care provider, whose task it is to be informed of what is or is not permitted in a particular state or licensing jurisdiction. The rules are no longer found in the published practice act. The regulations that are to accompany an open act may have been tied up in hearings for years after the act is passed. Or the regulations, even though decided on by the board, may not be published. Inquiries to different members of the same state board may result in different, in fact opposite, descriptions of what is legally allowable (Woodall, 1972). Yet, it is the health care provider's responsibility to *know* the law and then to obey it (Hall, 1960; Hall and Mueller, 1965). If the law is not knowable, that is a defense for the provider. However, the ambiguity of the scope of practice in many states is frustrating and a source of potential jeopardy for providers.

The problem is compounded when a health care provider decides to move to another licensing jurisdiction. Aside from the usual requirement that

he/she again prove competence to practice before a license is issued, the provider must begin anew the effort to determine what is or is not allowed in that state. Are all stipulations published? Is the state board in a period of indecision or disagreement? Are some published regulations not enforced at all because of the ensuing debate? What may the practitioner legally do for the patient?

With the state laws varying from each other as greatly as they do, and given the frustration many dentists and hygienists felt with the plodding process of having workable rules and regulations defined, many practitioners have chosen to stretch the law, or even completely violate it, in the way functions are delegated to dental hygienists and assistants. Despite the frequency with which the dental law may be ignored or "liberally interpreted," it is an extreme risk to join this group. State boards do investigate such cases and have taken disciplinary action against the violators. License revocation makes it impossible for the professional to practice; it is a great price to pay for ignoring the law (Dailey, 1983).

The issues surrounding the practice acts in various states are complex ethical, economic, political, and legal considerations. Earlier parts of this text discuss those issues more fully. But in terms of self-protection from prosecution, it is best to request the practice act and any accompanying rules, regulations, and interpretations *in writing* and then retain them with the issued license. If a request for written clarification is refused, one choice may be to secure the aid of an attorney or to at least retain the written refusal. This may be the only defense in a criminal case. Also, it is a wise policy to read professional journals to learn of any current discussion, proposal changes, or clarifications.

As described earlier in this text, the dental practice act is one of the major considerations in expanding the scope of care a dental auxiliary may provide (Manual, 1973; Woodall, 1972). It can be a major roadblock to change, or it can be

ing force to promote change. Regardless
le of the dental practice act in hindering
g change, the individual dentist or aux-

iliary is legally responsible to abide by it. And a
breach of that responsibility is a criminal act.

Review questions

True or false:

1. Civil law covers those rights and responsibilities owed in the contractual relationship between a patient and the health care provider. ___*true*___ p.84

2. Criminal law covers infractions against an individual patient when harm results to the patient. ___*false*___ p.84

3. The sources of criminal law are federal or state statutes enacted by the legislature. ___*true*___ p.84

4. Dental practice acts are written and enacted by the state boards of dentistry. ___*false*___ p.84

5. The state board of dentistry enforces the state dental practice act. ___*true*___ p.85

6. In an open practice act, all regulations are contained in the act as passed by the legislature. ___*false*___ p.86

7. The purpose of a state practice act is to protect the profession. ___*false*___ p.85

Indicate which of the following acts is covered by civil law (contract or tort) or criminal law, or both:

	Civil	Criminal
8. A dental hygienist places restorative materials in prepared teeth. Despite the fact that the services are performed well with no harm to the patient, the practice act does limit this activity to the dentist.		✓
9. A patient is injured by a dental hygienist administering a local anesthetic. Rules of the state board permit delegation of this function to the dental hygienist.	✓	
10. A patient is harmed by a negligent act of a dental assistant who is scaling teeth, despite the practice act's prohibition of this activity by dental assistants.	✓	+ ✓
11. A nurse prescribes and administers a medication. The state law prohibits the prescription of medication by nurses.		✓

GROUP ACTIVITIES

1. Consult a recent compilation of provisions included in state dental practice acts and compare and contrast four of them according to:
   a. Legally permitted functions by hygienists and assistants.
   b. Requirements for licensure
   c. Open or closed characteristics

2. If there is ongoing discussion for changes in the dental practice act, attend public hearings and prepare a summary of the issues addressed and state how resolution of the issues could affect the scope of your practice.

3. Conduct an "inquiry" regarding the provisions of the practice act in your area. Five or six students should familiarize themselves with the current act and its rules and regulations and play the role of the state board. The remainder of the class will play the roles of "interested consumers," hygienists, assistants, and dentists wishing to inquire about the provisions of the act. Questions prepared by the inquirers should reflect the role each has adopted for purposes of the inquiry.
4. Prepare a review of the literature surrounding the "best" way to structure a practice act.
5. Review the recommendations of the Council of State Governments for the structure of dental practice acts.
6. Attend a hearing or trial in the case of a health care provider charged with a violation of the practice act.

REFERENCES

Appeal of Beyer, 453 A.2d 834 (N.H. 1982).

Black, H.C.: Black's law dictionary, ed. 5, St. Paul, Minn., 1979, West Publishing Co.

Board of Dental Examiners v. Brown, Maine, 448 A.2d 881, 1982.

Dailey v. North Carolina State Board of Dental Examiners, 309 S.E.2d 219 (N.C. 1983).

Hall, J.: General principles of criminal law, ed. 2, Indianapolis, 1960, The Bobbs-Merrill Co., Inc.

Hall, J., and Mueller, G.O.W.: Criminal law and procedure: cases and readings, ed. 2, Indianapolis, 1965, The Bobbs-Merrill Co., Inc.

Kelley v. Texas State Board of Dental Examiners, 530 S.W.2d 132, 1975.

Manual for Consultants to State Boards of Dentistry, Chicago, 1973, American Dental Hygienists' Associations.

Megdal v. Oregon State Board of Dental Examiners, 605 P.2d 273, 1980.

Miller, S.L.: Legal aspects of dentistry, New York, 1970, G.P. Putnam's Sons.

Sarner, H.: Dental jurisprudence, Philadelphia, 1963, W.B. Saunders Co.

State Dental Council and Examining Board v. Pollock, Pa., 318 A.2d 910, 1974.

Strigenz v. Department of Regulation and Licensing, Dentistry Examining Board, Wis., 307 N.W.2d 664, 1981.

Woodall, I.: Changes in state licensing acts allowing for expanded use of dental auxiliaries. In Mescher, K., editor: Proceedings of a training workshop on adaptation of dental hygiene practice to changing concepts in delivery of oral health services, Little Amana, Iowa, 1972, Iowa Dental Hygienists' Association.

PART THREE

Ethics

It is easier to meet obligations when the details of what is expected are clearly stated. The law is helpful in defining many of these obligations. However, a health care professional has obligations that extend beyond what the law requires. The professional has ethical obligations. While the law and ethics overlap in many areas, there are attitudinal, frequently intangible, aspects of professional practice that the law cannot readily enforce.

The professions attempt to codify those expectations in their association precepts with varying degrees of success, and professionals are then left to decide for themselves in specific situations what is the "right" thing to do.

This section provides a rudimentary description of the philosophical and psychological views of ethics and morality that help shape our notion of ethics and the way the professions interpret ethics. Proceeding a step further, the chapters discuss how a professional code of ethics can be implemented in daily practice. It also points out current issues in dental ethics that pose serious challenges for dentists and hygienists.

Being an ethical professional person is not easily defined today because of the myriad of factors that affect our daily lives: economic, environmental, educational, legal, political, philosophical, and psychological. Finding the boundaries of openness and flexibility while maintaining important standards regardless of the tenor of the times continues to be the primary challenge of ethics.

Moral conduct

not socially enforced by law.

CHAPTER 12

Assessment of ethics and ethical codes

OBJECTIVES: The reader will be able to:

1. State at least one definition of ethics that is acceptable to the student.
2. Differentiate brief, simplified descriptions of the Judeo-Christian, existential-humanistic, and behavioral approaches to ethics, and identify at least one philosopher whose theory is compatible with one of each of the brief descriptions.
3. Describe Kohlberg's stages of moral development.
4. Identify and explain the basic components of the current American Dental Hygienists' Association Code of Ethics.
5. Differentiate an ethical code from a "patient's bill of rights."

moral conduct

A large component of philosophy consists of the various approaches to the concept and implications of ethics. Although the term can be superficially and simply viewed as knowing and doing what is right, it has much more complex and deeply rooted meanings for people. Who knows what is right? Can a particular situation cause some action to be viewed as right that in another situation would be wrong? Is ethics always directed toward the needs of the other person, or is there an element of personal integrity that prompts ethical actions? Is ethics a matter of obeying an absolute standard established by an external entity? Does it spring from an inherent goodness in each person and, given the proper encouragement, flourish?

APPROACHES TO ETHICS
Philosophy and ethics

These are but a few of the complex questions that are asked again and again in a consideration of ethics. The answers vary with the philosophical base of the respondent. The ancient Greek philosophers Plato and, particularly, Aristotle in his *Nichomachian Ethics* viewed ethics as a value to be strived for that is the basis of harmony in life and personal happiness (Durant, 1954; Veatch, 1962). The contemporary French existentialist philosopher Jean-Paul Sartre would scoff at such a projected view of ethics and focus on the dilemma it poses to the existential person in coexisting with persons whose needs may not always be compatible with his own (Barrett, 1962; Durant, 1954). The humanists, represented by Allport, Maslow, Fromm, and Rogers, see ethics among people as a key in expressing mutual respect and as a normal and expected phenomenon for persons whose environment has enabled the ethical values to emerge and develop (Nash, 1984).

B.F. Skinner, a primary figure in the behavioristic movement, sees ethics as a matter of a performance discrepancy, devoid of personal value and consisting mainly of activities that have to be learned by a management of contingencies (Skinner, 1971).

In Western culture people are almost exclusively attuned to the Platonic-Aristotelian approach, which posits that ethics is a definitive absolute value to be strived for (Johnson, 1946; Sabatier, 1957). Goodness is seen as an unalter-

Not easily enforced by Law.

able, specific form toward which humans endeavor to perfect themselves.

Thomas Aquinas in the thirteenth century Christianized Aristotelian ethics, translating the *absolute value* into the Christian God and redefining human behavior in relation to this God as *moral behavior*. The new religious view of Aristotelian ethics became the basis for the codes of behavior established by the Roman Catholic Church, the dominant theistic-philosophical forum in Western civilization at the time. The emphasis was placed increasingly on the division of body and soul—more specifically on the soul's struggle to override the body's "animality." Augustine in the fifth century had described this division as a matter of choice—an either/or decision to travel the rough road to heaven or the seemingly smooth road to hell. The matter of choice was definitive in its polarity. Behavior was right or it was wrong. The reward was heaven or hell. God was on one side; the devil was on the other. Good and evil were seen as the difference between light and dark. This simplistic view of behavior became known as dualism. Religious paintings depict a man deciding which pathway to follow at the fork in the road. The road to heaven could be managed by a "right soul" that was successful in meeting and fending off the body's temptation. To choose short-range pleasure, permitting the body its desires, meant long-range suffering at the end of life on earth.

With the Protestant Reformation in the Renaissance period of the sixteenth century, the either/or approach to ethics and morality remained basically intact (Sabatier, 1957). In fact, the matter of only two paths to follow was intensified by the fact that there was no provision for earthly absolution of sins and no provision for an afterlife to cleanse the soul of its impurities (purgatory) so that the minor offenders could move on to heaven (Bainton, 1950).

The Hebrew views of ethics followed similar patterns, reinforcing the either/or, light/dark, right/wrong approach to life and ethical behavior; Hebrew teachings were one of the wellsprings of Christianity (Pegis, 1948; Sabatier, 1957). Both elements of the Judeo-Christian tradition focused on the ultimate authority of God as father with mankind as the sometimes erring, sometimes obedient child.

With this cultural background guiding ethical behavior, people tend to search for external guidelines for right conduct and spend a good deal of energy identifying to whom it is they report their behavior (Johnson, 1946). Perhaps it is this cultural need that causes people to write codes of ethics and form ethics committees to enforce the codes.

To present the issues and their origins in such a simplified form does them injustice. Yet these issues are at the very core of a health care provider's professional mandate to behave in a manner that is in agreement with the service orientation and in response to patients' trust in the provider's good judgment and high ideals. A closer look at philosophical approaches other than the dualistic approach to ethics may provide health professionals with the understanding to fashion a more eclectic approach to professional personal ethics (Johnson, 1946).

Humanism, which can be either theistic or atheistic, focuses on the potential of the human spirit to "become." The phenomena that occur in a person's lifetime and the choices a person makes actually define what the person is in the here and now. This is quite different from the "true forms" of Plato and the subsequent Western views of man that see a person as having a predefined nature. Theistic humanists attribute the ability of a person to be unique, to make responsible choices, and to be free to self-actualize to the portion of the deity (god) in all of us that is the human spirit. Atheistic humanists proclaim the uniqueness and responsibility of the human spirit to perfect itself, regardless of the existence of a god (Herberg, 1958; Paterson, 1976).

For humanists, goodness and ethical behavior emerge if the person is given an environment to nurture them, and in some cases even when the environment would seem to preclude it (Johnson,

1946). For them, the human spirit is in many instances able to overcome seemingly insurmountable pathos.

Humanism is a continuing theme in Western civilization (Mukerjee, 1968). It is often seen as being in a tug-of-war with religious approaches to moral behavior. In this setting the humanist tends to view ethics as being comprised of the responsible choices a person makes in relation to the community and self. More religious approaches stress external authority; God's law is expected to provide the appropriate choices.

Humanism is found as a continuing theme in the religious philosophies of India and China. Although Western humanism deals primarily with the psychosocial integration of the human being and with the process of self-actualization, the Eastern philosophies go "beyond man himself to that transcendent realm of values and potentialities from which he unerringly chooses his conscience, moral aspiration and way of living" (Mukerjee, 1968). Eastern philosophies strive for a oneness with the commonality of mankind and cosmos:

> The most extensive and the most enduring human association without any boundaries, lapses or vicissitudes as it expresses the final depth and impeccable conscience of the self fused in the all-encompassing Being. This is the myth and *utopia* of cosmic humanism beyond humanity—the final, absolute and unchanging social category of which all human groups and societies are but faint shadows and reflections, deriving their authentic moral principles and standards from it (Mukerjee, 1968).

Thus contemplation and a tuning out of the noise of everyday life are an important aspect of the practice of Eastern philosophies.

The primary difference between Eastern and Western humanism is the notion of cosmos—as reflected in the degree to which Eastern thought focuses on oneness with the "being" that is defined by cosmos and Western thought focuses on temporal roles. Oriental versions of humanism are more cosmic. The following virtues are described in the *Bhagavad Gita:*

Purity of mind and understanding; fearlessness; forgiveness, steadfastness in knowledge and concentration; perfect control of speech, body and mind; habit of unbroken contemplation; complete absence of ego-sense, desire and possessiveness; equal-mindedness; love of solitude; truthfulness; vigour and courage; non-violence; faithfulness or reverence; universal altruism; compassion for all creatures in the universe (Mukerjee, 1968).

Contemporary Western humanism is often described as the philosphy of the "me generation" and thus is rarely described as cosmic. While the traditional Western religions aspire toward virtues, they emphasize the restraints of correct behavior. For example, the Christian tradition turns to the beatitudes ("Blessed are the meek . . .") for hope, but uses the Ten Commandments for its code of behavior.

The element of unity among the three surviving forms of humanism is their inclusion of the importance of responsibility for action in regard to, at least, the temporal society in which we spend our lives and to the importance of the human community for shaping and confirming our identities as they evolve. Martin Buber, an existentialist theistic humanist, defines this interrelationship in *I and Thou.*

Existentialism is a form of humanism, with its roots in twentieth century Europe. Wars, economic instability, and declining faith in the Christian God spawned a turning inward. Existentialism focused on the ability of the human spirit to cope with the despair of daily life and the inescapable knowledge of inevitable death. Most of the basic themes of existentialism are identical to humanism's notion of "becoming," which concerns defining one's own essence through existence rather than accepting a predefined nature. Existentialism is, however, typically characterized as resulting from despair, in which people recognize the fear they feel regarding death and the transience of life. Existential ethics, which relies on choosing freedom as the supreme value and the means of survival, is seen by some as being irresponsible. Eastern philosophers and many Western philosophers who are within the existentialist-humanistic camp see freedom as emerging from a responsible link with community and the cosmos. They disagree with the goal of temporal freedom, seeing it as a denial of human conscience (Barrett, 1962; Herberg, 1958; Muker-jee, 1968).

In-depth reading and discussion of the varieties of thought in humanism, existentialism, and the various Eastern philosophies are necessary before they can be fully understood. They are closely aligned and provide an interesting alternative to our traditional cultural views.

Behavioristic thinking in contradistinction to humanism takes a startlingly pragmatic approach. The behavioral premise is that an ethical or any other action is the result of learning through the positive and negative reinforcements and punishments received for similar actions taken by the person earlier in his/her life.

Psychologists who use Skinnerian principles, called behavior modification, focus on the specific behaviors that require change. They reward behavior that increasingly approximates the desired behavior until the goal is reached (shaping). They ignore and sometimes punish undesired behavior. The system of rewards helps the person in question learn what to do. Below is an example of how a behaviorist analyzes an undesirable behavior:

The deprived person who successfully steals is reinforced right away; if the alternative is to wait forever to save money while doing a menial (perhaps even degrading) job, then the immediate reinforcement of stealing may control behavior (Nye, 1975).

This point of view differs markedly from the humanistic analyses that could be derived from their philosophy of virtue and transcendence. Behaviorism is a here and now, problem-solving approach to ethics in which what is known about learning theory is practically applied to "improve" behavior (Nye, 1975; Sabatier, 1957). The rehabilitation strategies used in the novel *A Clockwork Orange* to reverse criminal behavior

are vivid examples of how behavior modification can be applied (Burgess, 1972).

Its principles are well tested and provide a scientific foundation for much of current learning theory. Its relevance in the context of this discussion of ethics is to show it in contrast with differing philosophical views of choice and morality.

Would the professions adopt a policy of teaching ethics by means of contingency management? Would they establish a program to identify the reward sequence and system that best produces ethical responses in people and then set out to improve the ethics of the professional membership?

The question of ethics for health care providers should extend beyond a listing of right or wrong actions that the associations of health care providers define as their codes. With the obvious changes in the late twentieth century of what is or is not morally, ethically, or pragmatically acceptable to society, the health care professions might do well to equip themselves with the ability to cope with change, retain the mandate of providing care for patients, and maintain the highest ethical values. Patterns of acceptable or unacceptable behavior are increasingly based on the particular situation in which the behavior occurs. Although many people still adhere to the clearcut definitions of right and wrong, many others have basically set aside most of the time-honored rules in favor of such a "situation ethics" approach. Perhaps somewhere between dogmatic delineations of proper behavior and the challenge of operating with no guidelines there is a reasonable approach.

Moral development

While the philosophers contemplate the source and role of ethics in human life and the behaviorists experiment with ways to alter "wrong" behavior, the human development experts spend their energies, in part, identifying how children and adults develop their sense of morality. Moral development occurs as children "adopt principles that lead them to evaluate given behaviors as 'right' and others as 'wrong' and to govern their own actions in terms of these principles'' (Vander Zanden, 1981).

Jean Piaget sees children as actively involved in their own moral development. As they interact with the world and modify the world, they observe and feel the consequences of their actions—how the world responds. They are not passive recipients of a moral code which they must internalize. The children move from a *morality of constraint* that occurs when they are subject to adult authority and are not equals with adults to a *morality of cooperation* that evolves as children become adults and have achieved the status of equals (Vander Zanden, 1981).

Lawrence Kohlberg has identified 6 stages of moral judgment, which categorize the kind of reasoning a person uses in solving a normal dilemma. According to his theory all humans go through the same stages, regardless of culture, and the main individual differences are how rapidly a person moves from one stage to the next and whether a person stops at a certain level, regardless of his/her age (Vander Zanden, 1981).

Kohlberg's stages (Vander Zanden, 1981) are:

1. Obedience-and-punishment orientation. The person obeys the rules to avoid punishment. The standards themselves are not internally valued. An example in dentistry is a dental hygienist who would gladly defraud an insurance company for monetary gain but who does not because the consequences of exposure are severe.

2. Naive hedonistic and instrumental orientation. The person obeys rules in order to obtain rewards and benefits. An example in this stage is a dentist who cites the laws restricting free market trade by dental hygienists and who supports them because they provide a measure of economic protection.

3. "Good boy"–"nice girl" morality. The person is interested in gaining approval of peers and superiors. A professional who is seeking acceptance and praise for impeccable behavior rather than accepting the reasoning and conditions supporting "right" behavior would be making moral judgments in this stage.

4. "Law-and-order" orientation. The person blindly accepts social conventions and rules. The emphasis is on doing one's duty. No matter how offensive the law, the person operating in this moral stage abides by the laws. An example might be a group of hygienists who refuse to assist a coprofessional in testing the law because the laws are to be followed, not tested.

5. Social contract orientation. Morality is seen as an agreement among individuals to conform to laws that are necessary for community well being. Since it is seen as a social contract, the laws are viewed as open to challenge and change as long as basic principles are not altered (e.g., liberty). Dentists and hygienists who worked for changes in the state practice acts to allow expanded functions would probably fit in this stage; so might hygienists who are attempting to change the laws regarding independent practice.

6. Universal ethical principle orientation. Behavior is guided by a strong set of internal principles. The person feels compelled to follow those principles even if it means violating set rules. Civil disobedience is acceptable if laws conflict with broad moral convictions. It is difficult to find an example in dentistry that fits this category. Kohlberg is reported as having difficulty finding people who operate in this category in everyday life. This category applies to the few who are active in human rights and peace initiatives where personal commitment and moral beliefs supercede existing laws (e.g., segregation, conscription into military service, illegal detainment, economic and political repression).

There are some adults, including dental professionals, who follow the laws only because they do not want to be punished. There are others who follow the laws because laws are to their own personal benefit. Some believe that they will gain prestige from doing what is right; others follow laws because it is their duty. Fortunately there are many who see the necessity of laws as defining behavior so that society can function in harmony and with justice. A small minority, at least according to Kohlberg's research, have a strong internal sense of the moral principles behind laws and "right" behavior (Vander Zanden, 1981).

People don't tend to function as immoral or unethical in all situations. There are some situations where an individual may meet the ideal in right behavior, while in one or two other situations, the standards of behavior do not appear to be as high. What a person sees as permissible or justifiable behavior frequently varies from what another person may condone (Vander Zanden, 1981). An honest discussion among students can produce an interesting array of perceptions about when it is "acceptable" to cheat, steal, tell partial truths, or "push the grey areas" of rules. Undoubtedly, an equally open discussion among dental professionals regarding topics that test their ethical fiber will result in an array of perceptions and attitudes, also.

Dental professionals can determine the moral imperatives behind laws and the principles of ethics by discussing the choices they are confronted with, expressing their personal responses, listening to the responses of peers, and perhaps altering their initial choices and interpretations. Thus a teacher or leader can play a Socratic role in ferreting out professionals' opinions and inclinations. Such strategies are collectively referred to as values clarification, where no one, including the leader, is set up as having the "right" answer. The purpose is to permit peers to hear one another's opinions and perhaps alter their own perceptions as a result.

According to Kohlberg, moral learning requires more than facilitating. In his opinion, it requires a stronger approach, where fundamental principles of "right behavior" are stated and defended

(Vander Zanden, 1981). While the 1960s and 1970s focused on discussion and nondirective approaches to teaching ethics, the 1980s reflects a trend toward a more doctrine-supported, directive strategy. With some of the basic principles of dental ethics under fire (the demise of antiadvertising codes and the requirement of silence regarding others' professional work), such an approach poses an interesting challenge. Can directive teaching regarding ethical behavior result in real changes or does it just provide the illusion of change?

Including a strong ethics component in dental and dental hygiene education programs and in professional continuing education courses is important if adults in the profession are to have their ethical perspectives enhanced and clarified (Cole, 1984).

A basic problem that persists despite the presence or absence of written codes is that a person will undoubtedly confront dilemmas in which two or more clear moral, legal, or ethical imperatives conflict (Davis and Aroskar, 1978; Paterson, 1976). No matter the choice, one or more standards or dicta will be compromised. In such situations it is up to the person to select the best choice apparent.

In medicine the dilemmas are sobering. Decisions that include informed consent for terminally ill patients, abortion, patients' rights and responsibilities, the right to die, and sterilization place an awesome burden on physicians, nurses, and other health professionals. In general they turn to professional guidelines and codes and to each other; then they turn to themselves for an answer that best fits their understanding of what is ethical (Basson, 1981; Davis and Aroskar, 1978; Paterson, 1976).

CODE OF ETHICS FOR DENTAL HYGIENISTS

Although the ethical decisions confronting them may not match those encountered regularly in medicine, dental hygienists do have choices to make. The ADHA has developed codes of ethics.

The first was in 1926, which stood until 1962. Others were written in 1969 and in 1975.

1926 CODE
The duties of the profession to their patients

Section 1. The dental hygienist should be ever ready to respond to the wants of her patrons, and should fully recognize the obligations involved in the discharge of her duties toward them. As she is in most cases unable to correctly estimate the character of her operations, her own sense of right must guarantee faithfulness as to gain the respect and confidence of her patients, and even the simplest case committed to her care should receive that attention which is due to operations performed on living, sensitive tissue.

Section 2. It is not to be expected that the patient will possess a very extended or very accurate knowledge of professional matters. The dental hygienist should make due allowance for this, patiently explaining many things which seem quite clear to herself, thus endeavoring to educate the public mind so that it will properly appreciate the beneficent efforts of our profession. She should encourage no false hopes by promising success when in the nature of the case there is uncertainty.

Section 3. The dental hygienist should be temperate in all things, keeping both mind and body in the best possible health, that her patients may have the benefit of the clearness of judgment and skill which is their right.

1962 CODE
Principles of ethics of the American Dental Hygienists' Association

The maintenance and enrichment of this heritage of professional status place on everyone who practices Dental Hygiene an obligation which should be willingly accepted and willingly fulfilled. This obligation cannot be reduced to a changeless series of urgings and prohibitions for, while the basic obligation is constant, its fulfillment may vary with the changing needs of a society composed of human beings that a profession is dedicated to serve. The spirit and not the letter of the obligation, therefore, must be the guide of conduct for the professional woman. In its essence this obligation has been summarized for all times and for all men in the golden rule which asks only that "whatsoever ye would that men should do to you, do ye even so to them."

The following statements constitute the *Principles of Ethics* of the American Dental Hygienists' Association. The constituent and component societies are urged to adopt additional provisions or interpretations not in conflict with these *Principles of Ethics* which would enable them to serve more faithfully the traditions, customs and desires of these societies.

Section 1. Basic Deportment. If and when a member of this Association is employed, she shall be associated with a member of the American Dental Association or with a dentist whose practice is in accord with the *Principles of Ethics* of the American Dental Association.

Section 2. Education Beyond Usual Level. The right of a dental hygienist to professional status rests in the knowledge, skill and experience with which she serves her patients and society. Every dental hygienist has the obligation to keep her knowledge and skill freshened by continuing education throughout her professional life.

Section 3. Service to the Public. The dental hygienist has a right to win for herself of those things which give her the ability to take her proper place in the community which she serves, but there is no alternative for the professional woman in that she must place first her service to the public.

The dental hygienist's primary duty of serving the public is discharged by giving the highest type of service of which she is capable and by avoiding any conduct which leads to a lowering of esteem of the profession to which she belongs.

Section 4. Government of a Profession. Every profession receives from society the right to regulate itself, to determine and judge its own members. Such regulation is achieved largely through the influence of the professional societies, and every dental hygienist has the dual obligation of making herself a part of a professional society and of observing its rules of ethics as defined by statute and ordinance in various states, territories and dependencies.

Section 5. Leadership. The dental hygienist has the obligation of providing freely of her skills, knowledge and experience to society in those fields in which her qualifications entitle her to speak with professional competence. The dental hygienist should be active in and available to her community, especially in all efforts leading to the improvement of the dental health of the public.

Section 6. Limited Practice. The dental hygienist has an obligation to protect the health of her patient by not taking upon herself any service or operation which requires the professional competence of a dentist. The dental hygienist has a further obligation to the patient of placing herself under the supervision of a dentist at all times, as prescribed by law.

Section 7. Consultation. The dental hygienist has the obligation of referring for consultation and diagnosis to her supervisor all patients, whose welfare should be safeguarded or advanced by having recourse to those who have special skills, knowledge and experience.

Section 8. Unjust Criticism. The dental hygienist has the obligation of not referring disparagingly to the services of another dental hygienist or dentist in the presence of a patient. A lack of knowledge of conditions under which the services are afforded may lead to unjust criticism and to a lessening of the patient's confidence in the dental profession.

Section 9. Advertising. Advertising reflects adversely on the dental hygienist who employs it and lowers the public's esteem of the dental hygiene profession. The dental hygienist has the obligation of advancing her reputation for fidelity, judgment and skill solely through her professional service to her patients and to society. The use of advertising, in any form, to solicit patients is inconsistent with this obligation.

Section 10. Cards, Letterheads and Announcements. A dental hygienist may not utilize professional cards, announcement cards, recall notices to patients of record, or letterheads other than as an adjunct to that of her supervisor.

Section 11. Office Door Lettering and Signs. A dental hygienist may properly utilize office door lettering and signs, providing that they are utilized as an adjunct to those of her supervisor.

Section 12. Use of Professional Titles. A dental hygienist may use the title of dental hygienist or letters of R.D.H. in connection with her name on cards, letterheads, office door signs and announcements, but only as an adjunct to those of her supervisor.

Section 13. Directories. A dental hygienist may not permit the listing of her name in other than professional directories.

Section 14. Health Education of the Public. A dental hygienist may properly participate in a program of health education of the public involving such media as the press, radio, television and lectures, provided that such programs are in keeping with the dignity of the profession and the custom of the dental profession of the community.

1969 CODE

The philosophical, practice science of ethics establishes, by reason and intelligent observation, principles to direct our human conduct. Professional conduct incorporates the knowledge of these principles into practice.

The following principles constitute a guide to the responsibilities of the dental hygienist to:

Self. The dental hygienist, supporting the laws governing dental hygiene, is individually obligated to assume responsibilities for professional actions and judgments when rendering services to the public.

The dental hygienist has an obligation to improve professional competency through continued education and research.

The dental hygienist functions harmoniously with and sustains confidence in all members of the dental health team.

The dental hygienist is obligated to report unethical practice to the appropriate authority.

Professional Organization. The dental hygienist has the responsibility to support and participate in the professional organization.

The dental hygienist participates in the study of and acts on matters of legislation affecting the dental hygienist and dental hygiene services to the public.

The dental hygienist through the professional organization participates responsibly in establishing social and economic status for the practice of dental hygiene.

The Community. The dental hygienist as a member of a community understands and upholds the laws of that community and has a particular responsibility to work with all allied health professions in promoting efforts to meet the general and oral health needs of the public.

1975 CODE

Each member of the American Dental Hygienists' Association has the ethical obligation to subscribe to the following principles:

To provide oral health care utilizing highest professional knowledge, judgment and ability.

To serve all patients without discrimination.

To hold professional patient relationships in confidence.

To utilize every opportunity to increase public understanding of oral health practices.

To generate public confidence in members of the dental health professions.

To cooperate with all health professions in meeting the health needs of the public.

To recognize and uphold the laws and regulations governing this profession.

To participate responsibly in this professional Association and uphold its purpose.

To maintain professional competence through continuing education.

To exchange professional knowledge with other health professions.

To represent dental hygiene with high standards of personal conduct.

Limitations of codes

Perhaps the most startling contrast is between the 1962 code and the others. None of the others dwells on the protocol issues of advertising or use of professional titles. And it is only the 1962 version that makes strong statements about the "obligation to the patient of placing herself under the supervision of a dentist at all times."

The tenor of this 1962 code seems to be one of setting limitations and defining propriety rather than of opening the hygienist to an increased scope of responsibility and discussing ethics. A case in point is Section 14. It seems unusual that a section dealing with the health education of the public would serve merely as an indicator that it is permissible to appear in the public eye and that the hygienist had best be careful that the programs are "in keeping with the dignity . . . and custom of the dental profession" (ADHA Code, 1962).

Nash points out that the professions' codes of ethics should be reviewed by an ethicist, partly to ensure that the percepts are not merely self-serving, "guild-protecting" guidelines and partly to ensure that the underlying assumptions of the codes include the ethical/contractual bond between a professional and society. Such a bond stipulates that the professional is "obliged to work for the fair distribution of the benefits and burdens of oral health among the populace" and

"to help faithfully to the limit of one's professional resources" when a patient is accepted by a health professional. The code should not promote paternalism in dealing with patients; it should not presume that "beneficence should take precedence over autonomy: literally doing perceived good to others in spite of their wishes." In general, the code should not set the profession apart as a special, elite group, but rather reflect an attitude of humble service and fidelity to society without a "conceit of philanthropy" (Nash, 1984).

If the code is based on this fundamental principle and avoids the mechanics of advertising, using degrees on letterhead, the acceptable size of a sign at the place of business, and other strictures, the code will be less subject to radical change. Abrupt changes, according to Cole, tend to demean the document. Time-honored precepts should form the basis for the code (Cole, 1984).

PATIENT'S BILL OF RIGHTS

Another approach to ethics, and perhaps one more in keeping with a consumer advocate role is the "patient's bill of rights" statement. Such a statement was adopted by the National League for Nursing (NLN). It includes three basic assumptions:

1. Nursing care encompasses health promotion, the care and prevention of disease or disability, and rehabilitation, and involves teaching, counseling and emotional support as well as the care of illness.
2. Nursing care is an integral part of total health care and is planned and administered in combination with related medical, educational and welfare services.
3. Nursing personnel respect the individuality, dignity and rights of every person, regardless of race, color, creed, national origin or social or economic status (Carnegie, 1973).

The actual differences between this patient's bill of rights and the various codes of ethics the ADHA has adopted are not very great. The reason seems to be that in both the ADHA and NLN codes, the elements focus on the *provider* of

'nursing care'' or ''nursing person-
than on the expressed wants, needs,
ons of patients. The title, which fo-
e patient, is appropriate for the age of
sm, but the content still clings to
ial self-centeredness: How *ought* the
provider act? A statement of wants, needs, and
expectations on the part of the patient could cause
each health care provider to be challenged with
patient-centeredness: How can the *patients'* rights
be met? The latter approach seems to be more
goal oriented, whereas the former is focused on
behavior or actions as ends in themselves. In
many ways the rights and responsibilities (outlined in Chapter 6) as an integral part of the patient–health care provider relationship provide a
better basis for drafting a patient's bill of rights.

It should be obvious that health care is in fact
patient centered and therefore should focus on the
well-being of the patient as the primary ethical
goal.

Below is an example of a patient's bill of rights
adopted by an educational program.

Patient's bill of rights

Patients can expect:

1. To be treated with respect and consideration for their medical, dental, and personal needs.
2. To be well informed of all aspects of their care.
3. A thorough assessment of their needs.
4. To be treated as partners in care, participating in goal setting and planning of treatment.
5. To be informed of appointment and fee schedules.
6. To have appointment times observed and a reasonable fee charged by the provider.
7. To receive current information and be assured quality treatment.
8. To receive treatment which will prevent further dental/oral disease.
9. To be taught to maintain oral health.
10. Reasonable continuity of care.
11. Appropriate and timely referrals for other needed services.
12. To be treated by providers who model good personal health and hygiene.
13. Confidentiality of all information pertinent to his/her care (University of Pennsylvania, 1977).

Review questions

1. True or false:
   a. Behaviorists see ethical problems as a matter of self-control that comes from choosing the ''right or wrong'' path. ___false___ p. 96
   b. Humanism is a strictly atheistic philosophy that relies on the human spirit alone for defining ethics. ___false___ p. 94
   c. Humanism has survived in three cultures: Western civilization, India, and China. ___true___ p. 95
   d. Humanism and existentialism see the person as defining his/her own essence by means of the choices he/she makes. ___true___ p. 95
   e. Eastern humanistic philosophies differ from Western humanism in that they are more ''self'' oriented. ___false___ p. 95
2. Match the following philosophers with their beliefs:
   a. Rogers, Maslow, Allport, and Fromm
   b. Skinner
   c. Sartre
   d. Buber
   e. Aristotle, Augustine

_D_ _1. Theistic, humanistic existentialism
_C_ _2. Atheistic existentialism
_B_ _3. Behaviorism
_A_ _4. Dualistic, theistic, authority-centered ethics
D + E _5. Humanism

3. Briefly state your own definition of ethics.
4. Which code (if any) fits best with your definition of ethics?
5. How does a bill of rights differ from an ethical code?
6. What are Kohlberg's six stages of moral development?
7. True or False:
   a. All people pass through each of the six stages of moral development and operate within the sixth stage as adults. _false_
   b. The main purpose of a professional code of ethics should be the enhancement of the professional image of the group. _false_
   c. According to Nash, a code of ethics should promote a caretaker approach to patients in need, providing service even when the patient is unaware of the need or when the service is not readily accepted by the patient. _false_

GROUP ACTIVITIES

1. Obtain the ethics code of the ADA and of two other health care professions. Evaluate each in terms of its either/or orientation, its emphasis on service, and its reliance on professional judgment for implementation. Find out whether the codes have an enforcement mechanism.
2. Draft your own patient's bill of rights that focuses on patients' wants, needs, and expectations.
3. Compare and contrast your individual definitions of ethics.
4. Read *Beyond Freedom and Dignity*, by B.F. Skinner, and discuss how this theory relates to the whole concept of ethics.
5. Read *Irrational Man*, by William Barrett, and trace the origin of existentialism and how its supporters view the issue of ethics.
6. Select two or three of the ethical dilemmas facing medicine, and discuss how you would apply your philosophy to their solution.
7. Review the latest version of the American Dental Association *Principles of Ethics and Code of Professional Conduct*. Read Nash's critique of the document (Nash, 1984). Discuss the meaning of "paternalism," "conceit of philanthropy," and "professional covenant."
8. Review this scenario: A student is caught passing notes to a friend during an examination. Both students were dismissed from school for violating the honor code which stipulates no assistance shall be given another student and no assistance shall be accepted from another student during examinations. Other students in the class were interviewed for their opinions of the situation. Review each response

and attempt to place the response in one of Kohlberg's 6 categories of moral judgment.
   a. The teachers expect entirely too much of us. If some of us don't help the students who have trouble remembering a million trivial points, they will have no chance of passing. I feel they committed no grievous error in what they did; it is a shame they are paying so dearly.
   b. If everybody cheats, then my grade won't reflect how much I know without cheating. They grade on a curve here, and I want credit for my hard work and my ability to learn quickly.
   c. It was my duty to report them. I signed the honor code statement last year, and I will uphold it no matter how tough things are.
   d. I think it was awful that they cheated. I would never do a thing like that. It is really important for professional people to be above cheating. You can check my work anytime you want, and you'll never find me stooping to such an activity.
   e. If I can get away with it, and I think I know the material pretty well anyway, I'll cheat just to raise my grade a few points. But I won't do it when it is clear that the teacher is looking; I sure don't want to be expelled.
   f. It is clear to me that cheating is wrong for people who are going to rely on that information when they are working with the public trying to be of service. If they never learned the material, how can they be expected to practice competently? I do think however that we have to change some of the grading policies and the expec-

tations of students that exist around here. I expect to form a group of interested students and approach the administration about what brought on this cheating.

NOTE: While some of the above statements clearly fit a specific category, there are some that are not as obvious. Discussing the way you view the response is more important than agreeing on which category it fits exactly.

REFERENCES

ADHA Code of Ethics, 1926, 1962, 1969, 1975.

Bainton, R.H.: The Reformation of the sixteenth century, Boston, 1950, Beacon Press.

Barrett, W.: Irrational man, New York, 1962, Anchor Books.

Basson, M.D., editor: Rights and responsibilities in modern medicine, vol. 2, Prog. Clin. Biol. Res., New York, 1981, Alan R. Liss, Inc.

Burgess, A.: A clockwork orange, New York, 1972, Ballantine Books, Inc.

Carnegie, M.E.: The Patient's Bill of Rights and the nurse, Nurs. Clin. North Am. **9**:557, 1973.

Cole, L.A.: Dentistry and ethics: a call for attention, J. Am. Dent. Assoc. **109**:559, 1984.

Davis, A.J., and Aroskar, M.A.: Ethical dilemmas and nursing practice, New York, 1978, Appleton-Century-Crofts.

Durant, W.: The story of philosophy, New York, 1954, The Pocket Library.

Herberg, W., editor: Four existentialist theologians, New York, 1958, Anchor Books.

Johnson, W.: People in quandaries, New York, 1946, Harper & Row, Publishers, Inc.

Mukerjee, R.: The way of humanism: East and West, Bombay, 1968, Academic Books.

Nash, D.A.: Ethics in dentistry: review and critique of Principles of Ethics and Code of Professional Conduct, J. Am. Dent. Assoc. **109**:597, 1984.

Nye, R.D.: Three views of man, Monterey, Calif., 1975, Brooks/Cole Publishing Co.

Paterson, J.G., and Zderad, L.T.: Humanistic nursing, New York, 1976, John Wiley & Sons, Inc.

Pegis, A.C.: Introduction to Saint Thomas Aquinas, New York, 1948, Modern College Library Editions.

Sabatier, A.: Outlines of a philosophy of religion, New York, 1957, Torchbooks.

Skinner, B.F.: Beyond freedom and dignity, New York, 1971, Bantam Books, Inc.

University of Pennsylvania School of Dental Medicine Department of Dental Hygiene, 1977.

Vander Zanden, J.W.: Human development, New York, ed. 2, Alfred A. Knopf, 1981.

Veatch, H.B.: Rational man: a modern interpretation of Aristotelian ethics, Bloomington, Ind. 1962, Indiana University Press.

CHAPTER 13

Changing ethical standards in society: practical application of principles

OBJECTIVES: The reader will be able to:

1. Identify at least one way in which an individual can fulfill each of the principles of ethics, such as those adopted by ADHA.
2. Given "touchy" questions asked by patients, express a response that reflects the following:
   a. Sensitivity to the patient's need.
   b. Respect for the limitations under which health care professionals provide care.
3. Identify examples of contemporary changes in ethical standards.
4. Redefine *professionalism* in terms of responsibility to patients.

CHALLENGES TO HEALTH CARE ETHICS

Current conditions challenge the health care professional's ability to chart a clear ethical course when meeting the needs of patients. These conditions are economic, social, political, legal, and technical. Dentistry, in particular, is undergoing a great deal of internal change that stresses the age-old maxims regarding ethical practice. Dental hygiene is suffering from its own internal stresses, both in relation to dentistry and to the external environment dental hygiene shares with dentistry.

As the 1980s come closer to becoming the 1990s, both dentistry and dental hygiene are emerging from the economic woes that plagued the whole country. Inflation took quite a toll on the ability of otherwise ethical dentists to make the "right" decision when it could cost them more and produce less revenue than an alternative, "less appropriate" business or clinical decision. It is difficult to be scrupulous when the standard of living is sliding toward the negative and dreams and aspirations are fading. Hygienists suf-

fered when dentists decided their partially empty appointment pages could be filled with the procedures usually performed by the dental hygienist and when the employer-dentist decided the hygienist willing to work for low pay could replace the well-paid hygienist who had worked for 15 or more years in that practice. Hard times prevailed in the early 1980s.

Many people who entered dentistry and dental hygiene had as one of their motives the aspiration to a good economic life and to the social respectability that comes from economic comfort and professional prominence. It is hard to feel socially accomplished when the flow of cash is impaired.

The political climate in the 1980s focuses on rugged individualism and each person carrying his/her own weight in society. This represents a huge swing from the mentality of the 1960s' Great Society, where less fortunate people would be given food, shelter, and an opportunity to reverse their situations, largely through federal subsidies. Health care professionals who have

105

learned about or grown up with the mandate of helping people who need help, regardless of their ability to pay, may find themselves in conflict with the current political stance. They may feel that they need to take up the slack and provide free care to those who are disenfranchised by federal subsidies, which creates an economic drain for the professionals. Or they may decide that it is up to the individual to move out of economic problems and that free care just makes that person more reliant upon outside help.

The legal pressures on health care professionals have become burdensome with the rise in the number and severity of malpractice claims and with the increased interaction with third party payers, such as insurance companies. Dentists and hygienists have to find a way to preserve their professional ethics while operating in an atmosphere of increased legal caution and when functioning with an impersonal payment agency. Insurance fraud has become too easy to justify for some clinicians who see deriving the maximum dollar benefit from carriers as a game or as the price the carrier should pay for having "interfered" with the doctor/patient relationship.

Even the technical advances of the era test the professional ethics of providers. New treatment options are available to clinicians, but they may carry a high price and provide a result that is only marginally improved over older, less expensive procedures that are perhaps less exciting for the clinician to perform. New research questions the need for expensive surgical techniques that cause pain and that cost the patient or carrier a great deal of money. Moving to a more conservative approach to care may in some instances be appropriate; but it is difficult to give up the sizable difference in fees that can be charged if the surgical choice is made. Even more critical are the technical advances that reduce the incidence of dental disease. Professionals are faced with encouraging the development and use of advances in disease prevention while realizing that decreased dental disease will change the face of dental and dental hygiene practice.

No doubt there are other environmental factors that test the ethical fabric of health care. There is little doubt that professionals need a firm grounding in professional ethics to make the choices that will confront the clinician in daily practice. Strategies for making sound choices based on a firm grounding of what is ethical should be a cornerstone in professional ethics.

FROM A CODE TO ETHICAL ACTION

Certainly the codes of ethics of the professional associations provide guidance in determining what is ethical. An important exercise is to turn to those codes and delineate how an individual clinician puts those guidelines into daily practice. What is critical is determining how each maxim translates into personal action, otherwise they are meaningless.

The first principle from the 1975 ADHA Code is "to provide oral health care utilizing highest professional knowledge, judgment and ability" (ADHA Principles, 1975). Does it have any message for how well a student attempts to learn what the educational process has to offer? Is "beating the system" to graduate compatible with this ideal? Does it perhaps offer the student in the clinical portion of the curriculum a guideline for the quality of care delivered to patients? It implies that the theoretical components of dental education have some definite relationship to the clinical components of care for people. Once the theory is linked with the practical, clinical functions, the student should take the time and energy to think about what plans for care are most appropriate and then act in the *best interest of the patient*.

The first ethical principle is the embodiment of the *service* orientation. It addresses itself to the well-being of the patient by focusing on the provider's need to know, think, and care. It should be easy to see how it applies to graduate clinical practice. It describes the graduate clinician as a knowledgeable, thinking, caring person who carefully assesses the patient's needs, plans care and appointments so that those needs can be met, and delivers the care to the best of his/her ability. The clinician avoids the monotony of repeated prophy-laxes and better serves the patient by never assuming that scaling and polishing are the automatic need of any patient. Beyond that the hygienist may ensure that the full range of dental hygiene services are available and may be selected as appropriate procedures for a patient seeking dental hygiene care.

The principle implies that the dental hygienist reviews the patient's medical history and alters care appropriately. It charges the hygienist with the responsibility for sterilizing instruments and otherwise ensuring that patients are not exposed to infectious agents from other patients who seek the care of the hygienist.

It suggests that the hygienist ought to place the patient first on the list of priorities.

The second principle of ethics reads "to serve all patients without discrimination." The intent of the principle is to encourage the dental hygienist to put aside any personal prejudices based on race, color, sex, ethnic origin, age, size, or other characteristic of another person (Motley, 1983). It is wishful thinking to say that people no longer have prejudices. Although prejudices are not as blatantly expressed today, low expectations of certain people or stereotypical ideas of what certain people value still exist in the mind sets of many people.

The degree to which these prejudices affect the availability or the quality of care people receive is of concern to the membership of the profession. Frankly stated, refusing care to a patient on the basis of his/her personal characteristics is unethical. Offering a lower standard of care is also unethical.

The ethical health care provider views the *needs* of the patient as the basis for offering care.

Once the patient is accepted for care, the health care provider is mandated "to hold professional patient relationships in confidence." This is the third ADHA principle of ethics. Keeping details of care provided to patients in confidence is not only an ethical duty; it is a legal duty (Miller, 1970; Motley, 1983). Casual statements about the nature of a patient's problems, information contained in the medical history, or any other information obtained about or from a patient in the course of treatment must be kept in strict confidence.

Sharing the process of the day's appointments with a fellow worker over lunch can be quite an embarrassment if the conversation is overheard, and the act may have legal repercussions. Analyzing patient data, such as evaluating a radiographic series or study models, in a public location where passers-by may see the name on the chart or even be able to read chart entries is a breach of confidence.

The only occasional exceptions in the ethical and legal mandate regarding confidentiality are cases of child abuse (Miller, 1970) or communicable disease that are discovered in the course of treatment (Motley, 1983). These may be expected to be promptly reported since they pose a severe public risk. However, it is best for a provider to consult an attorney for information about the precedents in the particular state in which he/she practices. Expectations concerning disclosure of such information vary from state to state; knowledge of the appropriate procedures to follow for reporting such cases is important.

Perhaps this whole concept of determining what to do when one finds oneself in such a predicament is a true test of appropriate judgment and due caution that are integral to ethical behavior.

"To utilize every opportunity to increase public understanding of oral health" addresses itself to the teaching role of the dental hygienist. This charge relates to the need for the dental hygienist to be "spreading the word" about dental health and the means to attain it. This applies to the one-to-one educational process that occurs in the patient–health care provider relationship. It also refers to educating larger groups of people through community activities. What does this ethical principle say about the practitioner who does not choose to include patient education procedures in his/her clinical routine? Is this principle an ethical matter or is it more a proclamation of the scope of practice of the dental hygienist? Perhaps it does suggest that ignoring this phase of clinical practice is a matter of ethics as well as definitions.

The Principles of Ethics take a stand with regard to professional isolation when it is made an ethical mandate "to cooperate with all health professionals in meeting the health needs of the public." In an era when the scope of practice of the dental hygienist has been defined as extending into hospitals, nursing homes, health maintenance organizations, and other sites where teams of co-professionals work together, it is a logical sequel that cooperation with the various health care providers in those and other settings would become a responsibility of the dental hygienist. The ADHA membership has made it an ethical principle. Cooperation is intended to extend to dental auxiliaries and dentists as well as to medical personnel in coordinating efforts to meet people's needs. It asks that the team approach be extended to its logical boundaries.

It may seem obvious that it is only proper "to recognize and uphold the laws governing this profession." However, in this era of change in the utilization of dental auxiliary personnel, there is a steady trend to implement what seem like logical changes in patterns of utilization *before* the laws are actually modified to permit those changes. Auxiliaries prepared educationally to perform various services legally allowable in one state may be tempted to provide the needed service in states in which the law says "no." Employer-dentists may ask an auxiliary to learn and perform functions that the law does not permit, or the employer may decide to substitute on-the-job training for the legal requirement of formal education to more quickly prepare support personnel for an expanded role.

The ADHA code implies that regardless of the state of flux of many laws, regardless of the person's skills or convictions, the individual must practice within the limits of the law.

If the individual is convinced that the law should be changed or that the scope of responsibility of the dental hygienist should be addressed, the professional membership of ADHA urges the individual "to participate responsibly in this professional association and uphold its purpose." The most effective way to facilitate change is to participate in a group with similar goals and objectives. Unity, strength, and logic are the keys to change. If the association does not appear to have all or perhaps any of the keys, then the place to direct energies is within the association first. Scattered, individual pleas for change have little impact in the long run. But the concerted efforts of dedicated individuals within the framework of an organization have far-reaching, tangible impact. The support network of the organization tempers wild-eyed idealism, disseminates ideas for membership discussion and possible action, develops the working knowledge of the members, channels energy into productivity, rejuvenates those who have fought for earlier causes, and creates a sense of belonging and accomplishment. Real change has occurred as a result of association effort, and each association member has the opportunity to help mold future changes.

The ADHA challenges the provider "to maintain professional competence through continuing education." Hygienists who have the keenest awareness of the need to make education a life-long process are those who were educated before the 1970s. A decade of technological advances and legal redefinition of practice has created a competency gap for graduates of that era who may have been unable to keep pace with the changes.

Dental hygiene is one of the professions that has experienced substantial change in scope of practice. Functions taught in the 1970s and 1980s often were not included in the curriculum of earlier years. Technological and research discoveries have been great, as well. To remain competent the health care provider must keep up with the present. Continuing education is one way of accomplishing this.

Closely related to the continuing education principle is the mandate, "to exchange professional knowledge with other health professions.'' *Sharing knowledge* is another way to keep up to date. It is an informal way of learning and a critical aspect of the societal nature of the professional association. A clinician who rarely ventures beyond the operatory walls is at a distinct disadvantage in terms of sharing experiences, techniques, ideas, and dreams. It should be clear by now that there is a great deal to be learned from nurses and the other allied health professions as well as from other dental hygienists and from dentists.

And finally, the profession asks the hygienist to strive ''to represent dental hygiene with high standards of personal conduct.'' The example that comes immediately to mind is a faculty person admonishing a student to stay out of bars when the student is attending a professional meeting and wearing a uniform. There are other concerns, however, that seem peculiar to the tempo of the times and probably better reflect the intent of this last principle of ethics.

In these times of tumultuous change and with the constant battering of ''old morals,'' few are shocked to consider members of one of the health professions engaging in premarital sex, experimenting with hallucinogenic drugs and chemicals, drinking alcohol to excess, choosing to live openly with a member of the opposite sex with no intention to marry, or ''associating with those who do.'' One opinion is that the only difference between 1957 and 1987 is the degree of openness. It is fair to say, however, that a 1957 ethics committee might have made some effort to discipline a provider who was found to have been involved in any of the listed activities. Today's ethics committees wonder if it is any of their business. So might the provider's lawyer.

Personal matters seem to have come to rest right back on the individual. Matters of personal decision cannot readily be assumed by anyone else for that individual (Purtilo, 1973). The ADHA, however, does address the issue through its stated principles and does hold that personal conduct often does reflect on the profession.

EXAMPLES OF ETHICS ISSUES
Fraud

Perhaps one of the most serious problems in contemporary society that relates to the professional ethics of the health care provider is the matter of fraud. With the tremendous dollar volume of the third-party payments for health care (medical and dental insurance), a few professionals apparently acquire payments for procedures never performed or performed so poorly that they might as well have never been done (Advisory Opinions 1980; Milgrom, 1978). It is important to note that the fraud is perpetrated against the insurance carrier, but the real victim is the consumer. Fraud in insurance payments is a significant factor in the determination of premiums. The consumer pays for the fraud through the higher and higher premium charges. This issue of personal conduct, which is also a legal one, is worthy of the attention of a professional association.

With advisory opinions of what is and is not ethical, the ADA has responded to the growing trend of submitting false and misleading claims. Fees charged to patients with third-party coverage should be the same as those charged for care delivered to persons who pay their own fees. Treatment dates must be accurate to prevent retroactive reimbursement for care delivered before the patient had third-party coverage. The dentist must accurately describe the procedures actually delivered so that proper reimbursement follows; describing a more costly procedure that was not delivered to secure a higher reimbursement is prohibited. The delivery of unnecessary care, given the patient's oral health status, to secure greater reimbursement is likewise inappropriate (Advisory Opinions, 1980). The filing of fraudulent claims is clearly unethical and is addressed strongly by the professional associations.

Can the profession monitor fraud and then report the instances to the insurance carrier? Organized dental hygienists in at least one state, appalled at their employers' outright theft, did create a ''watchdog'' system, and reports were made to insurance carriers that led to appropriate investigatory action (Michigan, 1974).

Advertising

Another area of ethics that has received attention in the past decade is advertising. The impropriety of advertising dental care has stood since the beginning of the formalization of the dental profession in the United States. Its prohibition was clearly stated in its ethics codes, and sanctions against dentists who advertised were definitive (Milgrom, 1978).

In 1977 the U.S. Supreme Court ruled that lawyers could advertise their routine services. It declared professional ethics codes that prohibited advertising as restraints of trade. Dentistry and medicine moved to change their positions on the role of advertising of their services as a result (Green, 1977). Since that time dentists who advertise are no longer banned from association membership.

In January 1977 the Federal Trade Commission filed a complaint against the ADA and several of its constituents for their restrictive practices relative to advertising of dental services (From FTC, 1979). In 1978 the ADA House of Delegates approved major changes in its Code of Ethics, including an allowance for dentists to advertise availability of services and fees charged. Their remaining restriction in the area of advertising was to disapprove "false, misleading, deceptive, or fraudulent representations" (ADA House, 1978). The FTC complaint was settled in February 1979 (From FTC, 1979). What was once considered unethical is now recognized as ethically and legally allowable, and no penalty may be issued to dentists who choose to advertise.

Many dentists disapprove of the idea regardless of its legality and subsequent rebirth as an ethical practice. Radio, television, and print media now have many advertisements for dental services. The messages range from sedate assurances of "quality" or "prevention-oriented care" to blatant appeals to the desire to be attractive ("If I'd known my teeth would get me this much attention and success, I'd have gone to [*Dental practice X*] a lot sooner!") and to the desire for low cost ("An upper and lower denture will cost you only $200, with three *free* adjustment visits!"). These examples of advertisements cause many self-respecting health professionals to wince.

Much of the obvious commercial-style advertising is sponsored by large franchises that have dental practices across the country, or at least in a given region. The name of the organization is used to benefit from the ads. Many of these network practices can be found in department stores and shopping malls. The network of practices or the right to use the name of the group is owned by a business group in many cases or by enterprising dentists. Again, many health professionals believe this trend is a sign of "deprofessionalism," which places emphasis on high volume and insufficient emphasis on quality and personalized delivery of care. Two important issues to separate in establishing a personal opinion about this trend are the professionalism associated with advertising and the professionalism associated with high-quality care. The two may well go together; the practice of advertising and the quality of care delivered are not by definition mutually exclusive.

Access to care

The issue of availability of services for the public continues to be an ethical issue even though the emphasis in health planning has shifted away from increasing health manpower (Nichols, 1981). Although the number of health care professionals has increased severalfold since the early 1960s, there are still geographical and economic areas in which people have little or no access to care. This continuing problem is compounded by economic woes. Health care providers are expected to meet the cost demands of inflation economy and the cost increases of the advancing technology in dentistry and particularly in medicine and still give the best care at the lowest possible cost (Robb, 1979). Some believe it is an ethical mandate to locate where the need for care is the greatest and to provide care for people regardless of the ability to pay.

The public has shown dentistry its discouragement with the profession's ability and determination to meet health care needs. The movement toward denturism, which is purported to provide prosthetic care at a lower cost for patients, is an example (Scholle, 1979). If the public is ever fully aware of the potential cost savings that could accrue from the use of EFDAs for restorative and periodontal care, it may also demand that auxiliaries be included in delivery systems, or at least that state dental practice acts that prohibit their use be changed.

Denying services

Another ethical problem relates to the refusal of some health care workers to provide care for patients receiving federal benefits for health care (Medicaid or Medicare). The intention of such financial assistance is to permit patients to seek the health care provider of their choice and to be the recipients of adequate care. However, some dentists do not wish to bother with the protocols involved or may have preconceived notions of the attitudes such patients will have regarding health care. In any case it can be difficult for a patient receiving public assistance to find a dentist who will even see him/her. Access to health care is a bigger problem than just providing funds for payment.

Some dentists may believe that patients who need federal assistance are suffering from low motivation and would be incompatible with their ideal of a practice consisting of "highly motivated" patients who immediately see the need for a comprehensive reconstruction of the dentition and who have been religiously practicing prevention on cue. In the 1960s there was a trend to classify patients according to their "dental I.Q." Class A patients were top, class B patients might make it someday, and class C patients were the uncaring group who either had to move up the

category ladder or go somewhere else. It was some dentists' view that a practice of all class A patients was *the* goal. That probably is not a poor goal, but it was sometimes achieved by eliminating the people who were classified otherwise as soon as the dentist could afford it. This is a clear case of stereotyping, which is also a questionable ethical practice.

Critical comments

A time-honored ethical principle in health care has been to refrain from criticizing the work of other professionals. The stated underlying rationale for this mandate was that it could not be known under what conditions certain procedures were performed, and therefore it would be unfair to comment adversely. This is referred to by some as the "conspiracy of silence" that was intended to protect the reputation of the profession by minimizing awareness of the errors its members commit (Milgrom, 1978). With the increasing emphasis on accountability in health care and the role that peer review now plays in assuring quality care, this principle has been revised greatly.

The ADA changed its stand to make it unethical *not* to report to the dental society any evidence of poor-quality dentistry (ADA Principles, 1979). The issue of what the patient should be told stands without comment. Therefore the dentist can feel comfortable in taking some official action when presented with low-quality dentistry but still must rely on his/her own judgment in determining how much the patient should know.

Dental hygienists frequently encounter situations in which the patient should probably know that the care he/she has received is substandard. This becomes particularly difficult when the hygienist works in a specialty practice since there is considerable opportunity to see the quality of care provided by a variety of dental hygienists and dentists whose patients are referred. The decision to inform the patient is a critical one that deserves careful thought and discussion with one's employer and co-workers.

BACK TO BASICS

Current writers in the dental literature have reiterated some of the major facets of ethical professional behavior. Reynolds focuses on accountability—moral, ethical, and social. He describes the ethical professional as having "persistence, integrity, compassion, veracity, fidelity, public spiritedness, humility, and dignity in appearance, speech, and demeanor." The greatest roadblock to consistent, ethical behavior is "an avaricious love of gain" which can "distort the practice and corrupt the practitioner" (Reynolds, 1984).

Griffiths explains that being highly competent and professional in providing clinical care is not synonymous with being ethical. A person can perform state-of-the-art clinical care and still be unethical. Patients could be taken advantage of, discriminated against, verbally or physically abused, or in some way neglected. Griffiths states that professionals must (1) keep up to date in their clinical skills and knowledge, (2) offer the highest order of care and refer those patients to others when the patients' needs exceed the clinician's ability, (3) make decisions based on what is "good for the patient," (4) "treat patients with respect and thoughtfulness," and (5) conduct one's personal life "in a manner which generates respect" (Griffiths, 1983).

These recommendations provide a sound, contemporary summary for generating a personal view of professional ethics in practice.

Contemporary ethics in dentistry wrestles not only with ethics in clinical practice but also with questions of ethics in research. Does the research purpose and protocol keep in mind the well-being of the subjects in the study regardless of the potential good outcome of the study? Examples of studies that did not follow this fundamental assumption are described in McHugh's discussion of research ethics (McHugh, 1984).

ENFORCEMENT OF ETHICAL PRINCIPLES

For the most part, ethical behavior is enforced by the individual practitioner and by the patients or clients who witness behavior that they will not support by continuing to seek care in that practice. Thus, the marketplace to a limited extent controls ethics.

Professional associations can enforce ethical behavior by reviewing charges made by patients or by other professionals and then censuring the person or expelling him/her from the professional association. Rarely, however, does this impose any real deterrence, especially if the unethical professional is not a member of the association to begin with. Furthermore, professional ethics committees leave themselves open to slander and libel charges if the member disagrees with the judgment and believes he/she can prove the review committee acted inappropriately and wronged his/her professional reputation (Feiler, 1983).

Enforcement of ethics has been taken up by the boards of dentistry in several licensing jurisdictions (Athans, 1980; Megdal, 1980; Moskowitz, 1984; Strigenz, 1981). In these instances, the state board reviewed evidence that the practitioner was practicing unethically and chose to impose penalties, including license revocation. Clearly revoking one's license is a penalty that catches the attention of potential wrongdoers. Clinicians who defraud or who are guilty of gross disregard for the well-being of patients may be reviewed by the state board.

It is the less noticeable, but still tainted, act of questionable ethics remaining under the sole review of the individual's conscience that separates the professional from the self-serving panderer in a professional's disguise.

CONCLUSION

Being a health care provider or a student preparing to enter a health field does carry with it an enormous responsibility to individual patients and to society. Patients depend on the provider's skill and caring attitude. They entrust the provider with their bodies. The enormity of that responsibility should be at the very core of professional, ethical behavior (ADHA, 1975).

Review questions

1. List five of the current ADHA Principles of Ethics and write out one practical implementation for each. *see p.100   1975 Code of Ethics*
2. Briefly explain each of the following contemporary ethical issues in health care:
    a. Fraud in billing practices. *billing for services not nec. or not done at all,*
    b. Continued limited access to dental care. *offering care to those is desolate areas & to those unable to pay.*
    c. Advertising. *the nature of some ads + growth of Lg. franchise dental clinics has some believing the profession is in decline.*
    d. Refusal to treat patients on medical or dental assistance. *Dr. discriminate or take loss on payment.*
    e. Informing the patients of poor-quality dental care they have received.
    unethical to downgrade previous dental work but must inform pt of their dental needs.

GROUP ACTIVITIES

1. Divide the group into subgroups of five people. Assign each group one or more of these terms from Reynolds's article on ethics: persistence, integrity, compassion, veracity, fidelity, public spiritedness, humility, and dignity. Each group should first define the term in relation to dental ethics and then identify and develop a clinical practice case where the term they were assigned was upheld or abandoned in the actions of the hypothetical practitioner.
2. Define *professionalism*. Identify examples of professionalism each participant witnesses every day. Cite examples of behavior that are not professional. What makes those behaviors unprofessional? If there is disagreement in the group, make certain persons on each side of the issue understand fully the viewpoint of the opposition.
3. Conduct a role-play session in which students playing the part of patients ask ''touchy'' ethical questions of students playing the part of health care providers. Discuss the ramifications of the spontaneous responses the group members gave to the questions.
4. Have a representative of a third-party payment organization speak on the incidence of fraud and how it can be combated.
5. Share, in a discussion format, your individual reponses to how you could implement each of the principles in the 1975 ADHA code.
6. Discuss the implications of the following quotation: ''A profession bent on self-righteous autonomy is bent on self-destruction, for it has ignored social approval. Obligations to the public must be met with ethical revisions that safely reduce, as much as possible, the differences between the interests of the profession and the needs of the public'' (Scholle, 1979).
7. Bring out the ''reasons for entering a profession'' and the ''measures of success'' lists that were generated during the group activity associated with Chapter 1. Use the group list that was compiled from individuals' contributions. Identify if and where the values and goals of the group members are in conflict with the ethical principles introduced in this section.

REFERENCES

ADA House approves major ethics changes, adopts policy statement on TV advertising, J. Am. Dent. Assoc. **97**:1065, 1978.

Advisory opinions on the ethics of deliberate irregularities in billings and performance of unnecessary procedures, J. Am. Dent. Assoc. **101**:304, 1980.

American Dental Association Principles of Ethics and Code of Professional Conduct, J. Am. Dent. Assoc. **99**:1003, 1979.

American Dental Hygienists' Association: Principles of ethics, Chicago, 1975, The Association.

Athans v. Arizona State Board of Dental Examiners, 612 P.2d 57 (Ariz. App. 1980).

Feiler v. New Jersey Dental Association, 467 A.2d 276 (N.J. Super. 1983).

From the Federal Trade Commission, the final order on ethical restrictions against advertising by dentists, J. Am. Dent. Assoc. **99**:927, 1979.

Green, D.: Dental advertising: where in the world will it end? Dent. Manage. **17**(11):33, 1977.

Griffiths, R.H.: What is ethics in practice? J. Am. Coll. Dent. **50**(2):9, 1983.

McHugh, W.D.: Professional ethics in dental research, J. Am. Coll. Dent. **51**(1):19, 1984.

Megdal v. Oregon State Board of Dental Examiners, 605 P.2d 273, 1980.

Michigan Dental Hygienists Association, Board of Trustees, minutes of meeting, East Lansing, 1974.

Milgrom, P.: Regulation and the quality of dental care, Rockville, Md., 1978, Aspen Systems Corp.

Miller, S.L.: Legal aspects of dentistry, New York, 1970, G.P. Putnam's Sons.

Moskowitz, D.P.: Professional disciplinary proceedings and the licensed dental practitioner, N.Y. State Dent. J. **50**:437, 1984.

Motley, W.E.: Ethics, jurisprudence and history for the dental hygienist, ed. 3, Philadelphia, 1983, Lea & Febiger.

Nichols, A.W.: Ethics of the distribution of health care, J. Fam. Pract. **12**:533, 1981.

Purtilo, R.: The allied health professional and the patient, Philadelphia, 1973, W.B. Saunders Co.

Reynolds, R.J.; Health care: changes, challenges, J. Am. Coll. Dent. **51**(1):35, 1984.

Robb, J.W.: Ethics and the health professions, Calif. Dent. Assoc. J. **7**(4):34, 1979.

Scholle, R.N.: The privilege of practice, J. Am. Dent. Assoc. **98**:159, 1979.

Strigenz v. Dept. of Regulation & Licensing, Wis., 307 N.W.2d 664, 1981.

PART FOUR

Selecting a practice setting

Embarking on a career in the health services is a time for dreaming, setting goals, looking for alternatives, assessing wants and needs, putting one's "best foot forward," and preparing for a lifetime of challenges, opportunities, and professional development.

Finding one's first employment setting is exciting. It is also demanding. Starting out in the wrong place can be demoralizing. It is essential to carefully assess the alternatives and make certain that plenty of appropriate preparation is carried out before applying for the "ideal" position.

This section lays out career alternatives and ways to select a career pathway. It suggests how the difficult decision of selecting a practice site can be made and offers tips for preparing a resume and participating in an interview. Finally, it includes a chapter on financial security and shows how the risks of responsibility can be supported by adequate personal and professional insurance.

CHAPTER 14

Career alternatives

OBJECTIVES: The reader will be able to:

1. Identify the practice setting in which direct patient care dental auxiliaries are most frequently employed.
2. Provide two reasons why the variety of practice settings for dental care providers is expanding beyond the usual sites.
3. List at least six alternative practice settings or roles that a dental hygienist could assume in delivering care.
4. Explain how alternative practice settings may call on the educational preparation and the willingness to assume responsibility to a greater degree than traditional settings and roles.
5. Survey the community for potential employment situations for direct patient care dental auxiliaries.

The majority of dental auxiliary students and applicants for positions in dental auxiliary programs describe the role of the dental hygienist and assistant in terms of routine provision of dental hygiene and assisting services in private dental offices. Usually such applicants have had their contact with dental hygiene and assisting within the confines of a private practice setting and see this site as the place to seek and find employment. This is understandable since the vast majority of active dental hygienists and other auxiliaries even today are employed in private settings in general dentistry.

A national survey of 21,847 dental hygienists in 1983 showed that 88.2% of dental hygienists practice in traditional settings—dental practices (Cohen et al., 1984). This percentage has, however, decreased from estimates of 95% just ten years ago (Lewis, 1972; Wyshak and Hoase, 1976). The greatest trend has been toward positions in community service, such as hospitals, long-term care facilities, day-care centers and nursery schools, home visits, government-supported clinics, and nongovernment clinics. Hygienists are also finding employment in retail stores, dental or dental hygiene schools, and in other situations, such as marketing and research for dental product manufacturers.

The trend away from a predictable job in a small dental practice can be explained, in part, by several trends. The first trend relates to the increase in the educational scope of the graduated dental hygienist, which does not always match the role in clinical practice. The employer-dentist determines, for the most part, the scope of practice of the employee-hygienist. Therefore, regardless of the freedoms permitted in the dental law, the dentist may opt for a more restricted practice for the employee. This can result in frustration.

Other trends relate to hygienists' longevity in practice. Hygienists are making dental hygiene a lifetime career (Malvitz and Mocniak, 1982). Nearly half of the hygienists who graduated in 1949 or earlier are still in practice. Graduates from the years 1950-59 and 1960-69 reveal 68.9% and 71.7% retention rates, respectively.

The percentage still in practice rises to 85.7% for 1975-79 and 92.1% for 1980-83 (Cohen et al., 1984). As a result, dental hygienists as a group may be looking for career advancement, relating to both professional and financial growth. Hygienists who recognize that the 1986 American dollar is worth approximately one third of its 1967 value can quickly calculate their current earning power and compare it to the salaries they received when first entering practice. In nearly all instances, it is obvious that salaries have not come close to keeping pace with inflation and do not reflect the growth in experience and the contribution to the goodwill value of a practice that extended employment brings. Therefore, hygienists look for more lucrative options—and often find them in sites other than dental practices. Also, hygienists may decide that professional growth is limited in a dental practice and opt for a position that builds new skills and that challenges an array of abilities.

CLINICAL PRACTICE ALTERNATIVES

An important goal for dental hygiene is to ensure that there are *clinical* opportunities for professional growth. If a practitioner's first love is clinical practice, direct patient contact, and helping people regain health, practice options need to be protected and established that can make such a goal a reality.

Hygienists and dentists need to work together to identify ways for *traditional private practice* to be attractive as a career option. There are, of course, tens of thousands of employers and employees who have identified how to make such an arrangement a true career endeavor. The dentist attends to the hygienist's need for professional growth by ensuring that the full array of clinical services can be provided to patients and by making it possible for the hygienist to attend continuing education and integrate new ideas into the practice. The hygienist ensures that the well-being of the practice is paramount, working to draw new patients, satisfy the current patient pool, and provide the best possible clinical care. Working together with reasonable patient fees and a rea-

sonable patient pool, the hygienist can realize an income that is more than acceptable and that grows with clinical ability and contributions to the growth of the practice.

Independent contracting is an alternative closely aligned to traditional practice, but shifts the responsibility for financial success to the hygienist. A hygienist can establish his/her own practice within a dental practice, thereby satisfying the legal requirements for supervision. Instead of receiving a salary, the hygienist collects patient fees and pays a percentage to the dentist for space, utilities, staff, and the privilege of supervision. This alternative is particularly attractive to a hygienist who has considerable clinical experience and who has access to capital to purchase equipment and start up the business. The arrangement is attractive to a dentist who has a spare treatment room and needs a dental hygienist, but has no funds to equip the unused space. The hygienist can purchase the equipment, provide the needed dental hygiene care, and usually realize additional income and a greater sense of practice freedom. No survey has estimated the number of hygienists functioning under such an arrangement.

A step further is to set up a dental hygiene practice entirely separate from a dentist and refer patients to a variety of dentists for more extensive care. While such practices exist, they are usually on the fringes of the dental laws which specify supervision requirements for dental hygienists. While this arrangement provides the hygienist with maximum freedom, it is a more difficult approach in terms of business management. Liaisons must be maintained with community dentists with regular, complete communication regarding patients being treated and referred. The hygienist must attend to business management as much as to clinical practice and compete with the typically low fees charged by dentists for dental hygiene care. Still, this trend may continue among experienced hygienists as dental laws are altered to permit independent practice.

Clinical practice can and does move beyond the traditional concept of an office. Nearly 10% of hygienists functioning in nontraditional sites work in hospitals, providing bedside care or care for medically compromised patients in the hospital dental service. The challenges in such an environment are many. Knowledge of oral medicine and diagnosis, modifications of routine care to meet special needs, and an affinity for patients who place extraordinary demands upon a hygienist's commitment are all essential for such a position. Often the hygienist has to look for and develop a position, but since the number of hospitals offering dental services has increased to 60%, such positions are less difficult to locate.

Hygienists can also use their clinical skills in a variety of community sites where patients with special needs are institutionalized or gather for social or medical reasons. Clinical dental hygiene can be provided for patients in centers for the physically and mentally handicapped, in penal institutions, in long-term care facilities, in hospices, and in community clinics. Care can be provided to senior citizens through nursing homes or through senior centers where the ambulatory elderly gather for enjoyment. Under special programs, dental hygiene can reach the homeless or the homebound. Visiting local sites that either have a fledgling dental program or none at all and proposing dental hygiene care can sometimes create new employment opportunities. Often a hygienist can write a grant proposal for private funding that can introduce such care to a needy population. Negotiations with an insurance carrier or other third-party payer may result in payments for preventive care delivered by a hygienist. In these ways, dental hygienists are able to extend basic clinical skills to groups that otherwise might not have access to care. In addition, the basic and behavioral sciences that support clinical practice are used on a daily basis as care is modified to meet the special needs of various groups.

MANAGEMENT AND PLANNING

It is also possible for a hygienist to find a position involving management and planning skills. Some hygienists can combine clinical practice with additional managerial responsibilities. Such roles are possible in large dental centers, particularly corporate-sponsored or franchise practices where managing the facility and staff requires a thorough knowledge of dentistry as well as basic management skills. Accepting such a role requires knowledge and skill beyond basic dental hygiene, since being skilled at clinical practice does not necessarily include prowess in planning, directing, coordinating, communicating, evaluating, and the other basic functions of a competent manager. Part Five of this text introduces the array of skills necessary for competent management. With additional expertise, management can be an important role opportunity for a dental hygienist, whether or not the position includes clinical functions.

Planning skills, in particular, can be put to use in community programs where large-scale educational or treatment programs are to be put into effect. A hygienist may spearhead a major project for detection of oral cancer or periodontal disease in a given community. A fluoride rinse program could be instituted in the school system. Hygienists and dentists in a community could be given intensive training in identifying child abuse. A hygienist could be in charge of a fluoridation campaign in a community that has repeatedly turned down the measure; or he/she could be in charge of rebuffing a challenge by anti-fluoridationists to remove fluoride from the communal water supply. Special skills are needed for strategic planning to be effective; a position involving planning usually calls for extraordinary leadership qualities including an ability to see a need, muster the forces to bring about change, and follow through on a project until a goal is attained.

MARKETING SKILLS

The dental products industry is employing hygienists to work as marketing agents to promote the use of oral irrigating devices, toothpastes and oral rinses, prescription agents, toothbrushes, and a whole array of products used by professionals and their patients. Those hygienists are often called upon to do presentations to professionals, to review marketing messages for ad campaigns, to bring products directly to dental professionals in their offices for discussion and review, and to perform other functions. A knowledge of the functioning of the business world is essential for such a position. Good public relations skills, an ability to accurately and succinctly communicate positive messages, and the ability to integrate professional commitment to high quality care and dental products with business goals must be developed. The opportunities for growth either in dental hygiene or in business widen with such a position.

Marketing skills can also be used to attract students to a dental or dental hygiene program. Recruitment offices in professional schools may employ a hygienist who can speak the language of prospective students and who embodies excitement about the profession and the school. Likewise such skills can be used in directing continuing education programs in institutions or operating independently of schools or other professional organizations. Hygienists can own their own businesses, offering quality education programs for area professionals.

RESEARCH SKILLS

A hygienist who sets his/her sights on research can find employment in a dental research center or university where clinical and basic research is usually found. It is also possible to secure a position in industry where dental products are evaluated for safety and efficacy. Skills in research design, statistics, and writing form the basis for competency in this field. One must, of course, have a solid science background to support the area of research, whether it is clinical, basic, or behavioral research.

Research centers and universities need competent people to carry out the research, manage the phases of the research, gather data, and work with statisticians to ensure proper development and interpretation of data. A hygienist working with a senior researcher can assimilate an understanding of how research is planned, conducted, and disseminated for colleagues' review and eventual inclusion in the literature.

TEACHING SKILLS

Clinical dental hygiene at the chairside includes a hefty portion of teaching. The hygienist's role includes helping the patient accept increased responsibility for maintaining oral health, and helping this occur is teaching.

Some hygienists see their career path as teaching others how to become hygienists or dentists. Nearly 36% of the hygienists who reported working in nontraditional roles indicated they were employed in a dental or dental hygiene school. Many of the management skills described above (planning, organizing, directing, coordinating, communicating, and evaluating) are necessary in education. Courses and clinical sessions need planning and other management attention on a daily basis. Special expertise in an area is important. The educator needs to know the recent research, select appropriate text materials, and plan activities that will help the students learn and retain the essentials. The educator must also decide what principles, facts, attitudes, and skills are necessary for the students to learn given resource limitations of time, faculty, equipment, and patient pool. Educators need to be able to market, too. They need to instill an excitement and energy in students that will help them continue growing long after graduation.

While employment opportunities in dental and dental hygiene education are not as plentiful as they were ten years ago, they offer reasonable stability, access to continual professional growth, an opportunity to stay young through continued contact with students, and a challenge that draws upon a wide variety of skills and interests.

PREPARING FOR ALTERNATIVE ROLES

Dental hygiene is described by some as narrow and restrictive. That is true if a hygienist's horizons are focused strictly on traditional clinical practice, and he/she is having difficulty locating an employer who chooses to integrate comprehensive dental hygiene care into the practice. Such a description is not accurate, however, when the myriad of positions in the community, industry, and education are recognized. A hygienist seeking an alternative role will need to develop advanced skills and look harder for opportunities that fit those skills, perhaps even creating entirely new positions and then working hard to blend professional values with those of the colleagues who now surround him/her.

Very often the hygienist needs advanced formal education in management, community dental health, teaching, research skills, the sciences, or some other area that requires special expertise. Hygienists often combine clinical practice with a gradual attainment of advanced degrees. Clinical practice forms a solid experience base for both patient care and participating in the work environment as a contributing team member. It teaches the clinician about working with co-workers and patients. Attending classes while working as a hygienist gradually moves the hygienist toward career alternative goals while rounding out the educational base of the *person,* regardless of the classes' direct relationship to dental hygiene.

As career goals become clearer, the hygienist can watch for or create career steps that add experience and responsibility and that bring the person in contact with people who work in the sought-after area. Eventually, with a few breaks and much diligence, career goals materialize.

Dental hygiene offers a broad spectrum of opportunities if the individual is willing to invest energy and then enjoy the challenges and growth that come from effort (Dreyer, 1985).

Review questions

1. In what practice setting do the vast majority of dental hygienists work?
2. What are two explanations for the gradual expansion of dental hygiene into nontraditional settings?
3. List six arrangements in addition to employment in a private dental office where clinical dental hygiene care can be delivered to the public.
4. What roles other than clinical practice can a hygienist develop for career alternatives?
5. Briefly describe how hygienists can prepare themselves for alternative roles.

GROUP ACTIVITIES

1. Contact local hospitals, nursing homes, day-care centers, and other institutions for the availability of positions for dental hygienists. Identify all employment opportunities in the community that could be available to dental hygienists to provide care to the population if money were available to fund such positions.
2. Design an informational program to demonstrate to each category of alternative practice opportunity how the employment of a dental hygienist could be managed financially and could provide needed care to the persons currently receiving other health care within that institution.
3. Invite a recruiter from each of the armed services to describe employment opportunities for civilian dental hygienists or for dental hygienists who wish to join the service for a number of years.
4. Conduct a survey of local dental hygienists to determine what functions they perform in their respective settings and to determine the scope of responsibility and the degree to which they call on their educational preparation in the daily activities they perform.
5. Prepare a career path for the next 10 years, projecting where you hope to be and what you will be doing. Outline how you can work toward that goal. Share individual plans in groups of three.
6. Read Regina Dreyer's book, *Career Directions for Dental Hygienists,* and discuss each of the career advances presented.
7. Review the past two years' issues of *RDH* magazine for hygienists' descriptions of their roles in clinical and nontraditional employment.
8. Invite hygienists who work in nontraditional settings to discuss their work activities, how they located the positions, and what special preparations were necessary to qualify for the positions.

REFERENCES

Cohen, L., LaBelle, A., Singer, J., Blandford, D., and Groeneman, S.: Prevalence of nontraditional dental hygiene practice. J. Public Health Dent. **44:**106, 1984.

Dreyer, R.A.: Career directions for dental hygienists, Holmdel, N.J., 1985, Career Directions Press.

Lewis, D.J.: A study of dental hygiene practice in the State of Connecticut: 1971, An essay presented to the faculty of the Department of Epidemiology and Public Health, Yale University, 1972.

Malvitz, D.M., and Mocniak, N.; Profile of dental hygienists licensed in the United States, J. Public Health Dent. **42:**54, 1982.

Wyshak, G., and Hoase, J.V.: Profile of dental hygienists, Dent. Hyg. **50:**497, 1976.

CHAPTER 15

Establishing priorities in selecting a practice setting

OBJECTIVES: The reader will be able to:

1. Identify at least ten factors that health care providers often express as important considerations in selecting a practice setting.
2. Select categories of concern that are important to him/her in selecting a practice setting.
3. Identify any additional categories of concern that should be considered in assessing how a practice setting meets his/her priorities.
4. Establish a decision making grid to determine what practice setting is most appropriate.
5. Explain how formal decision making applied to selecting an employment setting can clarify the strengths and weaknesses of each possible decision.
6. Describe goal orientation as a tool for planning change.

Often a new graduate of a health care program has unclear or idealistic expectations of what the practice of his/her profession will be. The educational environment focuses on the ideal in many instances and may not necessarily provide the person with an internship program that familiarizes the student with the economic and logistical realities of practice. The delivery of health care is rarely ideal. Each practice setting may measure up to some of the student's expectations and fall short in others. Each practice setting will be different in what it offers and in what it expects of the practitioner who is employed.

FACTORS IN SELECTING A PRACTICE SETTING

In a profession in which the scope of practice is changing and role delineation in practice is either not keeping pace with or is ahead of the educational preparation of the graduate, there are multiple factors that need consideration in seeking and accepting employment. These factors are both personal and professional. They are economic, emotional, logistical, and peculiar to each individual making the decisions and choices.

What kinds of factors do new graduates often consider in seeking employment? Basically, they fall into two main categories: personal need and professional opportunity. Often, for persons who have spent a large amount of time and money in obtaining their education, the personal need factor is the primary consideration. The new graduate is eager to earn some money for a change and to have a reasonably comfortable and secure position in employment. For others, the most important consideration is to identify a position where their professional commitment is valued and their need for continued professional growth can be fulfilled. These persons are willing to make sacrifices in the areas of personal need (or at least be willing to tolerate delayed gratification) in order to fulfill a service orientation (such as providing care to un-

123

derserved populations) or to participate in a practice setting where the opportunity to learn is much greater than the immediate financial reward.

There are numerous other factors that fit within these two main categories that make decision making complicated. Therefore it is often helpful to discuss the full array of considerations that contribute to a final decision. Each person needs to assess his/her own personal needs and values with regard to each factor before evaluating a practice site and before making a decision about which position to accept.

Salary and Fringe Benefits

Under the personal need category, there are many considerations that practitioners cite as important. The amount of the *salary* is a prime consideration. Is the salary offered commensurate with the amount the provider hoped to earn? Is it reasonable for the locale, for the degree of education required of the provider, and in relation to the economic income that will be generated for the practice setting?

Frequently a clinician will be paid on a percentage basis that fluctuates with the amount of practice income generated by the clinician (see Chapter 23). If this is the case, the applicant needs to determine what the percentage will be, what the average generated income is per hour, and the size of the patient pool. Even if the percentage sounds high, the position will provide little income to the clinician if the fees charged to the patients are unreasonably low. Furthermore, if the percentage and the fees both are good, income depends upon the number of filled appointments each day. If the patient pool is small, there is little opportunity to see patients, charge fees, and earn a percentage. It also is good to know if the employer will be moving patients out of the applicant's schedule into his/her own for care if the employer has a cancellation in the schedule. In addition, it is important to determine whether all services will provide the same percentage to the clinician and whether only low-paying procedures are to be scheduled for the clinician. In some

practices, exposing a radiographic series will carry a lower percentage for the clinician than an examination, charting, and prophylaxis, for instance. Also, some employers may opt to have root planing, curettage, and all expensive restorative care scheduled with them so that the percentage is based on the services that carry the lowest fees.

Closely related to salary is the amount of *fringe benefits* available to the provider. Often a low-level salary will be counterbalanced by a sizable fringe benefit package, including vacation time, sick pay, insurance programs, in-service training and opportunities for continued formal education, free personal and family health care, parking, professional dues payment, and other benefits. To assess the relative merits of the benefits package, the prospective employee should total up the dollar value of the benefits and add it to the salary before comparing it to a position that has a high salary but limited benefits. Insurance and any of the other items listed can be costly if paid out of the salary. Many benefits are not subject to income taxation, which makes them even more economically attractive. Therefore it is important to consider more than just the weekly rate of pay before making a decision regarding the economic benefits of employment.

Location

One consideration closely related to economic benefits but that has other factors related to it is the *location* of the employment setting. The farther away the practice setting, the more time and money it will cost to travel to and from work each day. If public transportation is available, how much will it cost each day? If the travel requires a car, how much will it cost in terms of gasoline and other mileage expenses? And how much is parking, if it is even available? Is there some likelihood that the car will be damaged while parked? Will insurance rates for the car rise?

Location can have other importance for prospective employees, too. If the position available is in a rural area, in the heart of a big city, or nestled in the suburbs, the location may have a different priority ranking for the people considering the position. The country lovers may be miserable in the city, whereas the city lovers may be stir-crazy in the mountains. Those providers who prefer the flavor of the suburbs may place little positive value on the other two locations. Isolation, crowding, atmosphere, availability of entertainment and services, and opportunity for rest and relaxation are all important considerations associated with the location of a practice setting. How far will the provider have to move to accept the position? Will the cost of living and availability of housing pose special problems? Whenever the opportunity requires a substantial change in location for the provider, these elements are important.

Security

Security is an important factor for many health care providers. What is the likelihood that the person will be able to retain the position? Is it a grant-funded (soft-money) position that may disappear from the face of the earth if the grant is not renewed or when the contract is complete? Does the employer have a high turnover rate among employees? Is there a union to protect employee's rights in an instance of unfair severance of employment?

Perhaps the most important consideration is whether security is an important consideration to the potential employee. Usually, security becomes an increasingly important factor as the provider assumes new responsibilities, such as raising a family, or as the provider ages. The loss of income and the inability to find another place to work can be frightening prospects when there is a family of three to clothe, feed, and shelter or when a provider is nearing retirement. It is true that some people seem minimally troubled by this factor when they accept employment, but they should consider that the relative importance of security may change. With time, security may be an increasingly significant factor for the provider,

but the benefit of security may not necessarily increase in the employment setting with longevity.

Opportunity for advancement

Opportunity for advancement and upward mobility are important factors for many health care providers, particularly if they view their profession as a lifetime career. Providers may wish to see possible opportunity to assume supervisory roles or to acquire education or skills that will enable them to move up the structure of the practice setting or prepare them for more responsible roles in other employment settings. Persons who are "upward oriented" may place a great deal of importance on how the offered employment will enhance their experience and improve their chances to succeed.

In many ways women struggle with this problem more than men because of the stereotyped approach to the ability or desire of women to stay in practice for longer periods of time and to function well as managers of people. Women until recently generally viewed professional life as a stopover between high school and marriage and as a source of security if the husband should turn out to be a poor financial provider. Women averaged few years of economic productivity and were willing to wear the label of short-term, low-commitment workers in a male-dominated professional world. These two factors have changed as women less and less fit the mold and do look forward to lifetime careers and opportunity for advancement.

Surveys conducted in individual states nationally and by educational programs tracking alumni employment patterns show trends toward more career orientation among dental hygienists. Women have shown a tendency to return to work after a family sabbatical.*

The applicant looking for career advancement needs to identify what kind of growth is expected,

---

*(Green and Jong, 1980; Lawson, 1980; Malvitz and Mocniak, 1982; Pitchford et al., 1981; Rubinstein and Miller, 1985; Woodall, 1986).

how that growth can be achieved in each of the settings, how long it should be before learning opportunities and promotions are likely, and the extent to which each position is likely to prepare the individual for other job opportunities. It is important to determine whether the employer expects to provide learning opportunities or whether he/she is hoping for an employee who wants to focus on being productive in a defined, basically unchanging role.

Role and responsibility

The *role* or position offered to the health care provider at the time of initial employment is even more often a primary consideration than opportunity for advancement. Will the provider have responsibility in decision making? Will there be an opportunity to exercise the judgment skills developed in school? Is there an opportunity to be creative and innovative? How well is the role defined, and what is the relationship between that role and the roles assigned to co-workers? Providing specific, predictable, often repeated services each day is ideal for some employees who view the predictability as ''security.'' For others, it is intellectual death. It may be wise to assess just how mentally stimulating and challenging a position may be for the individual provider in comparison to the stimulation and challenge the person was confronted with each day while in school. There is some chance that the daily routine of practice, if barren of responsibility and creativity, may be quite a letdown from the daily activities of succeeding in school.

Variety of services

Related to role is the amount of learning the provider will be able to draw on in practice. Will a relatively low percentage of skills be drawn on, or will the provider be able to provide a full range and *variety of services?*

It can be worthwhile to accept a position initially that is not completely drawing on the ability of the person but that can lead to a position that is more demanding and based on success in the performance of the practical, albeit banal, experiences of the lower-level position.

Interpersonal relations

While assessing the challenge of the position, it is also wise to assess the people with whom the health care provider will be working. Observing the cheerfulness and thoughtfulness of the personnel in the practice can provide some indication of how pleasant the *interpersonal relations* may be among the workers and how generally satisfied they are with their respective roles and responsibilities. In the majority of private practice settings, the number of employees is relatively small and relations among the workers must be good if there is to be some harmony. Generally there isn't room for avoidance of conflict and there is a great deal of opportunity for confrontation. Paying close attention to the communication frequency and the tone of the communication can provide a fairly accurate assessment of the ''group'' development among the team. It certainly can point out whether there is a team or merely a number of individuals who happen to be employed in the same setting and who perhaps are not pleased about it.

Working environment

In addition to the personnel in the office, there is the *physical working environment* itself. Is the equipment to be utilized in providing care adequate and operative? Is there adequate emergency equipment to handle medical or dental emergencies that may occur? Is the setting clean and neat? Are proper sterilization procedures observed, and is the space adequate to provide care?

It is amazing how the physical limitations of an area can affect the attitudes of the personnel and sometimes the quality of care delivered. For some people, physical setting can be a primary consideration in selecting a practice setting whereas for others, it may be a factor that can be outweighed by other positive elements.

Needs of people

One instance in which physical setting is often offset by another plus factor is the health care delivery setting located in a less than plush area, where care is being provided for people who usually would have little or no access to health care. Many government-assisted programs or programs carried out largely by charity donations and volunteer efforts are not located in high-priced quarters with the latest equipment. However, if the luxury of the setting is not the most important factor, it may be sacrificed in return for the genuineness of the caring of the personnel and for the satisfaction derived from *providing care where it is needed most.*

What other factors can be defined that will be looked for or expected in a practice setting? Others may be added to the preceding list of ten primary factors, preparing an individual to begin analyzing which are the most important, which are less than crucial, and which matter little if at all.

DECISION MAKING

Once the factors are identified, they can be weighted on a scale of 1 to 10. Those factors that are absolutely essential or very desirable are weighted with a higher number, whereas "nice to have" factors are weighted with a lower number. Once each factor has been reviewed for its relative importance, the potential employee is ready to compare the available opportunities in relation to those factors and make a decision regarding what practice setting is the most likely to satisfy the person. The perfect position probably exists nowhere, or at least it is unlikely that it will be found immediately by a new graduate. Unless it is possible to be among the ranks of the unemployed for some time, the health care provider may find him/herself in a position of accepting employment that does not satisfy all needs but that satisfies at least a reasonable percentage of the stated needs.

Refer to Table 1 for a quantitative analysis of a number of practice settings available to a health care provider. The potential employee has been interviewed by three employers and is awaiting their offers. Before the offers are made, the applicant decides to assess his/her own "druthers," weighting each preference on a numerical scale of 1 to 10. Salary, fringe benefits, and working environment are weighted equally at 5. A relatively low value is placed on security, whereas opportunity for advancement, scope of responsibility and role, personnel relationships, need of the people, and variety of services that can be provided are rated high. Location is only slightly more important than the salary and fringe benefits categories.

With each factor weighted, the three practice settings are weighted from 1 to 3 according to the degree to which each lives up to the hopes of the applicant as assessed during the interview. Opportunities 1 and 3 are in private practitioners' offices. One of them is a solo practice; the other is a group practice. Opportunity 2 is a government-funded health clinic operating on a grant due to be renewed in 1 year. It should be apparent from the weightings that the two private practitioners' offices provide the best salary, fringe benefits, and security as well as scoring well in the areas of personnel relationships (in one of the two offices) and working environment. They do not offer much in the category of opportunity for advancement nor in variety of services that can be provided by the interviewing provider. The role and responsibility that could be assumed by the provider also appear to be less than ideal in the private practices.

The government clinic offers the lowest salary, some fringe benefits, location in a less than ideal area, minimal security, and relatively poor physical working environment. Its plus factors include the opportunity for advancement, the role and responsibility the health care provider will be able to assume, personnel relationships, the need of the people, and the variety of services that the health care provider may actually perform. Because of the weighting of factors, the government

Table 1. Decision-making grid for selecting a practice opportunity

	Personal weighting		Opportunity 1	Opportunity 2	Opportunity 3
Salary	5	×	3 = 15	1 = 5	3 = 15
Fringe benefits	5	×	3 = 15	2 = 10	3 = 15
Location	6	×	2 = 12	1 = 6	2 = 12
Security	2	×	3 = 6	1 = 2	3 = 6
Opportunity for advancement	8	×	0 = 0	3 = 24	0 = 0
Role/responsibility	9	×	1 = 9	3 = 27	1 = 9
Personnel relationships	9	×	3 = 27	3 = 27	1 = 9
Working environment	5	×	3 = 15	1 = 5	3 = 15
Need of people	10	×	1 = 10	3 = 30	2 = 20
Variety of services that can be provided	10	×	1 = 10	3 = 30	2 = 20
PREFERENCE POINTS:			119	166	121

clinic earns more points than the two private practice settings. If opportunity 2 is offered and the health care provider was honest with him/herself in weighting the factors, the answer should be "yes." The quantitative assessment of the wants and needs of the provider match best with what the government clinic has to offer, and the health care provider will therefore probably be happiest in that position.

If opportunity 2 is not offered, but either opportunity 1 or 3 *is* offered to the person, the health care provider had best decide whether to look further for an opening more compatible with his/her personal wants or needs or to accept the job with the idea that he/she may be able to adapt to the position despite its drawbacks or find a better opportunity later. This choice is often a difficult one to make since the need for income may be the prompting factor to take the position and since a person's performance level may not be at its best in an employment situation incompatible with the person's goals. A lowered performance level seldom leads to advancements and hardly ever leads to good recommendations.

Given the same numerical assessment of the same three job opportunities on a scale of 1 to 3, a different person may arrive at quite a different conclusion regarding which setting is the most appropriate one to accept. For instance, a classmate of the first applicant for a position may also inter-

view at opportunities 1, 2, and 3, and could even arrive at the same judgments regarding their relative offerings in the same ten categories. Given a different personal weighting of the ten factors, in terms of their importance to the applicant, the numerical values ultimately tallied for each opportunity will be quite different.

In Table 2 the only significant difference between this ranking of opportunities and that described in Table 1 is the personal weighting. Notice that salary, fringe benefits, location, security, and working environment assume a much greater importance for this person than they did for the first person described. Opportunity for advancement, scope of role or responsibility, need of the people, and variety of services that can be provided are ranked lower on the scale of 1 to 10. As a result opportunity 3 appears to be the best opportunity for the potential employee. Opportunity 1 is almost equal, but opportunity 2 is less appropriate for this person. An offer from either opportunity 1 or 3 should be readily accepted, but an offer from 2 should be assessed in terms of how satisfied the health care provider will be. It is possible that advancement and challenge could make up for the shortcomings the facility and location have, but there is a large possibility that the person will continually be watching for a practice setting that better meets his/her wants and needs.

Not all people are alike in their respective

Table 2. Decision-making grid for selecting a practice opportunity

	Personal weighting		Opportunity 1	Opportunity 2	Opportunity 3
Salary	8	×	3 = 24	1 = 8	3 = 24
Fringe benefits	8	×	3 = 24	2 = 16	3 = 24
Location	10	×	2 = 20	1 = 10	2 = 20
Security	8	×	3 = 24	1 = 8	3 = 24
Opportunity for advancement	4	×	0 = 0	3 = 12	0 = 0
Role/responsibility	5	×	1 = 5	3 = 15	1 = 5
Personnel relationships	8	×	3 = 24	3 = 24	1 = 24
Working environment	8	×	3 = 24	1 = 8	3 = 24
Need of people	3	×	1 = 3	3 = 9	2 = 6
Variety of services that can be provided	4	×	1 = 4	3 = 12	2 = 8
PREFERENCE POINTS:			152	122	159

wants and needs in employment. It is important for each individual to carefully assess just what is important to him/her. Once this has been decided, it is relatively easy to assess how closely a potential employment site meets those wants and needs.

Honesty is, however, a crucial element in this decision-making process. Many persons would like to believe that they are altruistic and that a pleasant office with a fat salary is unimportant. If they rank their personal weightings based on how they wish they were rather than on how they really are, they will end up accepting a job that they are uncomfortable with, or they will abandon the decision-making system and simply accept the position they "really want" without realizing why. If a person's internal reaction is contrary to what turns up numerically on the decision-making chart, the tallies ought to be recalculated with an eye to greater self-honesty.

PLANNING CHANGE

Another important factor to remember is that a person's wants and needs do change with time. A person may have a more mature approach to the need for money after the first few years have seen the emphasis on material possessions lessen. It may be wise to reassess the individual's wants and needs periodically, particularly if the employment situation seems to be less than satisfying.

One sign that a person is not pleased with the current role or position in a practice setting is if he/she has little if any inclination to start work each day. Lying in bed wishing it were Saturday may be a sign of fatigue, but it may also be a sign that the challenge or the attractiveness of the person's employment situation needs a careful review. Sometimes a person can inject his/her own excitement into the job by developing some new approach to the daily routine or by generating some intriguing clinical study. The addition of a new employee who seems to be compatible with the health care provider can also spark new interest in a position.

However, the genuine reluctance to go to work each day is often the first sign that one ought to begin looking for a change in employment. The bored or frustrated employee is seldom viewed with a positive eye by the employer or by the patient, despite the provider's ability to perform. It is better to seek new employment on one's own than to be asked by the employer. This kind of self-imposed termination is difficult for most people, particularly if security is of high value. Employers often then do it *for* the person.

People often read termination (which is a nice way of saying "fired") as a failure, which is not always an appropriate interpretation. Being terminated from a position can often be the best thing that can happen to a person who has become fixed in a rut and finds little excitement in the current employment situation. Termination can actually rejuvenate a person giving him/her a new approach to life and success and can prompt a person to seek and find a position that is far more rewarding.

Some personnel advisors say that a person should change positions or working environment every 5 years to retain a dynamic, healthy approach to living. Others are content with changing some facet of their lives every 5 years, but not necessarily jobs. It is probably true that a person who is happy with his/her success and who is invigorated by the challenge of what he/she is doing will have opportunity for advancement far more often than every 5 years, so the person's need to single-handedly initiate a change in role or function may not be necessary. Perhaps the most critical point in all of this is that change is not necessarily bad—even when it is forced change. Change is often a very good thing. Planned change can be even better.

Planning for change is often termed "goal orientation." What is the person's goal for change? Are today's activities contributing toward the achievement of that goal?

For instance, it is quite possible that although a certain health care provider is excited about clinical practice and the current practice setting in which she is employed, she may have tucked away in her brain the idea that she would like to be a consultant for the efficient operation of health care facilities. While being employed in the facility, she may be observing how the practice is efficiently or inefficiently operating and she may have registered for one or two courses related to management and economics. The practice experience will help establish credibility for the person. The course work may provide a broader base of knowledge and lead toward a credential that will further establish credibility.

Attending appropriate professional meetings and establishing professional relationships with persons who are currently active as efficiency experts may establish some inroads to the profession and actually start the woman on her new career. The truly goal-oriented person assesses a large part of the activities of the current day in terms of how they build toward the future. Every request to assume a responsibility that can lead toward the goal is responded to with a positive answer. New challenges are exciting because they provide a broader range of understanding and because they can lead to even more exciting endeavors. With each new challenge the risk of failure is inherent, but the risk becomes less and less apparent with each new success. Perhaps the key is to assume those challenges for which the person is prepared, with a small edge of the unknown or the untested left to peak the brain power and logic of the person so that one continually adds to abilities with each new challenge rather than simply calling on old abilities again and again.

The goal-oriented person is growing intellectually and emotionally as each new experience adds to the person's ability and self-concept.

The antithesis of goal orientation is security orientation. The desire to remain in one secure position with minimal change and minimal challenge (minimal risk) results in a basically stagnant approach to life that can be devastating if the source of the security is taken away. A person who remains in one job position for 20 years performing the same tasks and learning few new things can be overwhelmed if that job is taken away by the death of the employer or by a physical disability that makes continued performance impossible. Women who remained homemakers for years and then were confronted with either the death of the husband or divorce have had to undergo tremendous change for which they often were not prepared because of the "security" of their unchanging worlds.

Generally the best preparation for such change is to build constant change into one's life so that the psyche is accustomed to the risk element and so that the prospect of risk is not so frightening as to impair the person's ability to respond to change and grow with it. Coping with change is a mental process that relies on a person's ability to see the growth that can come from it, how the change will improve the person's world, and how there is some element in change that is positive regardless of the short-term tragedy that may accompany it. Loss of a loved one is a change that deserves grief and a time of adjustment, but it also can be a spark that causes a person to find new sources of strength and the ability to succeed.

The goal orientation concept may be the best protection against the current tumultuous changes in technology, life-style, the family, acceptable behavior patterns, and the resultant demands on a person's ability to cope with each change. However, it needs to be tempered by a certain serendipity—or an appreciation of the natural flow of events and to accept the external forces that cause changes to occur, which may not be a part of the person's master plan for the future. Human beings have some control over the future, but not total control. So to avoid inevitable frustration and disappointment, the serendipitous element is a crucial aspect of coping with change.

Review questions

1. List ten factors that are often important considerations for health care providers seeking employment.
   a.
   b.
   c.
   d.
   e.
   f.
   g.
   h.
   i.
   j.
2. List the factors that are important to *you* and weigh each on a scale of 1 to 10.
3. Design a form that will permit classifying each of several job opportunities according to how well each meets the weighted preference factors.
4. What could be the possible difficulty if the total preference points in a decision-making grid point to an opportunity as the best selection contrary to the person's internal reaction?

GROUP ACTIVITIES

1. Discuss how individuals in the class weighted the ten critical factors in evaluating a practice setting. Explain why the factors were weighted as they were.
2. Describe what the "ideal" practice setting would be for each person, according to the factors.
3. Share long-range goals for employment, outlining how each person hopes to achieve his/her personal goals.
4. Debate the statements: "Change is always good," "To build toward a better employment position is a self-centered approach to daily work," and, "Women have a relatively short-term commitment to employment."
5. Invite a small panel of health care providers who have experienced considerable growth and change in their professional lives to speak. Ask them to describe how the changes occurred—whether they were planned, accidental, or forced. Assess how they are able to cope with change and make the best of each occurrence.

REFERENCES

Green, A.E., and Jong, A.: The role and responsibilities of hygienists and their association, Dent. Hyg. **54:**377, 1980.

Lawson, E.S.: The dental hygienist's perception of satisfaction in the private dental office, Dent. Hyg. **54:**74, 1980.

Malvitz, D.M., and Mocniak, N.: Profile of dental hygienists licensed in the United States, J. Public Health Dent. **42:**54, 1982.

Pitchford, T.F., Broski, D.C., and Reynolds-Goorey, N.: Job satisfaction in dental hygiene, Dent. Hyg. **54:**559, 1981.

Rubinstein, L., and Miller, S.: Dental hygiene practice behaviors and perceived decision making: report of a survey, Dent. Hyg. **59:**404, 1985.

Woodall, I.: Survey of dental hygienists' values, RDH **6**(2):44, 1986.

CHAPTER 16

Preparing a resume

OBJECTIVES: The reader will be able to:

1. Explain what a resume is and how it can affect an employer's decision to offer employment to an individual.
2. Specify the usual components of a resume.
3. Identify which items are by law not to be considered by employers in offering employment.
4. Prepare a personal resume for the following:
   a. Clinical practice employment.
   b. Employment within an educational institution.
   c. Employment in a public health agency.
5. Critique several sample resumes for their structure, completeness, and quality of preparation.

A resume is a concise statement of a person's qualifications. It serves as a formal written introduction of the potential employee to the interested employer. The employer is able to review the person's educational background, work experience, professional association activities, publications, and other pertinent information to assess how compatible the person's qualifications are with the requirements of the available work position. Since the resume is often available to the employer before an interview, it creates the first impression of the person. It can tell the potential employer a great deal about the applicant, including the person's gift for clarity, completeness, organization, and even the person's basic perception of him or herself.

What are the key components of a well-designed resume? How can it be structured so that vital elements of information are easily identified? What are some general guidelines that should be followed in preparing this statement of qualifications?

KEY COMPONENTS

The applicant's *name, address, and telephone number* should be conspicuously placed at the top of the resume so that the reader can readily identify whose statement of qualifications it is and so that the person's name is associated immediately with the contents. Its conspicuous location facilitates accurate filing so that it is not lost. This information also ensures that the potential employer will know how to contact the person for an interview or to at least acknowledge receipt of the resume.

Educational experience is a critical element in the resume, particularly in health-related fields in which specific credentials are required for a person to be accepted for employment. Usually only postsecondary education is listed in a professional resume unless some aspect of high school preparation is particularly relevant to the person's credentials. For instance, if a dental assistant received training or held a cooperative-education job while in high school, then it may be appropriate to include it. Each certificate and degree should be listed, chronologically, along with the institution from which it was received and the year it was earned. The major area of study or the discipline in which each degree is granted should be identified as well. Some resume forms recommend placing the most recently earned degree first on the list, then proceeding backwards chronologically to the first earned educational credential. This may be wise if the list of degrees is lengthy, but for the health care provider just beginning a career, the listing may include no more than one or two entries. In this case, reverse order is not necessary.

States in which the person holds licensure should be listed along with *professional certification status* as applicable.

Following the basic educational and practice credentials should be a statement of *work experience*. For persons with several years of professional experience, there is little need to list non-professional employment experiences. However, if the person is seeking a first professional position, it may be wise to include those employment positions held during high school and college years. Employers look favorably on a resume that shows that the person has been able to assume the responsibilities associated with employment and hold a position for an extended period of time. The statement of work experience should, again, be in chronological order. The places of employment should be identified, along with a brief statement of the nature of the position held and the dates of employment in each position. For instance, beneath an entry indicating clinical practice experience could be added:

Provided comprehensive dental hygiene services, including preparation of diagnostic information and assessment of nutritional status, oral prophylaxis and root planing, curettage, and plaque control and nutritional counseling.

The decision to add such explanatory statements is based on the kind of position being sought and on the amount of available space in the resume. For instance, if the position the applicant is seeking is a managerial one, the descriptive statements should focus on the skill and background in management and supervision with less description of other kinds of responsibilities. Furthermore, if the resume includes several entries for previous work experience, it may be cumbersome or even overwhelming for the prospective employer to have descriptive statements for each. Deciding what explanatory notes to include is a balance between providing adequate, relevant information and keeping the resume brief and clear.

Any time that such explanations are included, they should highlight the importance of the person's role. Contrast the sample statement above with the following:

Cleaned teeth and taught toothbrushing.

The prospective employer will probably be more favorably impressed by the first description, if the position to be filled calls for a competent dental hygienist with a full range of skills.

For persons seeking employment in a research or teaching institution or in a public health agency, it is best to subcategorize work experience into clinical practice, laboratory or clinical research, teaching experience, or community projects. For persons applying for an administrative or consultative position, the resume should specifically reference work experience that relates to administrative or consultative roles. These subcategories are usually not even necessary to mention in the resume of a person who is just beginning a career.

If the current employer is listed in the work experience category, state whether or not it is appropriate for the potential employer to contact the current employer as a reference. This can be a sensitive matter if the current employer is unaware of the employee's search for another opportunity. When the call is placed, asking for a reference, it may be met with a shocked response and the employee may be in a most uncomfortable position as a result. However, if the current employer is aware of the employee's intention to change positions and can provide a favorable recommendation, the potential employer should be aware that this is an appropriate reference to call.

Professional activities usually comprise the next category of information in a resume. Membership, committee activities, officerships, and special projects assignments in student organizations and then graduate organizations should be specified chronologically with a brief description of the positions held in each of the organizations. Having assumed a reasonable amount of responsibility within a professional association can be viewed as an indication of commitment beyond the day-to-day work activity of the profession.

Not all employers respond positively at first to obvious extensive involvement in associations. Some employers fear that association business will be conducted over the office telephone and that the political aspects of such a role may conflict with the goals of delivering care. Others view association activity as highly commendable and will offer to support such efforts with secretarial assistance, the use of the office telephone, and a limited number of release days for conducting professional association business. The point is that it is helpful to list memberships and leadership roles in associations and to follow up their entries at the interview with a candid discussion of the degree of commitment and with appropriate assurances that such involvement will not detract from the employment arrangement. If it appears that the level of involvement will affect daily employment activities, then expectations should be carefully described so that neither party encounters unpleasant surprises after the position is offered and accepted.

Clinicians may wish to list *continuing education courses* attended (and ones they have designed and conducted) and units (CEUs) earned. This may be particularly important if the clinician is in a profession in which role changes are occurring and newly delegated functions have been incorporated.

If the person seeking employment has partici-pated in *clinical or basic research resulting in publications,* the citations should be listed under that category. This category may be most relevant for persons seeking employment in a research or educational institution or a public health agency. It is a category most often applicable to persons who have had a research component in their master's or doctoral programs or for those who have extensive employment experience with opportunities for research.

Other items of information that may be included are *age, marital status, sex, number of dependents,* and *race.* A picture can be attached to the resume, also. However, many people now omit these items because they have been known to be factors that have tended to prejudice employers for or against an applicant regardless of the professional credentials described in the resume.

Some employers may automatically exclude male applicants, persons under 20 or over 45 years of age, black persons, or a married, childless woman. The laws now make it unnecessary for applicants to list age, race, or sex because of this prejudicial element, which places persons falling in the "wrong" stereotyped group at a great disadvantage. In fact, persons who can prove that they were discriminated against in being hired because of race, sex, creed, or national origin may prosecute.

If the applicant wishes to include that information on the resume, he/she may. However, it is difficult to identify how any of those factors should relate directly to the person's ability to perform the job as defined. It might be wisest to limit the resume content to relevant data.

The amount and kinds of information included in a resume can say a great deal about the person's ability to concisely state the essential elements to be considered in assessing suitability for a position. Detail regarding high school social club activities or church circle responsibilities may not offer the employer the information he/she is seeking and may detract from other, more pertinent items. Scant information regarding previous employment or missing chronological links because of failure to include time frames of school and employment may leave doubts in the reviewer's mind (such as "I wonder what happened between 1975 and 1980?").

References should be listed. Included should be previous employers, teachers, and other responsible adults who can attest to the applicant's expertise and character. Relatives and personal friends should not be included. The addresses and telephone numbers should be listed. Each person on the list should be contacted before being included as both a matter of courtesy and practicality. A prospective reference should have the opportunity to decline the responsibility. In addition, contacting each person allows the applicant to discuss the nature of the prospective position and explain what facet of the person's background is particularly important. This helps the well-intentioned spokesperson paint a picture that highlights the most relevant qualities of the applicant. No mention of references, or a limited range of persons cited as references, may prompt the reviewer to wonder what trail of havoc was left behind by the person. And it does not permit the reviewer to quietly follow up references before the interview.

At the end of the presentation of factual information, the applicant may include a brief description of his/her *professional goals*. Usually this is no more than a paragraph or two and is limited to career objectives and aspirations:

Within 5 years I hope to have established myself as a highly experienced, competent clinician. I expect to acquire additional responsibility in either personnel supervision or fiscal management. My goal is to move from a salaried position to a full partnership within 10 years.

It is important to remember the possible mind set of the reader when including a goals statement. If the goals sound too ambitious for the particular available position, this statement may actually work against the applicant. The prospective employer may conclude that the applicant will not stay with the position long enough to justify hiring him/her regardless of the array of credentials and the obvious achievement orientation shown in the resume. With this caution in mind, the applicant can prepare a goals statement that for many purposes adds a great deal to the resume. Many employers look for this kind of an inclusion and will follow up such information with further inquiry at the interview.

The happy medium is to include as much helpful data as possible without cluttering the resume with extraneous commentary and without presenting so much information that the prospective employer decides the applicant is too good for the job.

One way an applicant can reveal his or her personality is to include an *autobiography*. Usually placing a limit of 250 to 300 words on the length of the "life story" forces the applicant to decide what is relevant, what says the most about a person's successes, ambitions, roadblocks, and values yet does not cause the reader to doze off at "Chapter 3: When I Learned to Roller Skate." An autobiography says a great deal to the observant reviewer about the person's self-concept and helps to prepare for meeting the person in an interview situation. The reviewer gets to know the applicant on a more personal level before the session and has something with which to open the discussion.

In writing an autobiography, the applicant should let his/her personality show. The writer should use a comfortable style and mix personal and professional milestones as appropriate. It is important to remember the basic writing skills of coherence, unity, clarity, reasonable paragraph transitions, and grammar. This will facilitate the reader's understanding of what the applicant is attempting to express, and it is an obvious statement of the person's ability to think logically and use written communication skills, which are two qualities the employer may be seeking in an employee. Potential employers often focus in on these skills, particularly if the employment role calls for preparing charts and correspondence.

STRUCTURE AND GRAMMAR

People often evaluate intelligence in terms of writing skills and sometimes in terms of handwriting. Regardless of the applicant's view of the necessity of good writing skills, care and attention should be paid to the preparation of the autobiography in terms of its structure as well as its content. The autobiography should be neat and either typewritten or legibly handwritten. A reasonable mastery of the English language is also often evaluated in terms of the variety of the vocabulary and the appropriateness of word usage. So although it is not necessary to seek out unusual words in the thesaurus, it does help to have some variety in word selection.

The rules of clarity, neatness, coherence, unity, and good grammar apply not only to the autobiography but to the entire resume. It should be an attractive document that is easy to read and follow. The resume definitely should be typed and proofread. It should make use of headings and appropriate spacing so that the reader's eye can easily focus on relevant categories quickly. It helps to use plain bond paper (rather than the erasable bond) since it is less likely to smudge and leave its imprint on shirt cuffs and other papers on the reader's desk. It may be an obvious copy of an original (photostat or dry stencil product), but it should be readable and of high quality.

It generally is not necessary to use fancy folders or engraved letterhead. Sometimes these extreme approaches to the preparation of a resume speak more of frivolity and compulsiveness than of functionality and neatness. A well-prepared resume with a brief introductory cover letter is usually what an employer expects and wants.

COVER LETTER

The cover letter should briefly mention the attached biographical data and should specify the type of position for which the person is applying. If a specific position has been listed as available, it is wise to identify that specific job title and to mention where the position's availability was posted or listed. This assists the reviewer in matching resumes with openings.

The letter should specifically state an interest in obtaining employment, note whether the applicant wishes an interview, and suggest how contact may be made. For instance, the closing lines of the letter may say:

Please inform me of the availability of this type of position in your corporation. If you wish to arrange for an employment interview, I will be pleased to meet with you. Below are listed my address and telephone for your convenience.

The well-prepared cover letter makes the point immediately and courteously asks for a follow-up. It permits the reader to rapidly scan the page for the essentials and plan whatever follow-up is needed. It should invite the reader to review the attached resume, not only because it is referenced in the letter but because the cogent style says, "You want to know more about me."

It is a careful balancing act to be assertive without being demanding. Requesting a response and providing a ready means for the response to be made is a reasonable approach. Using phrases such as "I expect you to call me . . . ," or "I will call you for an interview . . . ," or "Have your secretary call me . . . ," are generally construed to be pushy. In contrast, the phrases, "I know you must be very busy, but I would be so elated if you could take a moment to answer me . . . ," and "I hope you will give me a chance . . . ," are too mushy and sound more like "begging" than requesting on an adult-to-adult level. Besides, these overqualified, modified, super-humble requests take up a great deal of space in a letter and add words through which the reviewer probably does not wish to wade.

While the resume may be a duplicate, the cover letter should be an original, single-copy correspondence. It should, if possible, be addressed to a specific person, and it should contain (as noted previously) references to the particular position available or the work setting. The mass duplication approach with only the reviewer's name and address typed at the top creates in the mind of the reader visions of resumes flooding the land in the hopes that someone will respond. It definitely helps to personalize the cover letter, even if it is only so that the employer feels some sense of potential significance in the applicant's life.

To whom it may concern:

     I am very interesting in persuing with you the possibility of a job in your hospital, if you will take the time to call me and arrange for an appointment sometime soon, at your convenience. I am sure there must be many opening for persons such as myself who are interested in employment. You could send me a list of what is open or we could discuss it at the interview. I have two years of education and have nursing experience. My currriculum vitae will be in the mail to you soon so that you may review it before our interview. What are the chances that I will be hired?

          Yours truly, Gerry Paddington
          281-0660

Fig. 16-1. An example of how *not* to initiate correspondence with a potential employer. The postcard is undated, contains little useful information, has a misspelled word and grammatical errors, includes only one method for replying, and does not have an accompanying resume.

Fig. 16-1* shows a cover letter that is not atypical of those received by potential employers. It is typed (at least) on a postcard and displays many of the no-nos that can cause the initial, albeit written, contact between applicant and reviewer to be less than favorable.

It is addressed to no one in particular. It is not dated. Nor does it have much useful information, despite the fact that it covers the available space. It refers to a curriculum vita (resume) that is to follow, necessitating that the reviewer hold and match arriving correspondence. Because it is on a postcard, it may well be lost in the paper shuffle on the desk top (if it is not purposely discarded) before the resume arrives. It refers to no specific available employment opening. And it does not offer much clue as to the category of employment for which the person is qualified. Besides that, it contains a misspelled word, errors in grammar, and only one means of contacting the person, without an area code.

*No entries in the cover letter and resumes shown in this chapter are to be construed as facts related to any actual person.

What is the likelihood for this cover letter to create a positive response in the reader?

Contrast this postcard variety of initial contact with the cover letter in Fig. 16-2. It is neatly prepared, concise, includes a reference to the specific job opening and how the person learned of the opening, and a reference to an enclosed curriculum vita (see Fig. 16-3). The letter's style is assertive but not aggressive, and it provides information for readily establishing follow-up contact.

A review of the resume shows good categorization of information, chronological order within each category, and a reasonable amount of data accompanying each entry.

Fig. 16-4 shows how the same information could be buried or missing in a poorly prepared resume. It is not difficult to predict the relative impact these two forms would have on potential employers. The latter version contains jumbled categories, incomplete data (including gaps in time), and extraneous information probably of minimal interest to the potential employer.

The safest way to prepare a resume that will be attractive to the reader is to write it using the guidelines (placed in checklist form in Fig. 16-5)

March 30, 1986

Mr. Dennis Griswold
Personnel Director
Rabash Hospital
5857 Main Street
Fordham, OH 55455

Dear Mr. Griswold:

I am a registered dental hygienist with three years'
clinical and supervisory experience in a hospital in
Pennsylvania providing routine preventive dental care for
extended-care patients and hospital out-patients.

Your advertisement in <u>Dental Hygiene</u> indicates that you
have a position open for a dental hygienist which would
include similar functions. I am interested in applying for
that position and have enclosed my resume for your review.

Should you find that I possess appropriate qualifications, I
would appreciate the opportunity to meet with you. You may
contact me at either of the numbers listed below.

Yours truly,

George Herrick

George Herrick
42 Marble Road
Bedford, PA 19002
Home: (626) 881-2262
Office: (626) 872-6437

Fig. 16-2. An example of a concise, informative, attractive cover letter for a resume. It refers to the specific position, briefly describes the applicant's qualifications, refers to an enclosed resume, suggests that contact be made for an interview, and provides information for contact to be established. It is assertive but not aggressive.

Resume

George Herrick, RDH, BS   March, 1986
42 Marble Road
Bedford, PA 19002
Home: (626) 881-2262
Office: (626) 872-6437

PROFESSIONAL EDUCATION:

    The University of Southern California   1972
      Certificate in Dental Hygiene

    The University of Pennsylvania   1980
      Bachelor of Science in Health Care
      Management (with high honors)

CLINICAL EXPERIENCE:

    Dental hygiene practice in   1972-1975
      periodontics (full-time)
      Dr. Linda F. Homan
      58 Westfield Drive
      Lindwood, CA 99210

    Provided oral prophylaxes, root planing and
    curettage for periodontal patients, maintained
    oral disease prevention program for patients,
    designed recall system

    Dental hygiene hospital practice   1980-1985
      (full-time)
      Bedford General Hospital
      61 Miami Blvd.
      Bedford, PA 19002

    Provided bedside dental hygiene care (oral prophylaxes,
    plaque control instruction, preparation of diagnostic
    aids) for long-term care patients in oncology, hemo-
    dialysis, and psychiatric units

    Dental hygiene practice in pedo-   1985-present
    dontics (full-time)
      Dr. Elmer Bloomquist
      78241 Randall
      Bedford, PA 19002

    Provided dental hygiene care (oral prophylaxes,
    fluoride therapy, preparation of diagnostic aids, and
    plaque control instruction) for normal and handicapped
    children, often within the hospital environment.

Fig. 16-3. An example of a concise, well-organized resume. It has appropriate categories, gives reasonable
amounts of pertinent information, grants permission to
contact references, and is basically unpretentious.

LICENSURE:

National Board Certificate	1972
California licensure (current)	1972
Northeast Regional Board Certificate	1977
Pennsylvania licensure (current)	1977

CONTINUING EDUCATION:

"Local Anesthesia"   3.5 CEUs 1976
   The University of Pennsylvania

"Expanded functions in   3.0 CEUs 1978
   Pedodontics"
   Temple University

"The Effects of Systemic   1.0 CEUs 1978
   Disorders on Oral Tissues"
   Montgomery County Community College

"Occlusal Traumatism: 6.0 CEUs 1979
   Recognition and Treatment"
   University of Medicine and Dentistry of New
   Jersey

"Radiologic Safety in Dentistry" 4.0 CEUs 1980
   Pennsylvania Dental Hygienists' Association

"Nutritional Counseling"   6.0 CEUs 1982
   Delaware Dental Hygienists' Association

"Dental Care for Special   6.0 CEUs 1984
   Patients"
   Philadelphia County Dental Hygienists' Association

CLINICAL RESEARCH AND PUBLICATION:

The effects of preventive measures on dental disease
as manifested in transplant patients medicated with
corticosteroids, RDH, 6(3): 22, 1986.

NOTE: Current and former employers may be contacted as
references.

Fig. 16-3, cont'd. For legend see opposite page.

```
                          Resume

     Education:

          H.S.  diploma in Anaheim              1970
          Cert. in dental hygiene              1972
          Penn. - B.S. degree                  1980
          Continuing education          1976 to present
             (total of 7.5)

     Work:

          Practiced dental hygiene for two dentists
                                        1972 to present
          Worked in a hospital                 1980-now
          Plaque control in hospital.  Got published.  1986

     Age: 35
     Married
     Two children: Amy-10
                   James-7
     Wife: Elissa, Age 32
          Unemployed
     Weight: 170
     Height: 5'10"                    Hobbies:  cooking,
                                                carpentry
                                      Novels read:
                                                Iacocca,
                                                Megatrends


     George Herrick
     (626) 881-2262
```

Fig. 16-4. An example of how a poorly prepared resume can underrate a person's competencies. Information is incomplete and jumbled. Extraneous data are included, but crucial items are missing. It should be contrasted with the resume presented in Fig. 16-3.

Content

1. Are name, address, and telephone number conspicuously spaced at the top of the first page? _____

2. Is education (beginning at the postsecondary level) listed chronologically? _____

3. Are certificates and degrees earned listed with the discipline or area of study identified? _____

4. Are licenses and/or certificates of competence listed, including state or region and date achieved? _____

5. Are places of previous employment listed chronologically with addresses and a brief description of the scope of activity or responsibility? _____

6. Are dates provided for each work experience with an indication of full- or part-time employment? _____

7. Are references that may be contacted marked (including whether or not the current employer should be contacted)? _____

8. Is a listing of continuing education courses with credits earned included? _____

9. Are research activities, publications, and consultant roles identified as appropriate? _____

10. Is an autobiographical statement of approximately 250 words attached (optional)? _____

11. Does it contain all (but only) necessary information? _____

Fig. 16-5. Checklist for evaluating a resume.

Form and structure

1. Are categories readily identifiable? _____

2. Is spacing appropriate to highlight main components? _____

3. Is it typed (neatly)? _____

4. Are words checked for accurate typing and proper spelling? _____

5. Is the finished product attractive but unpretentious? _____

Fig. 16-5, cont'd.

and then ask one or more people who are involved in making decisions regarding employment to review it and offer suggestions. With one or two drafts, a highly acceptable document can be prepared that may lead to the next step in finding employment: the interview.

Review questions

1. Why is a well-written resume an important part of seeking employment?
2. List six usual components of a resume.
    a.
    b.
    c.
    d.
    e.
    f.
3. Which biographical items are, by law, not to be considerations in selecting job applicants?
4. Often a resume will include brief descriptions of the responsibilities a person assumed in specific work settings. How should these descriptions be developed and selected for inclusion in a resume?

GROUP ACTIVITIES

1. Invite an employment agency officer to discuss the importance of resumes in obtaining positions and to suggest alternative styles.
2. Prepare a professional resume. Evaluate it in terms of the checklist in Fig. 16-5.
3. Write a cover letter to accompany the resume that could be sent to potential employers currently advertising positions in the professional journals or in the classified sections of the newspapers.
4. Critique each other's letters and resumes, offering suggestions for improvements.
5. Cover various actual resumes that have been received by the personnel office so that the writers are anonymous. Critique the style, content, and structure of each. Make suggestions for improvement.

CHAPTER 17

The interview

OBJECTIVES: The reader will be able to:

1. Explain briefly the purpose and significance of the interview in finding employment.
2. Describe the respective roles of the job applicant and the interviewer in the interview process.
3. Prepare for an interview session by using preinterview techniques including:
   a. Conducting a personal inventory of skills, characteristics, and goals.
   b. Analyzing the probable interests, expectations, and attitudes of the interviewer.
   c. Verbally "adapting" the findings of the personal inventory of these probable interests, expectations, and attitudes.
   d. Organizing key points for their greatest effectiveness.
   e. Practicing the interview and establishing a positive attitude toward the encounter.
4. List the four basic phases of the interview.
5. Describe briefly the interviewer's evaluation process.
6. Summarize basic methods for carrying out a successful interview, when:
   a. The interviewer appears to be experienced and the preinventory procedures were accurate with regard to the characteristics of the employer.
   b. The interviewer appears to be satisfied with minimal information.
   c. The interviewer "takes over" the interview.
   d. The interviewer plays a passive role in the interview.
   e. The interviewer appears to be less than eager to participate in the interview (appears distracted, preoccupied, or even angry).
7. Outline follow-up procedures that can enhance the effectiveness of the interview and perhaps increase the possibility of receiving an offer of a position.
8. List five guidelines for conducting an interview.

SIGNIFICANCE OF THE INTERVIEW

An appropriate resume and cover letter can do a great deal to create the expectations the employer may have of the applicant, but the greatest impact that will be made on the employer is the applicant's behavior during the interview encounter. The interview is clearly a time of assessment and evaluation. The reviewer begins the assessment process the moment the applicant arrives (or before that time if the applicant is late). And each successive moment of the interview allows the employer to focus on the applicant in an effort to determine if this is the kind of person he/she wishes to have in the practice setting, firm, corporation, or other establishment. There are some unique features about the kinds of employment interviews that health care providers are likely to encounter, but generally speaking, the interview process is quite similar from one situation to another. It is perhaps *the* "final exam," with rarely an opportunity for a retake. Based on a few minutes or hours of conversation, the employer will decide whether a position ought to be offered.

The interview also is a time for the applicant to learn as much as possible about the potential position so that he/she can make a reasonable decision about whether an offer from the employer ought to be accepted. It is not possible to use a decision-making grid for selecting an employment situation unless there is considerable information available about the characteristics of each position available. Therefore it is important for the applicant to make use of the interview to learn a great deal about the working environment, the scope of responsibility, and other factors determined to be of importance. As each bit of information is gathered, the applicant is assessing and evaluating the attractiveness of this particular employment situation.

ROLES IN THE INTERVIEW

The interview is a time for mutual evaluation. Both the employer and the potential employee are under scrutiny. The degree of scrutiny each feels will depend on how sought after the parties in the interview are for their skills (in the case of the interviewee) and in the opportunities they offer (in the case of the interviewer). If many applicants are seeking employment in a nearly ideal practice setting, for instance, each applicant may feel more in the role of the observed than in the role of the observer. When there are few employable, qualified people available for a position and the applicant is being interviewed by a number of potential employers, the employer may be wishing to put his/her best foot forward so that the applicant will look favorably on the situation being offered.

The ideal interview situation for both parties would be when the scrutiny element is about equal, that is, when both parties have a reasonable desire to receive a good evaluation and when both parties are interested in carefully assessing the other. In most interview situations the ideal is unlikely to occur.

In the realm of health care providers the interview situation was quite out of balance when there were only 9.8 active dental hygienists for every 1000 active dentists (Dentistry, 1975-76). This situation occurred in the early 1960s. A den-

tal hygiene program graduate could expect to choose from a flood of opportunities for practice. With four or more offers certain, the graduate could practically conduct the interview. Many dentists complained that they had little opportunity to interview the applicant because of the applicant's overriding interest in what each setting had to offer. The fact that a hygienist had a pulse often was considered sufficient qualification for that person to be offered a position. The situation was out of balance not only because of the few hygienists available but because many dental practitioners could plan on suffering great losses in time, energy, and money if the practice, which was often dependent on the presence of a dental hygienist, had to function without the hygienist. Patients expected regular recall appointments, and in practices in which a hygienist had practiced full time for several years, that meant a full schedule of recalls to be kept each month. For the dentist to perform those services would mean that little other care could be delivered. So recalls suffered and patients were not called for appointments, which meant some would go elsewhere for care, or those who did obtain an appointment would need more care than if they had been seen on schedule.

To avoid this problem, dentists were willing to accept the license to practice as proof enough that the hygienist would be an appropriate addition to the practice setting. This desire to hire also caused salaries to rise for dental hygienists. In an effort to keep the attractiveness of the employment situation high, the dentist would offer a slightly higher amount of money, which over a period of 5 years caused daily salaries to rise from an average of $18 to $20 per day to $50 to $60 per day. One dentist in the upper peninsula of Michigan advertised for several years that he would offer the services of his private airplane to bring a hygienist to his town to practice. Another advertised a mink coat, a Cadillac, and 4 weeks vacation each year to a hygienist who would practice in his particularly remote location.

However, the balance has shifted from being weighted in favor of the hygienist to being equal, to being in favor of the dentist, with signs of a trend back toward equal. Salary levels are starting to rise slightly after a long period of stagnation. The hygienist still is often the one feeling scrutinized. The potential employer now looks beyond the license and the pulse to the specified qualities and qualifications of the applicant. If the trend toward equality continues, the hygienist will once again be actively evaluating each prospective employer more carefully.

The evaluation skills the hygienist uses to assess a potential employment site are by necessity a bit more complex today than they were 15 years ago, also. With employment opportunities that go beyond the private solo practice dental office, the hygienist has a greater number of factors to evaluate in terms of how the practice setting meets his/her needs. One hygienist may have only three interviews, but one may be in a hospital setting, another in a penal institution, and only the third in a general dental office. With other hygienists also interviewing for each of those positions, the hygienist has to be well prepared to succeed in the interview in making him/herself the most logical selection for the position. The hygienist also has to have well-developed skills in ferreting out the needed information about the setting so that if more than one offer is made, he/she is in a position to make an informed decision.

Therefore the applicant and the interviewer serve a dual, simultaneous role—that of scrutinizer and the one being scrutinized. Fortunately, being an active, tactful inquirer (a characteristic necessary for a person to gain the needed information) is often a trait the other person is hoping to see. As a result, the dual roles are usually quite compatible or even complementary.

It is not the role of the applicant to sit back and "be interviewed" with the full responsibility of the discussion falling on the shoulders of the interviewer. It should be a mutual exchange of information, inquiry, and discussion, with the applicant having equal input with the interviewer.

PREPARATION FOR THE INTERVIEW

Being the expert applicant for a position requires some preparation. The best way to develop interview skills is to participate in a preinterview process, which includes careful analysis of what factors should surface during the discussion, which are likely to, and how to address each one (Amsden and White, 1974). How can the applicant's attributes best be presented? And how can those attributes be related to the functions and responsibilities the employer expects the applicant to assume?

The first step in the preinterview preparation is to assess carefully and honestly one's capabilities and qualifications with regard to the position available. The obvious, and perhaps easiest, qualifications to examine are the educational and work experience factors that are related to the position applied for.

A medical technologist with a special concentration of study and experience in blood analysis may find his/her credentials ideal for the position open at the newly established blood bank. But a nurse requesting employment as an administrator in a research center may need to more carefully analyze his/her credentials for the sources of expertise he/she believes are qualifications for the job. It is a helpful exercise to return to the written resume and jot down how each of the entries has helped prepare the person for the available position. Then the notes should be set aside, and the applicant should describe aloud, convincingly, how each component of education and experience relates to the job applied for. This can be done alone while the applicant is looking in the mirror so that mannerisms and other aspects of the delivery can be seen from the point of view of the other person.

Once the more professional aspects have been analyzed, the applicant should practice some introspection and analyze his/her personal characteristics. To focus on the positive, the applicant can begin by listing and describing aloud personal successes. Listing one or two successes each of early childhood (ages 1 to 8 years), adolescence, college years, the most current year, and the last week and describing aloud in the mirror why each of those is viewed as a success can be quite an experience. However, it is essential that the successes be explained *aloud*. Even though it is highly unlikely that such an autobiographical survey will unfold during the interview, certain elements of the success chain may be quite appropriate to reveal during the interview, and having already verbalized the vignettes may make it much easier to describe the events and the feelings the person has about them.

A step further is to analyze personal failings in terms of how they enhanced growth. Even what appears to be a major setback can have a positive effect, depending on how the person reacts. These so-called failures should be explained aloud in the mirror, also. This may be the most difficult portion of the process. It is usually difficult to rationalize away personal errors while looking in the mirror. It forces a person to see how easily self-deception can be perceived. Human nature often causes people readily to claim credit for their achievements and to place blame elsewhere when they perform below expectations. Explaining into the mirror that the reason for the failing grade in chemistry is that the teacher was "out to get me" can stimulate some second thoughts about self-honesty. It is better to view one's own self-deceptions and analyze them before parading them in front of a prospective employer.

An appropriate way to discuss weaknesses or failings is to admit them openly and then to cite how they have caused growth and how their "owner" is coping with their planned modification. No employer expects an employee to be perfect and he/she probably has little interest in hiring a person who has deluded him/herself.

Once the successes/weaknesses identification and analysis are complete, the applicant may follow a more conventional approach to preparing for the interview by rehearsing the following:

1. Describing, in general, what kind of person he/she is.
2. Stating whether his/her grades reflect real potential and explaining why.
3. Explaining what he/she considers to be the most meaningful part of formal education.
4. Listing and explaining his/her most important short-range goal related to personal and professional life.
5. Listing and explaining his/her most important long-range goals related to personal and professional life.
6. Identifying school, community, and volunteer activities in which he/she has been involved which reveal important personal characteristics, qualities, skills, abilities, or maturity (Amsden and White, 1974).

This more conventional series of problems should be answered aloud and in the mirror.

The applicant should then move on to analyze what the interviewer may be interested in knowing. What are the probable interests, expectations, and attitudes of the interviewer? This is not always easy to predict, especially if the interviewer is not a skilled conductor of employment interviews. The dentist an hour behind schedule may feel less than resourceful at the time of an interview and may ask questions related strictly to clinical skills and experience. With a little more time available, that same dentist may choose to initiate a discussion of how auxiliaries ought to be integrated into the practice of dentistry, along with a philosophical discussion of the political and legal considerations involved in such changes.

The verbal skills and tact required of the applicant are quite different in the two situations. In the direct-and-to-the-point interview, the applicant will need to offer considerable, positive input in a short amount of time. Every word spoken will count doubly, since the decision to employ will be based on a restricted amount of contact. The applicant will have to be certain that the crucial positive elements surface and that the information needed to assess the practice is obtained without having to fire a series of questions while being ushered to the door. In the latter encounter, more information than planned may surface. Also, the applicant will have to decide what game the employer is playing: Is he/she simply taking this opportunity to voice convictions with little expected response from the potential employee? Is he/she attempting to determine whether philosophies are compatible? Or is the employer attempting to measure the applicant's ability to think, articulate responses, and behave in an assertive yet nonaggressive manner in a face-to-face discussion? In addition to deciding the "game," the applicant will need to ensure that the crucial exchange of basic information occurs and that it is not subordinated to the philosophical discussion, regardless of how interesting it is.

It is relatively safe to assume that potential employers expect (1) evidence of competence (education, experience, and licensure), (2) a pleasant disposition, (3) an energetic approach to the potential position, (4) honesty tempered with diplomacy and a positive attitude, and (5) in instances in which the position includes contact with people, an ability to communicate easily both verbally and nonverbally. Experienced interviewers also expect that the applicant will have researched the background of the firm or practice and will be familiar with the goals, objectives, and accomplishments of the organization. A frequently asked question based on this expectation is: "How do you feel you will be able to contribute to the goals and objectives of our organization?" It should be obvious that such a question requires not only forethought but some homework on the part of the applicant before the interview.

The self-analysis process described previously should help prepare the applicant to meet the expectations related to items 1, 4, and 5. If the applicant learned to smile, sit up, establish good eye contact, and acquire a reasonably relaxed manner as a result of the conversations with the mirror, items 2 and 3 may have at least partial preparation.

The employer probably does not particularly desire to offer a position to someone who is "ho-hum" about the idea of functioning in the described role. He/she is more likely to hire the excited, energetic person who sees the position as an opportunity to accomplish great things. Some people need a great deal of practice in being excited. For those who have difficulty revealing their positive feelings, it is probably best to return to the mirror.

Sitting forward with eyes sparkling compared to slouching with lids at halfmast should provide at least one example of how nonverbal behavior can portray interest. In beginning a discussion of the actual available position, it helps to include statements such as: "I've always wanted to work in this kind of practice environment," "I'd love to try out some of the approaches to patient care you hope to introduce," "That would be an ideal way for me to put to use the skills I learned that I enjoy most," or, "The position you describe is really exciting. It would be a fantastic opportunity." Coupled with the nonverbal energy signals, these phrases can help the employer determine the applicant's interest in the position.

Employers have varying expectations of employees in terms of responsibility, management participation, and professional growth. Some view their employees as basically subservient support staff with strictly defined task-oriented roles. Others invite critical input, decision making, and signs of a need for increased responsibility. It probably is not wise to anticipate the expectations of the employer and slip into a role that is unnatural to the applicant. First of all, the attempt may backfire. Second, the attempt may be seen as an act. And third, if the applicant is hired as a "nice girl who knows her place" and then emerges in a few weeks as a real thinking human being, the applicant may be back at the mirror preparing for more interviews. In this category of concern, it is probably wisest to assess the expectations as they emerge in the interview and then decide how compatible or tolerable they are in terms of the goals and needs of the applicant.

The research element of the preinterview procedure includes acquiring some advance information regarding the employer's expectations of employees. This can sometimes be accomplished by means of a conversation with former employees. The gathering of background information may include an identification of the employer's goals and objectives. In an innovative group practice, an educational or research institution, or in a public health agency it may be fascinating to discover what the goals and objectives are, particularly if it is possible to compare them with measured results.

With a reasonably accurate idea of the employer's mission, the potential employee should begin identifying, first in writing and then aloud, how his/her interests and qualifications can match or contribute toward it. Interviewers are generally impressed by a person's desire to "join the effort" and to become a contributor toward attaining the mission.

Regardless of the ill-defined or simplistic nature of the goals, few employers will be excited about hiring a person whose range of interests is limited to hours to be worked, duties to be fulfilled, and money to be earned. The role of the applicant is to provide as much information and conviction as is reasonable and possible to help the interviewer see the merits of hiring the person. This can be done without affectation yet with a great deal of polish by means of the self-analysis, the analysis of the likely needs of the employer, and the matching of needs and expectations prior to the interview.

PHASES OF THE INTERVIEW

The presentation, however, needs some organization and timing for it to be effective. The matter of organization of the interview can be addressed in terms of its basic phases. There are four basic phases regardless of its length or sophistication. The first is the *introduction,* which includes the critical initial contact, the exchange of the basic amenities, and the establishment of rapport. The second phase is the discussion of the *candidate's background* when the interviewer asks questions and the applicant makes use of a great deal of the preinterview mirror talk. The third phase is the *matching of the candidate with the position* when the discussion of goals commences and the position itself is described. The last phase is the conclusion or *closure* when it will be apparent how successful the interview has

been. Plans for follow-up will be discussed, or there will be a definite farewell (Amsden and White, 1974).

With these phases in mind it is possible to plan the organization of presenting key items of information, asking key questions, and using nonverbal cues to best advantage.

During the introductory phase the applicant should do his/her best to establish positive, open communication. The tone of voice should be friendly yet gentle and respectful. The eye contact should be positive without being a stare and accompanied by a smile and an energetic approach during the walk toward the person and the handshake. There is no need to mazurka into the room or turn the handshake into an arm wrestle, but a hesitation-free walk forward with a genuine, firm handshake can do a great deal to assist the initial encounter. There is nothing quite so disgusting as a "dead fish" handshake nor anything so initially negative as a hesitant approach with a slippery slump to the most distant chair. The approach should not make the interviewer suspect that the applicant's mother forced the person to appear. And the handshake should assure the interviewer that the applicant is alive and possessing some nerve endings in the hands that are sensitive to other human beings.

A bit of excitement at the initial encounter is usually expected. It is softened by a "safe" discussion of the weather, the trip to the interview, or other recent events generally considered of mutual interest. It cannot be emphasized too greatly that the first 4 minutes are indeed critical (Zunin and Zunin, 1972). This is the time during which most people decide whether or not they wish to continue their relationship, based on nonverbal as well as verbal expression. It is difficult to undo these first impressions, especially if the less-than-favorable ones relate to honesty (really security) and encounters with obstacles (desire to succeed) (Zunin and Zunin, 1972).

The person who trips over the rug and knocks over an umbrella stand and speaks out, "Oh, I'm so glad I'm not nervous," may be met by a sympathetic, knowing smile or with a glance heavenward. The person who missed a train and was taxied ten blocks out of the way by a foreign-speaking cabbie and who can find amusement in the incident rather than rage may score points.

Trust is the key element that needs to be established. It may, almost magically, exist between two people from the first eye contact. Or it may take some time for it to be established. Sometimes it never happens.

Ideally, it will happen before the second phase. It is less than a comfortable position to be describing one's attributes while still attempting to establish trust. It is in this instance that the honesty of the mirrorside self-talks may be very handy. The start of the second phase is often marked by a question. The "small talk" shifts to a more interrogatory mode. And the applicant finds himself/herself describing the educational aspects, work experience, and interests that were carefully analyzed during the preinterview process. Questions such as, "Why did you leave that position?" "What did you like best about your clinical experience?" and, "Why did you decide to enter this field?" are likely. The responses should build on the trust established and avoid "cute" remarks or a degeneration into apathy. Information should be offered, and each question should be used as a springboard to provide the previous kernels of knowledge that were all explained in careful terms to the mirror.

It is important for the applicant to give the interviewer a clear sense of who he/she is and what unique skills, experience, and attitudes he/she could bring to the practice. An applicant can do this effectively by taking responsibility for the statements made and by not answering questions in the abstract. For example, a common interview question is, "How did you like your last job?" A good answer would emphasize the person involved in the job: "For me, the job was great because it gave me the opportunity to learn . . ." or "Although the job environment was nice, for me, it was not a good situation because . . ." Both of these answers connect the individual with a story line or a set of described circumstances and help the interviewer know the person better. On the other hand, a less effective answer emphasizes the circumstances: "The job offered many opportunities. It was a perfect learning situation." Another example: "The job was one of those dead-end situations." Here the answers do not tell the interviewer about the individual's reaction to the situation and therefore do not give much to be remembered.

When the attention shifts to career goals (short and long range), the third phase has begun. The employer is beginning the matching process of candidate and position. Well-thought-out personal objectives and careful research of the employer's needs become invaluable. The interviewer will probably describe the available position, or the applicant may ask about it—in a cautious, yet assertive, gesture of interest. If the match-up is apparent, the applicant should inject a measure of energy and excitement into the conversation, indicating interest, challenge, and commitment. This may be the key moment in securing the position if the overall interview has been positive (Amsden and White, 1974).

The applicant can make a favorable impression on the interviewer by showing an interest in the practice. Generally this must be done without asking probing questions and without making too many personal declarations such as, "I really like your office design." A more effective approach is to make a statement such as, "I'm interested in knowing a little history of your practice," followed by the question, "How long have you been at the current location?" This interaction conveys interest, and it gives the dentist a chance to talk about him/herself. It gives the interviewee a chance to learn about the prospective employer.

If the interviewer begins to "sell" the position by elaborating on its merits or by agreeing that it matches well with the applicant's credentials, it is usually an indication that the interviewer recognized the match, also.

The fourth phase begins with a discussion of follow-up procedures. The employer may offer a simple, ''We'll call you,'' or may suggest a second meeting and a discussion more related to specific benefits and discussion of roles. In any case it is essential that both persons agree to whatever the follow-up plans are. As the interview draws to a close, the applicant should reiterate or summarize those plans and seek the interviewer's nod of agreement. This can be accomplished during the final handshake, by pausing at the end of the summary and giving one last shake when the nod is given. If ushered to the door, eye contact at the parting should not be broken until the nod is obtained. It should be relatively easy to obtain the nod as long as what is being summarized is an accurate feedback of what the interviewer said. This is not time to put words in the mouth of the interviewer. If the interview reveals that personal characteristics and the position do not match, it is better to part with an honest good-bye and to maintain trust than to attempt a futile follow-up procedure.

SUCCESS WITH THE INTERVIEWER

The evaluator/interviewer is basically assessing the applicant from the first to the last contact, eliminating negative elements rather than building positive ones. If the applicant is on time, the interviewer crosses off the negative element of discourtesy or tardiness. If the person smiles and is generally pleasant to talk to, the interviewer eliminates grouchiness and dullness. If the applicant is interested, eager, and qualified, the traits of apathy and incompetence are erased. The key to success is to not fit the negative aspects that are anticipated and to have enough uniqueness and attractiveness that the interviewer remembers the person and the interview. A job offer may follow.

If the interviewer is a professional and the preinventory procedures appear to be working well, the secret is to relax and make the most of the success. Attentiveness to what is said and what is asked is important. If an item of information in the resume is misstated by the interviewer, tactfully provide the accurate information. To ignore the error may be a mistake if the

interviewer made the ''error'' as a means of evaluating listening and diplomacy skills. If a question is asked that is unclear to the applicant, he/she should ask to have it repeated by saying something similar to, ''I'm not certain I understand your meaning. Could you rephrase it for me, please?'' It is unwise to say, ''You didn't say that very well. What are you asking?'' If the meaning is still unclear, a simple feedback strategy may correct the situation. The applicant should say, ''What I understand you are asking is . . .'' If the applicant's interpretation is correct, the interviewer will agree and the answer can be supplied. If the interpretation is inaccurate, the interviewer can see where the misunderstanding lies then correct it (Amsden and White, 1974).

Timing for the inclusion of key elements of information is important. It is best to plan to include key elements according to the typical topics of the four phases. As each phase unfolds, the applicant can feed into the discussion the preplanned selling points and questions.

This is particularly important in instances when the interviewer doesn't request or offer much information. And in cases in which the applicant feels rushed as the fidgeting interviewer continues to glance at his/her watch, the tendency may be to blurt out a series of statements and questions at such speed that the impact of each is more negative than positive. In an obviously disastrously brief interview situation, it might be best for the applicant to suggest a second appointment. The interview requires the development of trust, and this is not possible when the introduction is limited to a ''hello'' and the subsequent components fly by like Keystone cops.

It also may be a feat to provide and gather the needed information in instances in which the interviewer seems to ''take over'' the session, conducting each phase in a directive manner. The interviewer asks the questions, moves the session from phase to phase, and may allow little opportunity for the applicant to initiate topics or ask questions.

The polar opposite is the nondirective interviewer who sits back and responds to how the applicant develops the flow of the interview. This is a technique that often is used to assess a person's ability to function in a structure-free situation. Some interviewers will begin in a directive manner and then adopt a nondirective style. The preinterview planning related to each of the four phases will help the applicant facilitate the development and the progress of the session. It will be possible to provide the needed personal background data, inquire about the position, match characteristics, and achieve closure with relative ease if it has been preplanned.

There may be times when the applicant finds a weary, distracted, or even angry interviewer. It is rarely the case that an interviewer approaches the visit with the same air of excitement and interest that the applicant has. So the applicant should prepare for at best a moderately interested person and at worst one who wishes to be somewhere else. When confronted by a harried interviewer, the most appropriate behavior is to be as positive as possible, with a continuous, warm smile. The objective becomes to be the highlight of the person's day. It may not be very difficult to compete with his/her earlier experiences if the mood is obviously a dour one. To fall into a grumpy state rather than to remain positive may result in the interviewer subconsciously heaping the blame for the day's catastrophes on the applicant. In any case few job offers are given to grumpy people on an already bleak day.

FOLLOW-UP OF THE INTERVIEW

Regardless of the outcome, it is appropriate to send a letter of appreciation to the interviewer thanking him/her for the time and the opportunity to share. The letter should contain whatever additional information the interviewer has requested. Even if the closing of the interview was not filled with hope, such a gesture may result in a second interview, particularly if other applicants did not perform much better.

The note of appreciation also provides an opportunity to add omitted or new information. The letter should, once again, be impeccably neat with a concise, coherent message. It should provide the interviewer with a pleasant reminder of the encounter.

The interview experience can be a rewarding one that leads to offers of employment if it is prepared for and conducted with a measure of self-assurance and honesty. To do otherwise may result in extended efforts at obtaining employment and plenty of opportunity for practice.

INTERVIEWING: REVERSING THE ROLES

As auxiliaries move into management roles that include supervision of personnel, they may be involved in the recruitment and selection of new auxiliaries for the practice. Although being a skilled interviewee is helpful in acquiring interviewing skills, the processes are quite different. Much of the previous discussion identifies the possible mind set an interviewer can have. This brief introduction builds on that information.

Before announcing the availability of a position, the employer or interviewer should specify the exact job responsibilities and desired employee characteristics. A job description should be prepared if the position is new; if the position has been previously filled, the description should be reviewed and updated. The interviewer should list all the traits hoped for in the candidate. The list can be broken down into essential skills and skills that would be nice to have. Keep the list brief, so that the lines of questioning that will develop can target those areas. It will be difficult to focus on a great long list during a relatively brief interview (Beinhorn, 1985).

An advertisement should be placed in local newspapers or in professional journals in which people fitting the desired characteristics are likely to see it. The advertisement should state the minimum qualifications and offer a brief description of the practice. It should request that letters of inquiry and resumes be sent to a specific address. It is also possible to take telephone inquiries, but the written contact can reveal some otherwise unapparent characteristics—such as neatness, spelling, accuracy, and promptness.

All applications should be screened so that time

spent interviewing is reserved for those most suited to the job based on their credentials and their letters of inquiry. Those not selected for interviews should be notified promptly.

Before each scheduled interview, the resume or application should be carefully reviewed. Questions about the experiences, strengths, weaknesses, and goals of the applicant should be formulated based on the application and the specific needs of the position.

The interviewer should check the candidate's references and determine how the person contributed to previous employment situations and how he/she was perceived by the other workers. It helps to remember the essential qualities and the nice-to-have qualities that are being sought when questioning references.

The interviewer should convey trust early in the interview. A person who feels a sense of personal worth in the presence of another will proceed further in offering candid information. A person who feels threatened or belittled will withhold controversial or more private information and supply pat answers to questions (Beinhorn, 1985).

One way to develop trust is to listen carefully to the answers the applicant gives and to reflect back and clarify much of what was said. This shows a genuine interest in the person and what he/she has to say. Plus, it enables the interviewer to check the accuracy of what he/she heard. This technique is called active listening. In its simplest form it paraphrases what the person says. In its more sophisticated form (reflective listening) it not only paraphrases but attributes feelings or characteristics to the person:

Applicant: "I left the last two positions because I performed the same duties day after day. I wanted to learn more but my employer was not interesting in helping me acquire new skills."

Interviewer: "So you left because you weren't challenged enough."

Applicant: "Yes, that's right."

Interviewer: "And you expect your employer to help you feel challenged. Is that right?"

In the above exchange, the interviewer moves beyond parroting what the person says to "reading in" what the person is all about and what he/she will expect. This reading in is done aloud so that the applicant can respond and clarify or agree. Being accurate in assessments of a person's feelings and paying attention to the meaning behind the words builds a closeness that grows into trust.

If the interviewer is constantly wrong in his/her assessments of the applicant's statements, this could spell trouble for the two people when they work together. It may take some doing to begin to understand each other accurately, which may be quite a hindrance in a busy work environment.

The use of active listening, observation, and carefully structured questions is critical in conducting an interview. As each question is answered, new follow-up probing questions should come to mind to get at the key information being sought. For instance, following the exchange described earlier, the interviewer should ask:

"What duties did you perform in the last practice?"

"What other duties would you have liked to perform?"

"Of the duties you did perform, which ones would you want to continue?"

Suppose the applicant indicates that she does not like giving patient education to children. The interviewer can follow up with, "What was it about that function that you disliked?" or more specifically, "Tell me how you gave patient education to the children. What exactly did you do?" Listening to the description of the procedure many may offer clues to the kinds of functions this person will do well and those that will be potential problem areas. The applicant may reveal in voice tone and emphasis that working with children is difficult for him/her. Or it may be that the difficulty came from insufficient materials and time to teach an adequate program.

It is important, particularly in the early stages of the session, to conceal the expected requirements for the job. For instance, if the position requires a person who is extremely dedicated to an active preventive program, this needs to be assessed for each applicant. Suppose the interviewer says, "This job calls for someone with a strong interest in prevention. Are you interested in developing a preventive program?" Anyone who wants the job will be effusively dedicated to prevention as soon as the question is asked.

The wise interviewer will note whether there is any mention of involvement in prevention projects in the application and casually ask about them. If there is no mention of prevention in the resume, the interviewer may ask what aspects of practice the applicant enjoys most. The interviewer waits to see whether prevention is mentioned. If it is not, the interviewer can then ask more directly whether he/she has ever worked with anyone who uses a lot of preventive techniques. It is important at this point to show no signs of support for the concept of prevention—a show of mild skepticism may be in order in some instances if the interviewer suspects the applicant is less than sincere with other answers. If the interviewer is an adept listener who follows key replies with probing questions to elicit further information, a bounty of information can be obtained in a relatively short period of time that indicates whether this person is a likely candidate for the position. In order for this to happen, the interviewer has to be able to listen a great deal and talk very little (Beinhorn, 1985).

As the interview proceeds, if the applicant is meeting many of the expectations for the job position, the interviewer may begin to reveal to the applicant that certain aspects of his/her experience and philosophies are compatible with the expectations for the position. This lets the interviewee know he/she is doing well. He/she begins to relax and be more open. Furthermore, there comes a time in the interview when a desirable applicant should begin to realize that this is the job for him/her. It is up to the interviewer to ensure that sufficient positive information about the practice is revealed so that the interviewee can see the match as well as the interviewer can.

Another important facet to evaluate is the degree to which the interviewee assumes control. Does the interviewee ask questions? Are they good ones? Does the interviewee use each question to give well-thought-out information? Or does the interviewee expect the interviewer to be in full command? If the practice needs an assertive worker, those traits should be watched for in the interview. Likewise, if the employer wants a quiet, unassuming worker, those traits should be observed.

Sometimes it is necessary to have a second interview if two or more candidates are well suited based on the initial encounter. It can be helpful to have others in the practice interview the prospectives as well.

In any case each applicant should be told when he/she will hear news concering the job. And each unsuccessful applicant should be informed promptly when the position is closed.

Interviewing is a skill that develops with practice. Ways to prepare are to be a good interviewee and to observe the style and skill of the interviewers encountered. When the time arrives to conduct an interview, it is helpful to remember how it felt to be interviewed and how important it was to have a fair opportunity to perform well.

Review questions

1. What is the purpose and significance of an employment interview?
2. List four ways in which the applicant can prepare for the interview.
   a.
   b.
   c.
   d.

3. What are the four basic phases of the interview?

   a.

   b.

   c

   d.

True or false:

4. The interviewer often assesses the applicant by eliminating negative elements rather than by building positive ones. _____

5. If an interviewer misstates some item of information about the applicant, it is best to ignore it. _____

6. An interviewer who seems satisfied with little information should be allowed to leave the encounter with whatever he or she chose to learn. _____

7. An interviewer who uses a nondirective approach is probably inexperienced in evaluating people. _____

8. The angry interviewer is a lost cause. The applicant should just get through the encounter and hope for the best. _____

9. A follow-up letter should contain no more than a thank you. _____

10. List five guidelines in conducting an interview.

    a.

    b.

    c.

    d.

    e.

GROUP ACTIVITIES

1. Role play several interviews as both employer and applicant.
2. Prepare a series of "trigger tapes" showing selected segments of interview discussion. Respond to each, discussing what guidelines for the applicant and interviewer were followed or violated.
3. Discuss the probable effects the various applicant responses may have on obtaining the desired position and how well the interviewer is prepared to hire or reject the applicant.
4. Review the cover letter and resume depicted in the previous chapter. Develop a job description and at least 10 interview questions that will help you evaluate the applicant's suitability for the position. Compare questions, critiquing each question as a group until a sound series of questions is identified and agreed upon.

REFERENCES

Amsden, F.M., and White, N.P.: How to be successful in the employment interview: a step-by-step approach for the candidate, Cheney, Wash., 1974, Interviewing Dynamics.

Beinhorn, C.: The right way to interview, Savvy **6**(12):18, 1985.

Dentistry and Allied Services, 1975-76, Manpower Analysis Branch, U.S. Department of Health, Education and Welfare, PHS-HRA, Bureau of Health Manpower, Division of Dentistry.

Zunin, L., and Zunin, N.: Contact: the first four minutes, New York, 1972, Ballantine Books, Inc.

Employment contracts and establishing a contractual relationship: the role of collective bargaining

OBJECTIVES: The reader will be able to:

1. Define an employment contract.
2. Construct a sample employment contract that could be utilized in an employment agreement in a health care delivery setting.
3. Explain the reason for preparing an employment contract.
4. Describe how an employment contract can be presented to an employer for concurrence.
5. Describe the basic rights to which an employee is entitled.
6. Define collective bargaining.
7. Cite examples of professional associations that include collective bargaining as one of their functions.
8. Explain how collective bargaining for dental health care providers is different from that which is used for health care providers in group settings such as hospitals.
9. Predict the effect collective bargaining could have on dentistry.

The arrangement that an employer and an employee agree to with regard to terms of the employment is a contractual agreement. It obligates both parties in the contract to some specific duties, and it is voluntary in nature. In many employment situations there is a written statement of those terms, which both persons (employee and employer) sign and agree to uphold. However, in the majority of employment arrangements, particularly with no union involvement, the agreement is oral. In some situations it is even implied.

The typical employment arrangement between the dental auxiliary employed in a practice and the employing dentist has been the verbal, express contract. The dentist offers a certain amount of salary or commission and specifies the numbers of days and hours to be worked. He/she may request that certain attire be worn and indicate whether there is any allowance for vacation or travel to professional meetings.

The applicant for the position either agrees to the terms or requests some other arrangement. He/she may request additional benefits or indicate that certain ones offered are not of use.

Once the two parties have reached an agreement, the contract is complete. One would then assume that the needs of both persons are well defined, and all that is left is a pleasant working relationship with predictable paychecks and predictable services in return for the remuneration.

Frequently, however, the employment agreement has been so lacking in specificity that the expectations of the two parties are not matched by the performance of their counterparts. The employee may expect that sometime during the first 6 months a raise will be provided. When no raise occurs, the expectation is unmet and the employee is frustrated. On the other hand, the employer may expect the employee to assist with other duties, such as radiographic processing, records maintenance, and the sterilization of instruments and supplies, when, because of cancellations, patients are not available for treatment. When, instead, the employee moves to the laboratory for a cup of coffee and chooses to read a journal for that 15-minute period, the employer may be highly frustrated.

THE EMPLOYMENT CONTRACT

A large source of misunderstanding and malcontent in a practice environment is the unexpressed, unmet expectations of the persons involved. One way to prevent that frustration is to have a written, preplanned employment contract that directs the two parties' attention to many of the typical concerns that can cause difficulty but that rarely surface in the employment interview. To use such a form may at first seem less than trusting—particularly if the presentation of the employment contract is done in a fairly chilling manner. Many employers confronted with such a document for the first time in their professional careers of hiring auxiliaries may be quite taken aback. An employer less than pleased with the new assertiveness shown by auxiliaries in recent years may decide to change his/her mind about the employment agreement. However, if it is used with some finesse and its advantages are pointed out to both participants in the agreement, it can be a valuable mechanism.

An employment contract generally has several categories to be addressed in discussing the terms of the working agreement:

1. Title of the position and a listing of basic functions to be performed.
2. Hours to be worked and, if appropriate, days of the week to be worked.
3. Amount of remuneration to be paid for the completion of the employment activities, as well as the following:
   a. Pay period schedule.
   b. Benefits to be deducted from the paycheck according to government schedules.
   c. Manner in which remuneration is to be calculated (including the precise formula if commission, or salary plus commission, is to be used as the means of calculating the payment).
   d. Identification of who calculates the paycheck amount and whether calculations are available for evaluation by the employee.
4. Schedule of review for raises (particularly if the raises are to be based on merit) and continued employment (probationary period).
5. Method of evaluation on which the raise reviews will be based. (What outcomes are expected? What criteria will be used? Who will evaluate? What will be the form of the evaluation?)
6. Fringe benefits available:
   a. Paid days for illness or bereavement.
   b. Paid days for participation in professional activities, including continuing education.
   c. Funding of travel or tuition for continuing education.
   d. Participation in insurance programs. (What type? What benefits are included?)
   e. Participation in profit sharing? (How often? How are shares calculated? Does seniority affect amount accrued?)
   f. Participation in retirement program. (Are funds transferable to another program if the employment agreement is severed?)
   g. Availability of cost-free health care. (In the facility? Or with the physician or dentist of the employee's choice?)
   h. Paid holidays. (Which ones?)
   i. Paid vacation. (How many days? Who determines when the vacation may be scheduled?)
   j. Uniform or lab coat allowance.

k. Parking allotment.

l. Days paid when the employer is not present in the facility (if the law stipulates the health care provider may not work without direct employer supervision).

7. Opportunities for professional advancement (if any) that exist within the setting for which the employee may at some time qualify.

8. Method by which employment contract may be severed (appropriate notice, reason for severance, etc.).

NOTE: This section should address the grounds for dismissal, an important protection for an employee who could, under current labor law, be dismissed at the whim of the employer despite the abilities of the employee.

9. Specific expectations with regard to the employment situation as perceived by the parties of the contract that are not covered above.

If all nine components of the employment contract or agreement are discussed in the course of the employment interview and both persons agree to these specified terms, it is a relatively easy matter to complete the contract form and share it with the employer as a confirmation of the discussion. The form doesn't have to be used during the interview, although it is helpful to have notes regarding the key items to be discussed in hand so that each area is covered and some agreement reached. It is more tactful to make brief notes and then prepare the contract after the interview is complete. Each category can be completed with the data agreed to and typed for review. If there are categories not yet agreed to, this can serve as a springboard for further discussion of those points and, it is hoped, their resolution. Reading the document together can be quite a symbolic act in establishing the employer-employee relationship on an even, professional ground.

It will serve to remind the employer of the agreed-on elements, and it will provide the employer with the knowledge that the employee is aware of the expectations that were discussed and that they are indeed in writing (a written contract). It may not even be necessary to require the signing of the document for it to be useful. If it appears that the employer is quite willing to do so, then it can be requested. Otherwise, simply handing a typed copy to the employer while folding one's own copy for safekeeping may assure the employee of a binding arrangement.

Many readers may feel that this procedure is unworkable, that there is little reason to go to such lengths to record the verbal agreement, and that to attempt such an approach to the employment aggreement would end in early dismissal from the job. However, health care providers have indicated that once there is a sufficient number of qualified persons available for any given practice position, the employer can become unscrupulous in the hiring and firing process and maintain an employment relationship with a health care provider only until another comes along for the position who is willing to work for less.

One suggestion for improving job security is to have hygienists in a specific region agree to work for no less than a suitable range of salaries. The employment contract can help frame those areas of agreement.

A series of federal and state laws may provide some job security for hygienists between the ages of 40 and 65 years who are faced with losing their jobs. The Age Discrimination in Employment Act of 1967 specifically prohibits discrimination against an employee on the basis of age. Given that higher salaries are generally paid to older workers with seniority, the courts could decide that firing an employee aged 40 to 65 years constitutes discrimination on the basis of age.

Federal and state labor laws as well as civil rights legislation provide further rights to dental auxiliaries both at work and if they should lose their jobs. For example, the Civil Rights Act of 1964 prohibits employee discrimination based on a person's race, color, religion, sex, or national origin. Title VII of this act requires that employers maintain working conditions that are free of sexist intimidation and harassment. Finally, the Occupational Safety and Health Act of 1970 requires that every employer must furnish each employee a place of employment free from recognized hazards causing or likely to cause death or serious physical harm. Dental auxiliaries who feel that their rights have been violated in any of these areas can contact the Equal Employment Opportunity Commission or the Occupational Health and Safety Administration for advice or to initiate a grievance procedure.

Dental auxiliaries who lose their jobs are entitled to compensation from the state for up to 6 months or as long as they remain unemployed. To initiate this compensation, individuals have to register with the state unemployment compensation office in their area. These are not welfare payments. They are designed to provide a person with a minimum income until another job can be located. The employer pays a specific amount per employee into a state unemployment tax fund. When a person loses his/her job, he/she can apply for unemployment payments drawn from this fund. The employer's unemployment tax rises as the number of employees apply for benefits over time.

Job security and an awareness of employees' rights in the employment situation are relatively new in the field of dentistry, largely because of the nature of the practice of dentistry. Most dentists are still housed in solo practice settings with little or no relationship with each other. Each practice setting is an entity unto itself, and each employs a limited number of persons or auxiliaries. For this reason, the employing dentist has been able to operate with little external control in paying employees and in upholding oral agreements.

Other health care providers are often housed in large practice settings such as hospitals and are a part of a system that may use contracts routinely in specifying salary amounts, benefits, and conditions for terminating the employment agreement. This procedure simply may be practiced for administrative record keeping of employee data and job descriptions. Other times it is because the employees within that large facility have unionized and through a collective bargaining process have been able to help formulate policy that governs the amounts of salary each category of employee is eligible for and that delineates the fringe benefits and working conditions for each category of employee.

COLLECTIVE BARGAINING

Federal laws give employees the right to bargain collectively with employers to determine terms of employment such as wages, hours, and working conditions. Employees must first organize a union and have either the state or federal labor relations board hold an election to certify the union as the collective voice of the employees. Once it is certified, the employer is legally bound to enter into collective bargaining "in good faith" with the representatives of the union. The union begins the process by presenting the employer with its demands; the employer responds with his/her offer and the bargaining begins. By threatening to strike and interrupting production or service, the union can encourage the employer to be more accepting of its demands. On the other hand, a strike interrupts the regular income to employees, and unless it has a good chance of obtaining concessions from the employer, a strike can do more harm than good for the employees.

In the United States, carpenters and roofers organized craft unions in the early 1800s. By the late 1800s in the large factories that grew up during this period, workers formed the first industrial unions. However, the industrial union movement received little support from state and federal government until the National Labor Relations Act of 1935. This act recognized the employees' right to unionize and the obligation of the employer to bargain collectively and in good faith with the representatives of the union.

As a result of this legislation the number of unionized employees increased significantly and workers through the collective bargaining process were able to increase wages and benefits and improve working conditions in their respective companies (Pelling, 1960). They also caused prices to rise since the companies had to pay for the increased salaries and the better conditions. Money for higher wages was rarely extracted from company profits; rather, it was collected from the consumer in the form of higher prices. So in many ways the people working in the factories who achieved the new benefits paid for those same benefits as consumers, when they purchased the goods and services made with their own efforts. Some economists attribute the inflationary spiral in this country to the increased costs to business caused by the demands of the unions. Others blame the employers for not permitting what they consider a more equitable distribution of the wealth by absorbing more of the cost of employee benefits.

With industrial workers, and later various service persons, earning higher and higher wages, the professional people, including teachers and nurses, began to examine collective bargaining as a way of increasing the benefits they were receiving. Professionally trained individuals such as nurses and teachers were surprised to learn that unskilled workers were earning more than they. The National Education Association and the American Nurses Association examined the role of collective bargaining in professional groups and opted to support such efforts. Special units affiliated with the state constituents of those associations worked to provide union opportunities for groups of professionals who voted to be represented in collective bargaining.

It is possible to belong to the professional association without being represented in a collective bargaining setting. The separate union unit of the association provides and promotes this opportunity for members who are interested.

As previously mentioned, after a group of employees petitions the state or federal labor relations board, the board holds an election that enables the employees to vote on whether to unionize or remain nonunionized. Sometimes the election will provide employees with an option regarding which group will represent them. The American Federation of Teachers, for instance, is a union of teachers competing with the constituents of the National Education Association. Those voting to unionize may cast their ballots for affiliation with one or the other group.

Usually the employer will vigorously oppose the unionization movement, citing how such a move will reduce the quality of employer/employee relations and increase the cost to the employee because of union dues. The employer attempts to demonstrate how well the employees have been taken care of in the past and to show that unionization will not improve the quality of their benefits or their working conditions (Power, 1980). Persons striving for unionization counter these statements with statistics showing how salary levels have not achieved the levels they should and how certain persons have not been fairly dealt with in the evaluation process or in the termination of the employment agreement.

If the employees vote in favor of a union, they elect officers and, for purposes of employment contracts, become an adversary of the employer. It is infrequent that the collective bargaining sessions have been warm, sharing, pleasant encounters. Usually they take on all the characteristics of an outright fight. The union pushes for everything it can win, and the employer fights to retain every cent and every right he/she could offer the employee. It becomes a game in many instances but may degenerate into all-night sessions, strikes, professional people resorting to emotional name-calling, and a general breakdown in trust.

It *can* result in higher salaries, better fringe benefits and working conditions, more clearly defined evaluation mechanisms, and a grievance procedure to protect the rights of workers in unfair severance of employment.

Unionization and dentistry

Union organization and collective bargaining for public service workers and professionals, including teachers, nurses, and in some cases physicians, have been growing in the United States over the last 20 years. Today it is not at all unusual to read of teachers striking and closing down public schools. Nurses or other allied health professionals cut back on services at hospitals, complaining that the hospital management refuses to bargain with their agents in good faith. In 1986 physicians in Boston agreed to stop working in selected hospitals in order to demonstrate their concern regarding a 60% increase in the cost of malpractice insurance. They were demonstrating their demands that the state legislation intervene to halt the growth of malpractice litigation and protective insurance (Stage, 1986).

In contrast, workers employed in the dental industry have not organized to any great extent. This is largely because dentistry is made up of cottage industry type of practices that on the average employ fewer than four people. The cost of organizing a union, hiring an agent to represent the employees in collective bargaining, and administering the agreed-on contract would be prohibitive for a group of four or fewer employees. To be even economically feasible for the smaller practices, unions would have to be supported by or affiliated with an association such as the ADHA or the ADAA. The law prohibits professional associations from conducting union activities, so local unions would legally have to be separate (Dolan, 1980). State nurses' associations have dealt with this problem by sponsoring panels to assist local groups of nurses to establish work rules and bargain collectively with their respective hospitals. Whether a similar institutional structure might work for dental employees remains to be seen.

Another reason that dental hygienists and auxiliaries have not unionized is because most of them are women, many working part time, who do not wish to face the perils associated with collective bargaining. Even if they feel entitled to a reasonable salary and better working conditions, some women still see their salary as a secondary contribution to family income and, as such, not that important. This, of course, has changed as

women developed a different perception of their roles in the family as financially responsible members who should be adequately paid for the work they perform. Another interesting quirk in the profession of hygiene that could affect the success of collective bargaining is that many women who are dental hygienists are married to dentists and work in their offices for no salary! An employment survey of hygienists in Michigan found this situation to be surprisingly frequent (Judge and Malvitz, 1976).

There has been periodic discussion among association leaders of the need to unionize for auxiliaries to earn respectable incomes for the vital work they perform in the provision of dental care. Efforts to work directly with dentists have not proved fruitful.

What might happen if unionization could be realized for dental auxiliaries? First of all, the labor relations board would be busy conducting hearings of reported instances of unfair labor practices involving the firing of persons active in the labor movement. That is prohibited by the law, but the widely distributed settings and the subsequent unlikelihood that each case could be investigated and resolved would tempt some employers to react harshly, putting many auxiliaries out of work immediately. Some might do this because they are unfamiliar with the law governing such acts.

Secondly, the adversary relationship that would be established between dentistry and the dental auxiliaries would quickly negate many of the efforts to establish interdependent programs of mutual interest and concern. Auxiliaries have been attempting to demonstrate a new assertiveness in planning their own futures and in refusing to rely on what they see as the fatherly leadership of dentistry. This new assertiveness has in itself been met with quick, authoritarian-style rebuttals. Any headway that has been made to demonstrate cooperation and a desire to work toward common goals on a common ground could be overshadowed.

Thirdly, the success of any collective bargaining activities would certainly drive up the cost of health care. There is little reason to suspect that the dentists would be willing to absorb the cost of increased benefits from their own profit. The cost will be passed on to the consumer, as it has been in most other industries.

Dental auxiliary professional associations may be faced with the decision to unionize—regardless of whether it is a local union or a national movement. The costs and the benefits will have to be measured carefully before such a decision could be made.

The costs of unionization will be high, if collective bargaining is to be successful. Dues assessed each participating member must be sufficient to cover the cost of employing collective bargaining agents—ones who fully understand the needs of the client and who are successful at winning important benefits. When collective bargaining requires 10 hours each week for 2 months, the hourly cost of such an agent (often $100 or more) can amount to a great deal.

Dental auxiliaries may acquire a great deal of practice in decision making if this issue surfaces soon. It may well be a key issue in the decade ahead.

An interesting and related issue involves the formation of professional unions by dentists and physicians. These so-called unions have organized from time to time since the late 1970s.

However, they were not started because of poor working conditions or low salaries among dentists but primarily to resist the influence of dental insurance companies and other third-party payers on dentistry. The ADA has formally stated that "unions have no appropriate role to play for dentists," but local professional unions continue to crop up. The primary action these groups have taken is to encourage members to boycott specific dental health insurers. On at least one occasion the Federal Trade Commission has ordered a dental union to disband, calling it a front for an illegal conspiracy against dental insurers (Szanski and Hickox, 1980). In 1981 the attorney general of Pennsylvania filed suit to stop a local dental association from encouraging its members not to treat patients covered by Blue Cross dental insurance.

Obviously, the dentists see a possible benefit if they can organize and collectively negotiate with an insurance company that pays a major portion of their income. As of early 1982 the courts had not supported dentists in this type of organized effort to improve their economic well-being. However, having recognized how collective organization can be a benefit, dentists in the future may be more receptive when their employees seek to work collectively to improve their economic well-being and professional status.

Review questions

1. What is an employment contract?
2. Why is it wise to prepare a written employment contract when individuals agree to an employment situation?
3. Identify five key components in an employment contract.
   a.
   b.
   c.
   d.
   e.
4. What is collective bargaining?

5. Identify two professional associations that sponsor union activities, including collective bargaining.
   a.
   b.
6. What primary difference exists between dental care delivery and other forms of health care delivery that make unionization in dentistry more difficult?
7. What are three costs that dental auxiliaries may suffer if they elect to implement collective bargaining?
   a.
   b.
   c.

GROUP ACTIVITIES

1. Invite a representative of a local professional union to discuss the procedures involved in collective bargaining. Request information regarding how unionization has affected salaries, fringe benefits, working conditions, and the cost of professional membership.
2. Request information of the national professional associations regarding their recommendations for employment contracts. Determine whether the association has addressed the issue and if they recommend any particular format for practitioners seeking employment.
3. Outline the procedures that are followed (in detail) in organizing a union and in beginning contract formulation through collective bargaining.
4. Analyze the power sources in the collective bargaining processes of negotiations at the table, the strike, the lockout, the work cutback, and other tactics. How does each power act affect the economic well-being of the employer and the employee involved in the struggle?
5. Introduce the idea of collective bargaining at a local component meeting of the dental hygiene or dental assisting professional association. Record the responses of the group with regard to the interests they see will be enhanced or undermined by such a move.
6. Simulate the formation of a union with the group, agreeing on minimum salaries that will be accepted (upon graduation), minimum fringe benefits, and other specific employment characteristics. Analyze what could be gained by such a group agreement. Describe aloud any reasons for being reluctant to form such a group.
7. Investigate the move toward independent contracting for dental hygienists. Read the interview and articles in *RDH* 1(3), 1981, and discuss how establishing an independent contractual relationship differs from establishing an employment contract.

REFERENCES

Dolan, A.K.: The legality of nursing associations serving as collective bargaining agents: the Arundel case, J. Health Polit. Policy Law **5**:25, 1980.

Judge, S.P., and Malvitz, D.M.: The survey of dental hygiene in Michigan, Dent. Hyg. **50**:463, 1976.

Lentchner, E.: Professional unions: a counterproductive concept, N.Y. State Dent. J. **40**:406, 1974.

Pelling, H.: American labor, Chicago, 1960, The University of Chicago Press.

Power, J.M.: Guidelines for dentist employers faced with union organizational activities among their employees, N.Y. State Dent. J. **46**:500, 1980.

Stage, M.: Boston physicians strike, National Public Radio, February 4, 1986.

Szanski, A.M., and Hickox, R.F.: Capitolgram, Dental Economics **70**(11), 1980.

CHAPTER 19

Insurance

OBJECTIVES: The reader will be able to:

1. Identify the basic reason for purchasing insurance coverage.
2. Explain briefly how insurance is financed.
3. Describe the reason for and the benefits of the following:
   a. Malpractice insurance.
   b. Health insurance.
   c. Disability insurance.
   d. Life insurance.
   e. Retirement programs.
   f. Personal liability insurance.
   g. Household and other personal property insurance.
4. Describe some key variables in coverage that should be assessed in the written policy when purchasing insurance.

Insurance is an investment in security against undue financial loss in events of modern life. As individuals and as members of organizations, everyone runs the risk of financial hardship and even disaster as the result of malicious or accidental acts of others, random natural events, and his/her own activities. The purchaser of insurance is attempting to guarantee financial backing in case of certain events. His/her purchase along with those of others provides a pool of money available for use in case of such events. Insurance companies manage these investments, administer disbursements, and control the cost of the insurance according to the likelihood of the events occurring. The likelihood varies according to a number of factors.

Our society recognizes financial risk by requiring, in some cases legally, that we insure ourselves. As providers of professional services, health care delivery personnel are subject to additional risks. Errors in judgment and accidents can cause legal action and carry costs beyond what an individual can ever earn. Therefore the health care professional must consider the possibility of malpractice insurance, in addition to life, automobile, mortgage, home-owner's, and other normal coverage.

Insurance should be considered carefully. A large insurance investment against an extremely unlikely event can be a serious financial error as can the failure to be insured. It is nearly impossible for even the most self-reliant individual to operate without insurance. Thus it is important to understand the components and basic kinds of insurance.

A *premium* is the amount of money a person pays to purchase insurance. It may be paid monthly, quarterly, yearly, or at some other interval depending on the arrangement made with the carrier. The premium paid varies with the amount of coverage purchased and with the degree of likelihood the carrier will have to pay a claim.

For instance, in the case of malpractice insurance, if a dental hygienist requests $100,000 coverage (the maximum amount of the carrier would need to pay if he/she were to lose a malpractice suit with damages of $100,000 or more to be paid the plaintiff), the premium payment will be higher than for $50,000 coverage. The insurance company may charge a higher premium to a dental hygienist working in an area in which malpractice suits are frequently filed against such health care providers, since the risk may be higher. The carrier may refuse to insure a provider who has already been sued, or worse yet, who has lost a suit, because the risk is considered too great. Insurance companies advertise their services on the basis of "needed protection" and hope to attract large numbers of premium payers who will not need to file claims. To be successful they must collect enough premiums to more than offset payouts on claims. To remain in business they must insure against the possibility that premiums they collect do not cover the claims against them. State and federal regulations require that insurance companies maintain reserve funds to cover an unexpectedly high level of claims. The companies invest these reserve funds in a variety of ways and the dollars earned are used to reduce policy premiums or increase profits of the company.

MALPRACTICE INSURANCE

As mentioned previously, one type of insurance that should be considered by professionals is malpractice insurance. Purchase of malpractice insurance protects the person against financial loss from a successful negligence or technical battery suit or, with certain limitations, against a charge of breach of contract. Costs that may be covered are damages paid to the plaintiff, court costs, and attorney fees. The policy offered by the insurance company should be evaluated in terms of actions covered and maximum benefits in each cost category. Some policies maintained by physicians or dentists will also cover persons acting as their agents (assistants, hygienists, nurses, or other personnel), if both the employer and the agent are

sued. However, it may not cover the agent who is sued separately. Or the maximum benefit allotted to the agent may be relatively low. Therefore it is a wise precaution for allied health personnel to carry their own malpractice insurance. For a dental hygienist, the annual premium for $1,000,000 coverage purchased through ADHA in 1986 was $43, which most hygienists consider a great deal of security for the dollars spent.

HEALTH INSURANCE

A second kind of insurance frequently purchased by health care providers is health insurance. Health insurance protects the person against the costs of illness, usually physician's costs, hospital fees, and, sometimes, medications. The policies vary with regard to their coverage of office calls to the physician, the length of hospitalization and the daily rate that will be paid, the kinds of illness or surgical treatment, and the amount allocated to cover various procedures.

A policy may have a "deductible amount," which is a threshold amount the patient pays before the insurance company begins covering costs. It is deductible from claims paid to the insured. For example, the policy may specify a $50 deductible amount for all physician costs. If the insured person incurred $150 in covered expenses, the company, subtracting the deductible amount, would pay only $100. Depending on the policy, the deductible amount might apply only once to a specified period of time (the more common arrangement) or it might be required with each new treatment. In other policies there may be a provision in which a flat percentage of the cost is paid. If the policy specifies that it covers 50% of hospital costs, the patient will need to pay for the other half. The type of shared-cost arrangement is known as *coinsurance* or *copayment*.

Another variation among policies is the kind of services for which the insured is covered. It is important to determine which health care services are covered and which are not. Some policies cover dental care and corrective eye lenses. But the premiums are high because so many people have a need for these services, which means the carrier is going to be paying out a great deal in claims. Most policies do not cover preventive services such as physical examinations or nutritional counseling.

The dental auxiliary should ask whether a policy provides major medical or catastrophic event coverage. The cost of treatment and rehabilitation associated with a debilitating accident or a chronic disease can easily cost $25,000 or more in physicians' fees and hospital costs. Obviously, the cost can have a devastating effect on the finances of most families without insurance that covers this type of expense. Even though the probability of facing such an expense is low, the premium for major medical coverage is inexpensive, and the amount of financial security per premium dollar spent is undoubtedly a worthwhile health insurance purchase.

It is wise to carefully assess the policy to see what is being purchased with the premium cost. Policies do vary greatly. The worst time to find that out is when the hospital bills are astronomical and the benefit payments are minimal.

DISABILITY INSURANCE

Closely related to health insurance is disability insurance. When a person is ill, financial burdens of getting well are compounded when the income of the person drops or stops. There may be a certain allowance by the person's employer for sick days when the usual salary continues, but it may be financially impossible for the employer to pay full salary for 2 weeks or more. So how does a hygienist with a broken wrist earn income for the 8 weeks it takes to heal? Or what if a skiing accident strains the back muscles of a nurse so that he/she must spend an extended period in traction? What if the person is disabled for life by arthritis, a brain tumor, or an accident?

Insurance carriers do offer insurance against disability. After a certain period of documented disability, the carrier begins paying regular dollar amounts to the insured. The amount for which the

person is insured should be at least equal to the regular income of the person so that financial hardship is minimized. If the health insurance purchased does not cover medications or the cost of a home nurse, it might be wise to purchase a level of disability insurance that would cover these costs as well as providing the usual income level.

LIFE INSURANCE

The career person who has a family dependent on his or her income ought to purchase life insurance. Even if no other person is specifically dependent on the income, a person may consider purchasing insurance sufficient in amount to cover funeral costs. Such a topic is often unpleasant to consider since purchasing life insurance is an admission that the person will die. Most persons prefer to forget that fact. Young persons in particular readily scoff at the idea of life insurance, which is financially unfortunate. The annual life insurance premium of a 40 year old is a great deal higher than that of the 20 year old. By purchasing coverage at an early age, a person may secure the lower rate, which—for a so-called whole-life policy—will remain constant throughout the entire term of the policy. Furthermore, life insurance may become less available for a particular individual as his/her age increases.

There was a time when women were rarely encouraged to purchase much insurance. Typically, a family was supported financially by a man. A woman with children and no career was lost financially if her husband died leaving no insurance or only a small amount. It was presumed that the man, already the financial provider, could carry on after the death or disability of his wife.

With women acquiring greater financial responsibility in the family, two changes have occurred. The more obvious change is that women are purchasing larger amounts of insurance. The second trend is that the amounts purchased by each will be more modest, since the death of either person will not drive the family into poverty. When both earn a reasonable salary, the continued income from the remaining partner can feed and clothe the family even if one partner dies. The risk remains, however, that both partners could die, leaving children with bare essentials and little aid for educational costs if little or no insurance is provided. The orphaned toddler will require a great deal of money to survive before reaching adulthood, and the charity level of the extended family should not be relied on to provide it. The wisest route is to assess the financial needs of the greatest disaster that could strike and plan reasonable insurance coverage on that basis.

Shopping for the amount and type of life insurance to buy can become complicated for the average consumer. A detailed and recommended guide for the serious insurance consumer is *The Consumers Union Report on Life Insurance: A Guide to Planning and Buying the Protection You Need,* ed. 4, Mount Vernon, N.Y., 1980, Consumers Union. This book provides a formula for determining the amount of coverage one needs and helpful comparisons of the advantages and disadvantages of different types of policies. The Consumers Union was preparing to publish a fifth edition as this text went to press; be certain to work with the most current edition.

Two types of life insurance are available: *term* and *cash value.* Most people choose renewable term insurance over cash-value insurance because in the event of death, their benefactors receive 6 to 7 times more dollar coverage for a dollar of premiums. Term insurance is insurance that pays off only in the event of the purchaser's death. Premiums increase or benefits decrease with the insured person's age. If the policy is a renewable term policy—which is highly recommended—it can remain in effect even if the health status of the insured declines.

Cash-value insurance, which is often called whole-life insurance, is a combined savings account and insurance policy. However, the rate of return on whole-life savings is low compared to other savings plans available in today's market. For example, the return on whole-life savings held less than 5 years is actually negative, whereas the same savings invested in money market funds could return 8% to 10% per annum. The premiums on whole-life insurance remain the same throughout the life of the policy.

In spite of its limitations, cash-value insurance is purchased by a small percentage of consumers as a means of forced savings. However, in recent years commercial banks and other government-insured financial institutions are making it easier to save regularly by offering individual retirement accounts (IRAs). As will be described in greater detail later, these accounts enable savers to deposit in a tax shelter up to $2250 of income that regularly earns higher rates of return than that available from whole-life insurance. Given these alternatives, its is expected that even fewer insurance consumers will purchase whole-life policies in the future.

RETIREMENT PROGRAMS

Life insurance can provide for retirement. However, there are other retirement programs designed specifically to provide regular income after leaving full-time employment. Pension plans can be available through the employer. Professional associations may sponsor such opportunities. While retirement may seem remote to a beginning professional, its financial realities are best considered early. Social Security may provide basic retirement income, but for most people it is not sufficient for them to maintain their "before-retirement" life-style. The cost of living will likely be higher in years to come, and income should be sufficient to meet that inflation. For a savings plan to be a minimal drain on current income yet a sufficient allotment to pay for retirement living, the habit of allocating some income to retirement should be practiced as soon as employment begins. Long-range planning is essential, especially when retirement programs are not provided or encouraged by the employer.

Many employers do provide such programs. However, accruing sufficient sums may depend on longevity and continuity of employment. Some plans pay back lump sums of retirement savings when the employee changes places of employment, causing considerable temptation to spend the money rather than to reinvest it. In some pension plans the employer matches some portion of the employee's investment in retirement. That portion of the savings may be lost when employment is severed for reasons other than retirement.

There are retirement funds that are not tied to work with a specific employer. For example, Teachers Insurance and Annuity Association–College Retirement Equities Fund (TIAA-CREF) is a retirement fund for employees of educational programs accepted by numerous institutions throughout the United States. Thus employees who move from one participating school to another can contribute to the same retirement fund. Although much smaller than TIAA-CREF, the ADHA offers members a similar retirement program that enables hygienists who move or work for more than one employer to maintain a continuous savings program (ADHA, 1986).

Before the 1960s physicians were not able to incorporate their practices and gain for themselves—and their employees—the favorable pension benefits that business corporations can make available to their employees. In 1962 the Self Employed Individuals Tax Retirement Act (the Keogh Act) was passed by Congress, allowing all self-employed persons to establish a tax shelter for a limited portion of their incomes and thus to build up retirement trust funds somewhat like the corporate pension plans. The individual retirement plans authorized by the Keogh Act—often referred to by its prepassage bill number, H.R.10—were not as beneficial to employees as corporate plans, but they were a first step toward equality of treatment for physicians and their employees. To obtain the benefits of a Keogh plan, the physician is required to make contributions into the plan on behalf of all employees as well.

Several changes have been made to the original Keogh Act since its passage, making the self-employment plans very similar to the plans which are allowed to corporations. Initially, the maximum contribution a person could make under a Keogh plan was $2500 annually, with only half of that deductible on income tax. The Employee Retirement Income Security Act (ERISA), the Tax Reform Act of 1976, the Economic Recovery Tax Act of 1981 (ERTA), the Tax Equity and Fiscal Responsibility Act of 1982 (TEFRA), the Deficit Reduction Act of 1984 (DEFRA), and the Retirement Equity Act of 1984 (REA) modified the law making self-employment an attractive alternative to incorporation.

Starting in 1984, dentists, physicians, and other sole proprietors and partners were allowed to contribute up to $30,000 to a qualified plan. The actual allowable amount for an individual is calculated by taking 25% of earned income (gross earnings minus business deductions) minus the amount contributed on that amount prior to passage of TEFRA. For instance, $25\% \times [60,000$ (earned income) $- \$12,000$ (pre-TEFRA contribution)$] = \$12,000$.

The full amount put into the retirement plan is deductible. Therefore, if the sole proprietor is in the 50% tax bracket, the contributor can be spared $15,000 in taxes (50% of the $30,000 maximum contribution). The amounts put into the plan are not taxable until the money is withdrawn from the plan, usually in increments after retirement. The person's income is naturally lower after retirement, so the tax bite is less. In addition, the interest earned on the contributions is tax free.

If the plan is terminated or if the person receives a lump sum at a certain age (usually 65), the tax laws allow the person to roll over the entire sum into an individual retirement account (IRA), without a tax penalty.

Beyond the basic deductible amount (up to $30,000), a self-employed person can also elect to contribute an additional $2000 to the Keogh plan or to an IRA. This amount is raised to $2250 if the self-employed person has a nonworking spouse. Thus, the total maximum amount that can be set aside without short-term taxation is $32,250.

As a result of these provisions, self-employed persons can rapidly accrue tax-free money. Because less short-term out-of-pocket tax is paid while the working income is high and subject to a greater percentage tax, additional amounts of cash are available for contribution to the retirement plan. Depending upon the person's income, his/her age when the plan commences, interest rates, and the age at retirement, substantial savings for retirement can be generated.

Until 1984, the Keogh Law required that all employees with 3 or more years of service in an employment setting be vested in the plan, if a Keogh plan was available to an owner-employee. The TEFRA changes eliminated that requirement. Plans no longer need cover all employees with 3 years of service. Usual corporate vesting rules apply. TEFRA changes also state that if a plan provides for 100% vesting (full participation) after 3 years of service, the employer can defer participation until an employee has put in 3 years of service. Thus an employee receives no retirement accrual until having demonstrated longevity in the organization. The law also states that persons within 5 years of usual retirement age do not have to be included in the plan.

Certain requirements must still be met in order for a Keogh plan to be qualified with regard to employee vesting. The employee must be able to receive the normal retirement benefit upon normal retirement age. In other words, the employer cannot withhold the amount due. Also, all of an employee's accrued benefits (based on the *employee's* contribution to the plan) must be nonforfeitable; they cannot be denied to the employee. The *employer's* share of the accrued benefits can be withheld based on years of participation in the plan. The IRS has specific rules to prevent discrimination against lesser-paid employees and has specific rules to test the qualifications of the plan (How to, 1985).

Participation in such a plan as an employee can be a major benefit, particularly if the employee expects to work in that setting for an extended period. Sizable amounts can be accrued for retirement depending upon the size of the contribution, the matching amount contributed by the employer, interest rates on the investment, and years of contribution to the plan.

Individuals who are not covered by a retirement plan (and even those who are) can establish an Individual Retirement Account (IRA) and contribute a maximum of $2000 per year, or $2250 if the person's spouse is not working. When both the husband and wife work, each person's contribution is calculated separately for a maximum contribution of $4000. The amount contributed can be deducted from taxable income; taxes are paid when the individual begins to receive retirement benefits (usually on a lower tax base) or if the person withdraws the sum prematurely (an unwise practice in terms of taxes since there is a 10% penalty for early disbursement). Withdrawal from the account must begin no later than the taxable year during which the individual reaches 70.5 years of age (*U.S. Master Tax Guide,* 1986).

Between the possible qualified Keogh plan contributions and IRA contributions, an employee has the opportunity to shelter considerable income and accrue investment income for retirement. Such plans should be thoroughly investigated with a qualified planner who can review current law and recommend the most advantageous steps. The related laws have changed several times in the early 1980s and can be expected to change again.

The tax laws were under revision by the legislature in 1986. The tax shelters provided by these plans were being challenged. Consult a tax advisor to determine current law and rulings before investing.

PERSONAL LIABILITY AND PERSONAL PROPERTY INSURANCE

There are other kinds of insurance that persons may wish to purchase regardless of their employment status. One kind is personal liability insurance; the other is household and personal property insurance. Often the two will be included in one policy. Personal liability covers a person against damages for having harmed another person or property through negligence—outside of professional activities or the use of a motor vehicle. The person who falls on the snowy path left unshoveled or the person who falls in an unmarked trench in the front yard may incur harm for which the property owner must pay.

Such policies may also pay for damage to the insured's house caused by fire, wind, flood, or other natural disaster. Coverage can be purchased for loss by theft. Usually a comprehensive householder's policy covers all these needs related to the home. Also, many people just entering a career do not realize how much it will cost to replace personal property if an apartment burns. A renter does not need to have insurance on the dwelling itself but will need coverage on contents. Coverage can include burglary and vandalism, but it can be expensive in city areas in which such incidents are frequent. Automobile insurance packages also may cover liability, theft, and damage related to the auto. Savings can sometimes be realized by purchasing all personal liability and property insurance in one package. Once again it is important to read what is covered and under what special circumstances, what dollar limits are imposed, and whether there is a deductible or percentage of coverage clause.

PURCHASING INSURANCE

Virtually anything can be insured if the purchaser is willing to pay the premiums. The important point is to decide what risks the health care provider should or should not be willing to take in terms of potential financial loss. In the areas in which a risk-come-true is devastating, it is probably wise to purchase coverage.

Some forms of insurance (malpractice, health, disability, life, and retirement) are often available through professional associations at lower premiums than would be available through individual plans. The ADA, ADHA, and ADAA offer major medical, term life, and professional liability insurance to their members.* When a large group of people is purchasing insurance, the carrier can usually offer the coverage at a lower cost, because marketing costs are lower than if the company were to sell to numerous individuals. A large source of potential insured persons may lead to a large number of premiums. Professional associations take advantage of this fact and offer package group insurance benefits to members.

Insurance coverage is frequently a negotiable item for fringe benefits. It may be wise to accept insurance as a fringe benefit in place of some monetary compensation. A side benefit is that tax laws may exempt the dollars spent on insurance benefits by the employer from taxation as income to the employee. Tax laws are constantly changing and should be consulted for the current applicable provisions. There may be some tax advantage for the employer. It may be wise to investigate whether such provisions could be implemented and discuss this with the employer.

Regardless of what procedures and special packages are available, it is in the interest of a career person to establish financial security. Insurance is one way of accomplishing that.

---

*More information can be obtained from The American Dental Association, 211 E. Chicago Ave., Chicago, IL 60611; the American Dental Hygienists Association, 444 North Michigan Ave., Chicago, IL 60611; and the American Dental Assistants Association, 666 N. Lake Shore Dr., Room 1130, Chicago, IL 60611.

Review questions

1. What is the basic reason for purchasing insurance?
2. How can an insurance company afford to pay the insured amount when a claim is filed?
3. List seven kinds of insurance coverage that may be purchased.
   a.
   b.
   c.

d.

e.

f.

g.

4. Describe why each of the above kinds of coverage might be a reasonable purchase for a health care provider.

a.

b.

c.

d.

e.

f.

g.

5. Identify three key variables that should be kept in mind in assessing policies when an individual purchases insurance.

a.

b.

c.

GROUP ACTIVITIES

1. Invite an insurance representative to discuss various insurance programs, including the options available in policies, how claims are paid, and how premiums are determined.
2. Define personal needs for insurance and compare several policies that could provide coverage. Select the policy that best meets the stated needs.
3. Compare regular individual commercial coverage and rates for insurance with comparable coverage and rates available through a professional organization package.
4. Investigate IRA programs offered by local banks, and project how beginning such a savings program can affect current tax savings and long-term security.
5. Invite a tax consultant to explain how an employee is vested in a corporate retirement plan and in a Keogh plan.

6. List your rights and responsibilities as an employer and as an employee under both plans under current law.

REFERENCES

American Dental Assistants' Association: Personal communication, 1986.

American Dental Association: Personal communication, 1986.

American Dental Hygienists' Association: Personal communication, 1986.

How to make the most of Keogh plans, pension and profit sharing, Bulletin 14, Section 2, Englewood Cliffs, N.J., 1985, Prentice-Hall, Inc.

U.S. Master Tax Guide, Chicago, 1986, Commerce Clearing House.

PART FIVE

Organization management

Every member of an organization has an obligation to help the organization in which he/she works be effective in achieving its mission and be an enjoyable place for people to work together in harmony. This is true whether the work site is a dental practice, a school, a hospital, a health care maintenance organization, or any other place where a career leads.

The obligation takes on a new meaning if the member becomes a leader or manager within an organization. The new manager has a major responsibility to the organization that includes good judgment and action in:

- planning,
- organizing,
- directing,
- controlling, and
- communicating

while continuing to use his/her technical expertise.

The manager needs to be able to deal with the technical aspects of management including operations, facility design and utilization, problem solving and decision making, management information systems, finance, and marketing.

He/she also needs to be able to work effectively with people, inspiring dedication to the mission and tasks, resolving conflicts, recognizing and reducing stress, encouraging and using good interpersonal skills, and developing team effectiveness.

This section provides a rudimentary introduction to these aspects of management with three goals in mind:

1. The development of an understanding of what one's manager (or boss) must do in order to effectively assist an organization, no matter what its size or mission.
2. The development of a personal sense of responsibility for the well-being and development of one's work group when one is in the role of an employee.
3. An introduction to the areas of skill and responsibility a career move into management could require.

CHAPTER 20

The basics of management

OBJECTIVES: The reader will be able to:

1. Describe the purpose of planning in managing an organization.
2. Differentiate *mission, organizational goals,* and *project objectives.*
3. Write an organizational mission for a dental office and a set of related goals.
4. Given an assignment to plan a project, list specific, measurable, time-based objectives and work assignments that will ensure the attainment of its overall goals.
5. List eight components of good organization.
6. Given a project plan, develop a chart for organizing the efforts of the project team.
7. List seven important functions the manager performs when directing a project or work activity.
8. Describe how "controlling" fits among the management functions.
9. Identify a list of problems, select the most critical problem, and construct a "fishbone" diagram identifying contributing factors.
10. List five guidelines for planning a meeting.
11. Conduct a meeting using the basic guidelines for meeting management.
12. Explain why it is important for a manager to have technical expertise in the area he/she is managing.

PLANNING

An organization relies on good planning for its continued existence. Planning is deciding in advance what must be done in the future (Gaskins, 1985; Numerof, 1982). Members of the group need to take the time to determine what needs to occur, what steps are necessary to bring about the desired result, and who will do what, with which resources, in order to carry out the steps and evaluate progress. Such planning occurs when any family, church group, school, agency, professional practice, hospital, corporation, or country needs the direction to keep moving or to bring about a specific change.

The first key to organizational effectiveness is effective planning that keeps the people working together with a reasonable sense of direction, timing, and harmony.

Not all planning is effective. Some is too late. Some is accomplished when aiming at less-than-ideal purposes. Some is poorly designed, so that the wrong people are doing certain tasks or so that resources are squandered. Most poor planning is probably due to a lack of overall purpose, or to poorly articulated goals and objectives.

Good planning is more likely to occur when the leaders and the followers have a good sense of the overall mission. In other words, the people know why the organization exists, what its overall aim is, and what major accomplishments make it successful (Gaskins, 1985; Numerof, 1982). A business may have as one of its goals the earning of money; an additional mission may be the production and distribution of a high quality product that improves the lives of people who purchase it. The business is saying something about itself if the

177

former or the latter of these two aspects of its mission is more important or essential to the planning and decision making of the business.

A dental office provides another example. A mission could be to provide high quality care; to bring prevention and self-help to every patient; to provide complex, reconstructive dentistry to patients with serious problems; to provide comprehensive care for children or handicapped persons; to provide low-cost, conservative care; or any other focus that a professional practice sees as fundamental to its existence. The mission statement should clearly define the overall purpose or orientation of the practice. This will make it much easier to define projects and programs with specific goals and objectives that fit with the mission. It helps people understand what is important and work together to achieve it (Numerof, 1982).

Once the mission is defined, the organization members need to decide what needs to be done to achieve that mission—to make it come true. This is done by specifying projects and programs that fit with the mission, with measurable, realistic goals and objectives delineated for each (see Fig. 20-1). For instance, a dental practice that has decided to alter its mission to include meeting the needs of the handicapped has determined that it has three important projects to carry out before the mis-

Fig. 20-1. Relationship of mission, goals, and objectives.

MISSION: Overall purpose for the existence of the organization; one or several emphases within the organization that makes it special among all other similar organizations.

GOALS: Concrete outcomes that fit with the mission and that suggest changes, projects, or ways of handling everyday business

OBJECTIVES: Specific statements of performance that are time-based and measurable that lead the group participants toward achievement of the overall goals and the fulfillment of the mission

---

sion is possible. One is the physical alteration of the practice and the equipment so that patients can have access to the treatment areas. A second is hiring personnel who are eager to work with the handicapped and who perhaps have experience with their needs. A third is informing the community of the availability of this special service.

When the planners specified what the overall outcome should be (i.e., a practice that attracts and appropriately cares for handicapped persons, increasing the number of patients in the practice by 20%), they then brainstormed all the possible things that could and should be done in order to achieve that overall outcome. Alternatives were discussed, constraints or limiting factors identified, and a "best" procedure specified. Fig. 20-2 details the goals and objectives associated with each. Notice how (1) the goals for each project fit with the overall mission, (2) the objectives delineate how the goals can be met, and (3) each of the objectives is specific, measurable, comprehensive (taking into account its impact on other areas of the practice), and time-specific.

Notice also that associated with each objective is an assignment to those who will carry out the tasks, and a target for when the tasks are to be completed. Notations regarding how the objectives and the overall goals will be measured should be included and referred to at each step of the plan. Any project requires specific assignments and specific ways to evaluate success, or the best-laid plans will fail or lead to a less-than-ideal result.

Taking the time to carefully plan a project makes its implementation easier. Steps are clear, obvious roadblocks are anticipated, resources are identified, and a timetable is posted to which project participants can refer.

One important note about planning is that many leaders take full responsibility for planning and then simply delegate the functions to employees. While this certainly speeds up the process, it denies employees the opportunity to contribute as thinkers as well as doers. Employees can improve a plan by offering ideas, projecting outcomes, volunteering for responsibilities, and watching its

MISSION: To provide high-quality preventive and therapeutic dental care to adults and children, especially those with physical and mental impairments. To maintain a busy, productive practice that earns the owner and each employee a good living.

PROJECT GOALS: To prepare the practice to accept handicapped persons
To draw sufficient numbers of the handicapped population that the size of the practice patient pool rises 20%

PROJECT OBJECTIVES: To redesign the current office to accommodate handicapped persons.
1. Consult with designers familiar with such needs
   • Call local hospitals, universities, design agencies to determine who is skilled in this area (M. Taylor, Week 1)
   • Meet with design experts individually to select an appropriate team, individual (G. Govalle and M. Taylor, Weeks 2-3)
   • Review and coordinate plans with dental equipment personnel (G. Govalle and M. Taylor, Weeks 5-7)
2. Change appointment scheduling to accommodate renovations (N. Derring, Weeks 6-7 for weeks of renovation)
3. Monitor renovation orders and construction (M. Taylor, Weeks 6 through completion [7-8])

To hire two additional personnel (1 dental hygienist, 1 dental assistant) to work with the handicapped patients
1. Prepare advertisements for local newspapers and regional dental journals (N. Derring and G. Govalle, Week 1)
2. Develop interview application form and screening procedure (N. Derring and G. Govalle, Weeks 1-2)
3. Contact dental and dental auxiliary programs for recommendations for appropriate staff (N. Derring, Week 3)
4. Review applications, make interview appointments (N. Derring, Week 3)
5. Interview applicants (G. Govalle, N. Derring, M. Taylor, Weeks 4-6)
6. Select new employees (N. Derring, G. Govalle, M. Taylor, Week 6)
7. Orient/train new employees (M. Taylor, Week 8)

To draw new patients into the practice who need special services due to a mental or physical handicap
1. Prepare news releases for local newspaper (G. Govalle, Week 5)
2. Contract for photographs of renovations in process and at completion (N. Derring, Week 5 for Weeks 6-8)
3. Prepare announcements to send to physicians, centers for the handicapped, senior centers, local service organizations (G. Govalle, Week 5)
4. Send announcements (N. Derring, Week 6)

EVALUATION: Target for completion is 8 weeks; facility should be renovated, staff should be hired and ready for new patients; all appropriate media should be used to announce the new availability of the services for special needs patients.

Fig. 20-2. Relationship of planned project to mission, goals, and objectives.

Fig. 20-2. cont'd

Facility must allow ready access for special needs patients.

Facility must be workable, allowing good traffic flow and ensuring good space utilization.

New employees should have background in work with handicapped persons as well as being skilled as dental personnel and able to work well with the team.

Two new patients should be added each week due to special referrals and to the news publicity; overall rise should be 20% within 6 months.

CONSTRAINTS: Availability of consultants and construction personnel to complete the project on schedule

Cost of renovations

Ability to easily remodel current facility to accommodate handicapped personnel

Financial loss while renovation occurs due to lost practice time

Availability of interested, qualified personnel for new positions

Salary requirements of new personnel

Interest of community in supporting the special target of the practice

Response of current patients to the change in the practice focus

Space availability of local media to cover the project

Time required of current personnel to carry out the projects while carrying normal full workload

Consider: Lengthened time-line

Adding a temporary worker to carry a portion of the team's workload during project implementation

Finding temporary quarters to provide dental care while the office is under renovation

Conducting the bulk of promotional and personnel hiring/orienting during the time the facility is being renovated

---

progress. Involving the people who will carry out the plan enhances their feeling of "investment" in its success. While not every program calls for such involvement, this is an important aspect of planning that is often indicated (Gaskins, 1985).

Not all planning is related to major projects such as those described above. Planning is also part of the day-to-day operations of a practice. People plan how appointments will be scheduled, how a recall system will work, how to bill patients, how to manage a day's activities, and how to sequence procedures within a given appointment. Regardless of how large or small the task, planning makes the subsequent steps flow smoothly and gives the members of the group a predictable direction for their work.

Clearly, planning is the main function and skill of a manager who does more than shepherd the status quo. Being a good, consistent planner who

can forecast what the future will (or should) look like adds the dimension of *leadership* to management.

ORGANIZING

Once the plan is defined, the detail work of organizing the project becomes paramount. Organizing "is the process of grouping the necessary responsibilities into workable units, determining the lines of authority and communication, and developing patterns of communication" (Massie, 1979). It is not enough to lay out the hoped-for outcomes. Someone needs to take responsibility for:

- identifying a complete sequence of tasks,
- specifying contingency plans for each step,
- assembling the appropriate staff to carry out the tasks, matching work assignments with workers' strengths and interests,

- ensuring the availability and organization of resources (budget, raw materials, consulting or agency assistance, etc.),
- using appropriate, established lines of communication for information and decision making,
- specifying when activity and outcome reports are necessary,
- establishing tracking methods for task completion and outcome measurement,
- delegating authority for decision making to people who carry responsibility for various aspects of the plan.

In large organizations, where more than a few people (sometimes hundreds) are involved in project implementation, organizing is an awesome responsibility that requires considerable skill and attention to detail. Tracking diagrams known as PERT (Program Evaluation Review Technique) charts or CPM (Critical Path Method) charts are frequently used to organize the efforts of several segments of an organization so that they are well-timed and coordinated (Liebler et al., 1984).

Fig. 20-3 shows an organizational tracking chart to follow the implementation over an 8-week period of all three plans mentioned in the section on planning. Notice that the projects are being carried out simultaneously (rarely does one project operate in isolation of others) and that the people carrying out the projects are often working on more than one at a time. The chart defines who is doing what and when. This tool is extremely valuable in organizing how tasks will be accomplished. A good practice is to develop such a chart when the plans are organized and post it for everyone's reference. As contingency plans become necessary, they can be entered on this chart along with changed assignments, time lines, etc.

DIRECTING

Once the start date comes, someone needs to be in charge of directing the project. It may be the same person who was in charge of planning and organizing, or it may be a person who has inherited those plans. In its simplest terms, the directing manager makes certain that people are doing what is best to help the group meet its objectives. The directing manager follows the plans outlined in the organizational phase and helps the team of workers carry out the steps in the plan.

Assuming that the people who are to carry out the tasks have been identified in the planning and organizing phases, project direction ensures that these people have the training and orientation needed to perform their assigned functions. This is particularly important if a worker has new responsibilities. If there are vacancies or new positions identified, the directing manager must define the skills that are required and secure persons to fill those roles.

Project direction includes making fair assignments. No person should be overburdened while others carry a light load. In addition, the director should observe how tasks are being carried out, participate in doing some of those tasks, and coach the workers on improved work methods that help people "work smart." A good manager helps people find ways to improve their performance and asks for their suggestions on how work methods can be made easier and more productive.

When a problem arises, a good manager asks people who are directly involved with the task for suggestions and an analysis of the problem before attempting to solve the problem. The manager should have and use sound logic in listening to problem analysis and selecting among the possible solutions. He/she should also have good skills in creative problem solving that use nonlinear approaches to identifying and sorting through a problem and its remedies.

Additional management direction involves gaining cooperation among the individuals working on a given task and among individuals working in different departments or on discrete tasks. People involved in different phases of a project need to feel that they are all working toward the same goal and that they should help and encourage one another. The good manager fosters open, constructive communication. For instance, the

Fig. 20-3. Project tracking chart

Project	Week 1	Week 2	Week 3	Week 4	Week 5	Week 6	Week 7	Week 8
Office redesign	Call local resources for design experts (MT)	Meet with design experts (GG & MT)			Review, coordinate plans with dental equipment personnel (GG & MT)	Change appt. scheduling (ND)	Monitor renovation orders and construction (MT)	Orient/ train new hires (MT)
New Personnel	Prepare ads (ND & GG) Develop application and screening procedure (ND & GG)		Contact dental education programs for recommendations (ND) Review applications, make appointments for interviews (ND)	Interview applicants (GG, ND, MT)		Select new employees (ND, GG, MT)		
Attract new patients					Prepare news releases (GG) Schedule photos for weeks 6-8 (ND) Prepare announcements to send to physicians, centers, etc. (GG)	Send announcements (ND)		

manager in the dental practice which is expanding to include handicapped persons should encourage staff members working on the planning for physical changes in the practice layout to suggest pictures to be included in a new advertising brochure for distribution at hospitals. Their interests and ideas can be shared more fully while maintaining good morale.

A good manager follows up on decisions and questions and makes timely inquiries and adjustments. It does not help to review a suggested change in wording or photos in a flyer a week after it has been sent to the printer.

Also, decisions regarding task implementation should follow and support the organization's policies and decisions. Changes should not undermine the original intentions and desires of upper management or the planning committee. However, a good manager does work to adjust policies and decisions that hamper productivity and cooperation.

CONTROLLING

Project control is closely aligned to project direction. Control involves carefully comparing project plans and decisions with actual work-group progress. For obvious reasons, there should be a great deal of similarity between what was planned and what gets done. Work-group achievements should be compared with the targets that were set and the standards that were to be met.

For instance, is the final design for physical renovation completed on time? When the work is completed, does the carpentry, plumbing, floor covering, and all the other details match the agreed-upon specifications? Controlling involves asking these questions during the project in addition to at the end of the project. It requires monitoring work as it progresses, matching expectations with the observed progress of each phase of the overall job.

Once again, the good manager asks the project workers what they think of the progress being made and how well the outcomes match their expectations. People working with the project or those who will rely upon the changes being made will have good opportunities for close scrutiny as the project unfolds.

Several organizations use quality circles for problem solving and evaluation (Goldberg and Pegels, 1984). The workers gather in small groups to list current inefficiencies and obstacles to productivity. They agree upon the most troublesome problem and focus on it. They use "fishbone" diagrams to detail all the contributing factors that bring about the problem. The workers then use measurement techniques to quantify the current status of each of the contributing factors to establish a baseline. The workers set a goal for improving that certain condition and implement changes to alter each contributing factor, one at a time, until the problem diminishes and a different problem can be tackled (Deming, 1982; Ishikawa, 1980).

Fig. 20-4 shows a fishbone diagram used for problem identification and analysis in a dental office. Notice that the dental team identified seven current problems that need solving. One problem, time overruns in dental hygiene appointments, was selected as being the most critical; it became the focus (the head) of the fishbone. All the little fishbones detail how factors within the practice are contributing to the problem of a poorly kept schedule.

Table 3 shows how three contributing factors affected time overruns, measured at baseline and at weeks 2 and 3, after changes were made in appointment control procedures for the dental hygienist.

COMMUNICATING

An important, ongoing function of effective management is ensuring accurate, timely, caring communication through every stage of project management and in day-to-day work activities. None of the good things that should come about from good planning and organizing will be easily accomplished if the plans and directions are not communicated.

The good manager explains decisions, plans, problems, needs, and feelings thoroughly to the

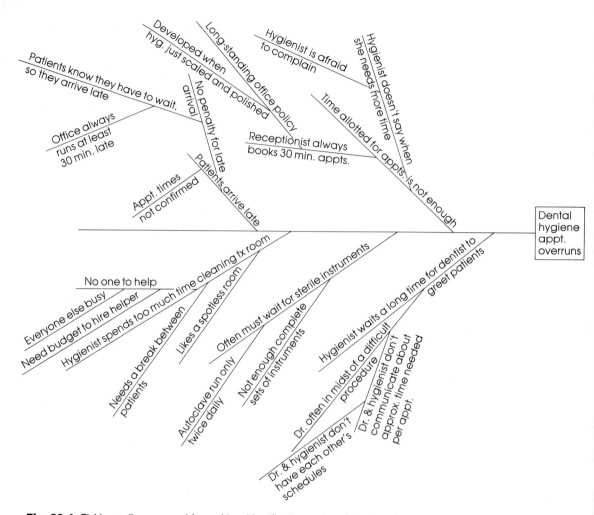

Fig. 20-4. Fishbone diagram used for problem identification and analysis in a dental office.

Table 3.

	Baseline	Week 2	Week 3
Doctor time*	18 min	12 min	6 min
Appointment schedule accuracy†	45%	68%	88%
Time spent in operator preparation‡	6 min	4 min	2 min

*The number of minutes (average per appointment) the hygienist waited for the dentist to leave her patient and greet the hygienist's patient.

†The percentage of appointments scheduled within five minutes of the actual time it took for the hygienist to provide care for the scheduled patients.

‡The number of minutes (average per appointment) the hygienist spent cleaning and setting up the treatment room for each patient.

people who work with him/her. Sound management requires careful clarification of policies, plans, and procedures when workers are uncertain why they are to work a certain way. Workers need to be told what they have to know in order to do their work. Closely related is the necessity of providing reliable, timely information regarding the organization, its goals, policies, and plans as they change with external and internal needs. Most plans are not static; they are altered in sometimes subtle but critical ways when some unexpected change or factor indicates an alteration is needed. Workers need to know what these changes are and why they are happening.

Most project communication is on a one-to-one basis as the manager observes how the tasks are progressing. But a method used nearly as frequently and perhaps with greater effectiveness is the group meeting. Depending upon how fast a project is moving along, a task-group should meet for a 1 hour progress-and-regroup meeting for major decision making weekly or every two weeks. These can be reserved for major decision making if there is a brief (5 to 15 minutes) "stand-up" progress meeting every day where all people on a task gather together to discuss short-term project progress and assignments.

Planning and conducting a meeting require specific skills. Without these skills the meetings are unproductive, boring, and may produce anger. Regardless of the time required for a meeting, the manager calls the meeting, sets a time and place, makes certain all the necessary people are invited, describes the purpose of the meeting, lists the proposed agenda, and starts the meeting on time (Metzger, 1981).

Managing a meeting requires a special set of skills. The leader should *open the agenda* for possible additions but must take responsibility for limiting the agenda to the topics that are appropriate for the time and setting.

The leader *opens the discussion* with brief announcements and a review of the activities of the day (for the stand-up meeting) or overall status on the project (for lengthier decision making and

project review meetings). The leader then *asks for and waits for* comments, suggestions, and questions. The leader needs to *accept questions and comments* readily, without becoming defensive or jumping on a person who has trod on the "thin ice" of a project. Workers need to be encouraged to candidly discuss work-related problems and plans.

The leader should play a major role in *clarifying* what the questions and comments mean to ensure accurate interpretations. The leader should also accurately figure out what a person is feeling as he is contributing to the meeting. Is it a cool, objective observation? A joyful evaluation of a major accomplishment? An angry commentary on poor performance? The leader will need to clarify the accuracy of those interpretations and then *decide what to do* in response to the feelings as well as the content of the message. The members of the group, in many instances, should be contributors in deciding what action should follow.

A person in distress should receive careful attention and not be left to suffer alone in the meeting. A person who is celebrating a major accomplishment should receive the manager's and the group's encouragement and support.

The manager needs to recognize when the work group is not getting along and then develop a strategy to help the group acknowledge this fact and resolve it. If such strategies are beyond the ability of the manager, he/she needs to know enough to get help in how to plan and implement such an intervention. Likewise, the manager needs to help people confront one another when there is a problem and use sound methods of giving constructive feedback (see Chapter 22).

Basic interpersonal skills are vital. They include such common-sense habits as making eye contact with a person when speaking and listening, stopping what you are doing when someone is talking to you, showing respect for what another person says and feels, and caring about the well-being of each person, regardless of whether or not you share agreement with his/her comments. People who sense a sincere interest, con-

and respect will follow and accept manage-
more readily than those who sense
___ erest, paternalism, or distrust (Metzger,
1981). This will be discussed further in Chapter
22.

In addition to using astute group management
and listening skills, the manager needs to attend
to the progress through the agenda and move the
group along, sticking to the initial time frame and
making certain that critical topics are discussed
and decisions made.

EXPERTISE ON THE JOB

Another fundamental aspect of being a manager
is knowing *how* to do what the workers are doing,
in addition to knowing *what* they are doing. A
manager needs to know what it is like to perform
the functions of the people being supervised, otherwise helpful input and direction is sparse. If a
person is promoted to a management position, often it is because he/she did exemplary work in the
department and is being recognized for that service. People in that situation need to learn management skills. However, often a person who has
no particular skills in an area is made manager
because he/she is good at planning, organizing,
etc. That person's responsibility is to learn, as
quickly as possible, the procedures and overall
functions being performed by the work-group he/
she is supervising. Credibility with those being
supervised rises and falls with technical expertise
and the empathy and understanding that come
from that awareness.

FOLLOWING THE MANAGER

The basic skills of management—planning, organizing, directing, controlling, communicating,
and using technical expertise—form the backbone
of successful change and organizational develop-

ment.* This is true in any organization, be it a
small dental practice or a 700-bed hospital. The
successful manager needs to develop skill and
judgment in each of these areas. Development can
come from additional coursework, opportunities
to manage projects with appropriate guidance,
and observation of managers as they go about
their jobs. Not all role models are good managers.
Therefore, a person who aspires to be a manager
can learn by identifying the strategies and habits
that work and those that fail. The learner can develop good judgment by assessing what he/she
would do differently and why a certain strategy
worked well or failed.

In the meantime, a person who is interested in
becoming a manager, or someone who intends to
be a loyal follower for years to come, can help a
project along by being an ally to the manager and
other group members rather than a hindrance.
Good followership includes:

- doing one's job to the best of one's ability
  (giving 110% in effort and attention),
- pointing out alternative strategies to the manager while showing due respect to that person's skill and feelings,
- assisting co-workers in solving work-related
  problems,
- listening carefully to the ideas and feelings of
  co-workers and the manager,
- helping the manager move meetings along
  successfully by helping summarize major
  points that have been made, staying within
  time guidelines for agenda items, knowing
  when to drop an issue, and clarifying misun-
  derstandings between the manager and a
  group member.

---

*Fayol, 1949; Gaskins, 1985; Liebler et al., 1984; Numerof,
1982

Review questions

Effective way to plan for the future

1. What is the purpose of planning in organizational management?
2. Label each of the following as *mission, organizational goal,* or *objective:*
   a. To provide readily available dental care to the elderly. ___mission___

b. To increase the number of patients who have meticulous preventive home care.
Goal

c. To schedule at least 85% of all patients due for recall within the month they are due for an appointment. _Objective_

d. To establish a bonus system for employees who perform in an exemplary fashion.
Goal

e. To reduce accounts receivable by 35% within 6 weeks. _Objective_

f. To develop a staff which has outstanding technical skills and enjoys working with people. _goal_

g. To increase the dental health awareness within the community. _mission_

3. Organization is a primary function of good management. What are eight of its components? _P. 180-81_

4. Assigning people to specific tasks, coaching people to work smart, solving work-related problems, and encouraging cooperation among workers are a few of the tasks a manager performs while _directing_ a project or daily work activities.

5. A _fishbone_ diagram is used as a tool in helping a group identify problems and their causes.

6. List five guidelines used when planning a meeting:
   a. _call the meeting_
   b. _set a time & place_
   c. _invite the right people_
   d. _describe the purpose & list an agenda_
   e. _start the meeting on time_

7. Why is it important for a manager to have technical expertise in the area he/she is managing? _p. 186_

GROUP ACTIVITIES

1. Analyze how the family "manages" a major activity that requires planning, organizing, directing, etc., and report how each of these functions was delegated and to what extent family members were involved in the management and implementation of the project. Examples: Thanksgiving Day activities, a vacation, going out to dinner, redecorating a room, doing the laundry, planting a garden, buying a car.

2. Write an organizational mission for the group (class, study club, component) which states in simple, direct terms the purpose of your group.

3. Given a mission, such as the one prepared in activity 2, identify one major goal that the group should accomplish in order to make the mission a reality. Specify measurable, specific, time-based objectives that will help the group achieve the goal.

4. Given a mission, a goal, and a set of objectives, divide into groups of five people, and plan and organize how the goal can be achieved.

5. Take turns leading the planning and organizing meetings, using the guidelines described in the text. Critique each other's meeting leadership techniques, offering constructive suggestions for improvement.

6. Identify a problem facing the group and prepare a fishbone diagram that specifies the contributing factors that cause the problem.

7. Observe meeting leadership and problem-solving techniques used in nondental groups, e.g., church or synagogue, civic organizations, volunteer groups.

REFERENCES

Deming, W.E. Quality, productivity, and competitive position, Cambridge, MA, 1982, Massachusetts Institute of Technology, Center for Advanced Engineering Study.

Fayol, H.: General and industrial management, London, 1949, Pitman. (Translated from the 1916 French publication.)

Gaskins, L.E.: A primer on dental practice management, Reston, Va., 1985, Reston Publishing Co.

Goldberg, A.M., and Pegels, C.C.: Quality circles in health care facilities: a model for excellence, Rockville, Md., 1984, Aspen Systems Corp.

Ishikawa, K. Guide to quality control, Tokyo, 1980, Asian Productivity Organization.

Liebler, J.G., Levine, R.E., and Dervitz, H.L.: Management principles for health professionals, Rockville, Md., 1984, Aspen Systems Corp.

Massie, J.L.: Essentials of management, ed. 3, Englewood Cliffs, N.J., 1979, Prentice-Hall, Inc.

Metzger, N.: Communications. In Metzger, N., editor: Handbook of health care human resources management, Rockville, Md., 1981, Aspen Systems Corp.

Numerof, R.E.: The practice of management for health care professionals, New York, 1982, AMACOM.

CHAPTER 21

Technical management skills

OBJECTIVES: The reader will be able to:

1. Summarize the five steps in problem definition.
2. List the five steps in problem solving that follow problem definition.
3. Arrange in order, from authoritarian to laissez-faire, examples of decision-making strategies.
4. Identify three variables that are critical in deciding how much decision-making authority to give workers.
5. State the cardinal rule if decision making is to be shared with workers in varying degrees depending upon the situation.
6. Define a flow of work for a sequence of tasks.
7. Explain how time and motion analysis can help improve work flow and productivity.
8. Given a space configuration, dimensions, and a number of work spaces with their dimensions, draw a facility that meets the basic criteria for good design.
9. State six criteria for a well-designed dental office.
10. List the four primary management information systems that should exist in a dental practice.
11. Describe the role of computers in management information in a dental practice.
12. Differentiate *marketing* and *advertising*.
13. Describe the steps for implementing a marketing program in a dental practice.
14. Describe the consultant's role in the technical management of an organization.

Technical management skills are skills that help the work team operate efficiently and effectively once a plan is in place and the basic goals, objectives, assignments, and evaluation schemes are established. The manager needs to know how to make daily operations and special tasks work more smoothly by standing back and observing

- how work progresses,
- what physical barriers are impacting the flow of work and what resources are being used,
- what information needs to be collected,
- and how the quality work of the organization can be presented in a way that will encourage consumers to seek out what the organization offers.

Overlaying all of these responsibilities is the ability to define problems, solve problems, and make decisions. These are skills integral to all of the other functions of management presented in this section of chapters.

DEFINING PROBLEMS

Careful planning reduces operations problems, but even the careful planner spends time sorting through and solving problems that were not anticipated or that arose despite the best efforts of the team. Therefore, being able to identify and solve problems is a key skill that a good manager must have.

Many people err by spending time attempting to solve problems before they even know what the problems are. Some people try solving problems that don't even exist! People are often too quick to assume that a problem has occurred and that they know exactly what it is.

The good problem solver *listens* to what is going on in the organization. Some people refer to this ability as having finely tuned antennae that pick up complaints, notice slowdowns, detect errors in quality, and sense distraction or dissatisfaction. Thus, rarely is the good manager sequestered in some remote office, unaware of the daily functions of the organization. He/she is on the job, helping, watching, asking, evaluating, and supporting.

A good manager knows there is a problem brewing, preferably before the conditions are so obvious that he/she practically trips over it. The good manager does not discount or ignore a problem, hoping it will go away. He/she at least monitors the problem for a day or two to gather more information and see if conditions change. If the manager does not see an obvious problem that someone else has brought up, or there is an uneasy feeling in the pit of the manager's stomach, he/she had best attend to problem definition.

The steps in problem definition are (Fig. 21-1):
1. Identify the *feeling* (anger, fear, worry, depression, frustration, tension), especially if the problem is elusive to begin with.
2. Specify the events or circumstances that bring about that feeling, naming as many as possible and being as concrete as possible for each.
3. Fit the events together so that the source(s) of the problem can be identified; gather information.
4. Try to work from the obvious sources backward until the real roots and nature of the problem are more certain.
5. Once there are three or four hypotheses identified about the problem, take time to validate those hypotheses by watching the work group in operation and by asking for the opinions of those working with and around the problem; formulate the problem (Schein, 1969).

An example of a problem in a dental office that was defined this way is a slow but steady increase in accounts receivable—the amount of money

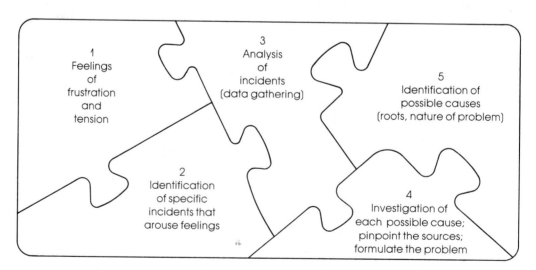

Fig. 21-1. Problem formulation.

owed to the practice by patients who had not yet paid in full.

The office manager noticed that despite the fact that productivity was up and prices for the goods they purchased to keep the practice running were stable, there was less and less cash available to pay the office bills. The manager first noticed it as a sinking feeling she got when she would reach the last of the checks that needed to be written. There just wasn't as much in reserve. So she sat down with the financial reports of the past 6 months and noticed that accounts receivable had risen from a very healthy 4% to 4.8%, 5.4%, 6.0%, 7.5%, and 8.2% in each of the following months. She showed the figures to the owner-dentist and they began to speculate what the problem could be. They listed five possible causes of the sudden change:

1. The new receptionist was not encouraging people to pay immediately after their visits.
2. Statements were not being prepared accurately so people were delaying payment or paying less than their full owed amount.
3. Overdue accounts were not receiving follow-up from the billing clerk.
4. The general downturn in the local economy was making it difficult for people to pay their bills.
5. People were dissatisfied with the care they were receiving and were withholding payment.

The manager and the owner agreed to investigate the problem further by watching how the receptionist handled exiting patients, by spot-checking statements being sent, and by examining the billing clerk's records about delinquent follow-up procedures. They agreed to examine the last two possibilities if their earlier investigations were fruitless. The observations continued for about a week, with everything working smoothly. The manager decided to meet with the staff to ask their opinions. She presented the problem, explained what she had done to try to investigate its causes, and presented the results. Then she said, "Why do you think the accounts receivable percentage is up this way?" After about a minute of silence (which seemed like 10 minutes) and 10 minutes of speculation, the receptionist said that she "really hates to bug people for money when they are leaving," but she forces herself to do it when the manager or the other staff are listening. Thus, the real problem was identified—or at least a contributing problem. The manager spent time in the following weeks coaching the receptionist on how to ask politely and how not to feel guilty about it; the manager told the receptionist that if she really felt uncomfortable with that role she could move into a different position in the practice.

It could have been that the problem would continue to worsen even if the receptionist was able to ask for payment. It could have been that it was not the real problem. Therefore the manager monitored the accounts receivable closely for several more months. The problem had been identified correctly.

It is possible that a different manager would not have taken as much care or time in defining the problem. A different manager may have assumed the cause and acted to correct it—leaping from assumed problem identification to immediate problem solving. Such a leap may have caused more problems than it solved, which is frequently the situation when a manager acts impulsively without good investigation.

PROBLEM SOLVING

As soon as a problem is recognized and there is some concurrence or corroboration among team members that the real problem has been uncovered, the manager then moves on to problem solving, which has its own set of steps. In the example above, the "solution" eventually arrived at was for the manager to work with the receptionist to help her. But how did they arrive at that solution? They followed this sequence (Fig. 21-2):

1. They brainstormed a variety of steps to take in order to solve the problem.
2. They analyzed the likely outcomes of each of those suggestions, looking for the new problems each "solution" would create.

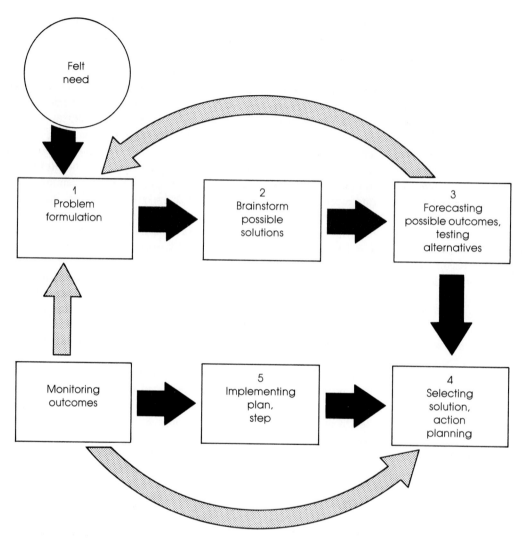

Fig. 21-2. The problem-solving cycle. (Adapted from Schein, PROCESS CONSULTATION: ITS ROLE IN OR-GANIZATION DEVELOPMENT, © 1969. Addison-Wesley, Reading, MA. Fig. 5.1. Reprinted with prmission.)

3. They selected the solution that was the most likely to target the problem while creating few new problems, and planned action.
4. The action was implemented.
5. The outcomes were monitored (Schein, 1969).

The "solutions" they discarded included moving the receptionist into a different role and having someone else (the dentist, the manager, or the assistant) tell the patients to please pay; telling the patients ahead of time (on their appointment reminder cards) what their charges would be and asking them to bring their checkbooks; and having a form prepared on which the receptionist could simply write down the fee and pass it to the patient silently.

Most of the solutions probably would have created new problems—the receptionist feeling like a failure, the need to train someone all over again if the receptionist were relieved of that role, the complication of having a different person relay the fee amount, the impersonal nature of the reminder card or the silently passed charge. So the group chose to have the manager help the receptionist feel comfortable with her task. Eventually she did.

These problem identification and problem solving steps can be used in everyday life. They often help sort out complicated problems and point the direction for good solutions. They are essential skills for managers and should be practiced until they are second nature. They will be put in use daily in most managerial positions.

DECISION MAKING

Decision making is, of course, closely related to problem solving. It is a part of problem solving, but is also a part of planning, organizing, directing, controlling, and communicating. It shares center stage with problem solving as an essential skill for managers.

Decision making involves weighing alternatives, looking for the good and bad outcomes likely to accompany each alternative, and selecting a path to follow that is most likely to yield good outcomes and few bad by-products. Decision making ensures that contingency plans are in place if the path selected proves to be unsatisfactory. Good decision making should not lead the organization into a box it cannot escape.

The way in which decisions are made is highly reflective of a person's leadership style and his/her overall attitude toward co-workers. At one end of the continuum is the authoritarian, a person who never consults the workers and who believes they generally have little to offer to decision making. At the other end is the laissez-faire leader, a person who lets the co-workers make the decisions as a group and who believes that co-workers are essential to making good decisions and should have that authority. In between are

democratic leaders, managers who structure the input of co-workers and who recognize that certain decisions require more worker input than others (Katz and Kahn, 1978).

Each decision to be made has a proper place on the continuum. There are some decisions that should be made unilaterally by the manager; there are others that should have worker input but still be made by the manager; and there are others that should be made by the workers as a group decision.

Time is a major function in selecting a strategy since the more group input obtained, the more time will be required. A second major factor is *compliance* since the more the group input obtained, the greater the probability of worker agreement and eager compliance with the decision. A third factor is how much *control* the workers should have over a given decision. If the manager carries major responsibility for the outcome, giving away decision making control is ill-advised.

For example, a dental office manager decided how much control the workers should have over each of the following decisions in this way (Tannenbaum and Schmidt, 1958):

Make the decision and announce it: bonus distribution for the quarter, change of banking institution

Make the decision and ''sell'' it: new benefits package

Present ideas and ask for questions: new location for practice

Present tentative decision subject to change: new equipment for sterilizing instruments

Present problem, get suggestions, make decision: update recall system, vacation scheduling for coming year, layout for new office

Define limits, ask group to make decision: new surgical soap, schedule for computer in-service training

Permit workers to function on own and make decision (with a few limitations): plan holiday party, select colors for their work areas, update emergency-response protocol

While not all managers would agree with the assignment of each of these decision areas, it should be apparent that decisions that just should not have much input were reserved for the manager, while others that could benefit from group input were introduced to the workers with varying amounts of freedom to decide.

A cardinal rule for a manager who chooses decision making based on the nature of the situation is that the *workers must be informed, from the start, of the extent of their control* for each situation. Otherwise, the workers may function as though they have some control and then learn they do not. This creates anger. Conversely, if they do not believe they have much say, they will not expend much energy to come up with good suggestions. Fledgling managers, and authoritarian managers experimenting with more participation from workers, experience such failures regularly if they are not clear about their intentions and if they do not give the team sufficient time to think, discuss, learn, and carefully decide. The new manager may think he/she has a group of impossible followers. The authoritarian may revert to old ways, having proven to him/herself that the team really doesn't have the ability to help make decisions. It takes group members time (sometimes weeks) to understand what the manager wants and that they have input that is valued and used.

OPERATIONS: WORK FLOW, TIME AND MOTION

A good manager can describe in detail the flow of work performed by the people he/she manages. The flow of work is the series of activities that occurs from start to finish in delivering a service or producing goods. It is the process that people follow; it is the sum total of everything that happens to the person receiving the service (consumer, patient, or client) or to the raw materials that are transformed into some usable item for purchase.

The flow of work in a dental office includes how (1) the phone is answered when a patient calls for an appointment, (2) the appointment is scheduled and confirmed, (3) the dentist or hygienist prepares for treating the patient, (4) the equipment and room are prepared for the patient, (5) the patient is greeted and treated, and (6) the patient is given a later appointment, billed, and dismissed. Clearly, the dental office is an organization comprised of smaller subsystems that make the whole organization work smoothly. Patient care doesn't just happen; it occurs within an organized, well-planned environment (Cooper and DiBiaggio, 1979).

One of the manager's functions is to set up and monitor the work flow. Once the subsystems are planned, usually with the help of the people who will implement them, the manager watches to see how they function.

Two variables that are scrutinized when monitoring the flow of work, which go beyond how hard and well people are working, are the physical arrangement of work (such as work layout and facility design) and time and motion (the complexity and time consumption of movements people must make in order to accomplish a task).

An example of a work layout problem that could be encountered in a dental office is the instrument cleaning and sterilization work flow. The instruments flow from the treatment rooms to the area where they are cleaned, packaged by tray setup, sterilized, and allowed to cool. They are then moved back to the treatment rooms as stock for future patients. This can work smoothly or it can be a time-consuming, bottled up, inefficient, unreliable fiasco.

Problems could include: (1) instruments accumulating in the sink instead of being moved to the cleanup area, (2) instruments that are inadequately cleaned requiring repetition of the cycle, (3) bags that are not large enough to hold an entire tray setup, (4) an autoclave or oven that is not large enough to handle the flow of incoming instruments, (5) the sink being across the room from the autoclave or oven, (6) bags that are stored out of reach, and (7) no one being assigned the task of restocking the instruments in the treatment rooms. A good manager would watch the work flow of instrument sterilization, identify these problems, and work with the team to identify solutions, such as using instrument cassettes, finding larger and more efficient instrument cleaning and sterilizing equipment, relocating the equipment and supplies, and making clearer work assignments.

The study of work flow includes time and motion evaluation, often termed work simplification. Its ultimate goals are to provide the highest quality care with the most efficient utilization of the resources available to the team for the ultimate benefit of the practitioners in terms of fatigue reduction, longevity in practice, and increased income (Kilpatrick, 1974). An additional important benefit is the reduction of the cost and fatigue factors of procedures for the patient.

The objective is to increase overall productivity. However, this is not accompanied by hurrying through the procedures at breakneck speed. Time and motion management seeks to reduce delaying factors and improve the usefulness of energy spent (Kilpatrick, 1974). The increased efficiency must not diminish the quality of care; likewise it must not depersonalize the practice so that it takes on an "assembly line" atmosphere (Roberts et al., 1977). It is a systems approach to what happens in the facility viewed in terms of increments of activity: Who will perform the procedure? How long will it take to perform? Where will the procedure take place? The systems approach analysis determines the following:

1. Which team member with which skill level is performing the procedure.
2. The number of motions made.
3. The function, distance, and complexity of each motion.
4. The amount of time needed for each motion.
5. The surrounding environment that has an effect on the procedure's efficiency, such as:
   a. Illumination and color of area.
   b. Sound control.

A reasonable sampling of health care procedures is necessary to focus on each person's contribution in terms of time and motion (Kilpatrick, 1974).

In a typical dental examination, for instance, the analysis starts with which of the team members ushers the patient to the operatory, prepares the patient for dental care, obtains needed supplies and records, enhances the patient's comfort by making friendly conversation and by determining the patient's primary needs for this appointment, and performs the procedures such as medical and dental history, blood pressure and other vital signs, soft and hard tissue examination, dental examination, periodontal assessment, and nutritional assessment. These various steps may involve several different members of the team or only one or two. The analysis should point out when highly skilled personnel could delegate particular functions to other personnel without jeopardizing care or patient comfort yet improving efficiency (Cooper and DiBiaggio, 1979). It may also point out which procedures could be sequenced so that the number of providers involved is reduced.

Each of these providers is assessed in terms of the total *numbers of motions* carried out during the examination. Each motion is categorized as a *transportation* motion, an *inspection* motion, an *operation* motion, a *storage* motion, or as a *delay* (waiting for something else to happen) (Kilpatrick, 1974).

Then each of those motions is categorized in terms of *complexity.* Motions involving walking from one area to another are most complex. The entire body is physically moved from one area to the other, drawing on the energy of the person. Walking from the door to the dental chair, then to the sink 6 feet away, and back to the dental chair is an example of how complex movements are related to transportation motions.

A slightly less complex movement would be walking to the dental chair, being seated, swiveling on the stool to the sink (located much closer), and swiveling back to the table. Swiveling from one position to another involves less energy and less stress than walking to a position 6 feet away.

Stretching to reach supplies and twisting at the waist are only slightly less complex movements. They place considerable stress on the body and can result in extreme fatigue if they comprise a large portion of the day's activities, particularly if those positions are held for long periods of time. Holding a mouth mirror inside a patient's mouth while twisting around to reach supplies is an example. Supporting a weight while leaning is another.

Simply bending at the waist is less complex than bending at the neck. The "hanging" or "drooping" head can place considerable strain on the neck muscles, which can cause genuine pain. The bending at the waist seems to be more easily maintained for long periods, particularly if the spine is kept straight, and an abdominal support can be used to limit the acuteness of the angle and to ease the stress of leaning forward. Placed just below the rib cage, the abdominal support facilitates body posture and balance.

With the body in a basically static position (such as seated in an operator's stool at the side of a dental chair) with good posture and balance, other movements can be assessed in terms of complexity.

Arm movements can become the point of focus. The greater the distance of arm movement and the more arm muscles involved, the more complex the movement. Movement from mouth to instrument tray is more complex than moving the instrument from the lips to the teeth. Reaching up is more complex than reaching downward. Lifting a foot to a pedal is more complex than sliding it to the side.

Time and motion management assesses all these movements for complexity and then adds the dimensions of distance and time consumed. Having even a rudimentary knowledge of these components helps a manager sharpen awareness of weaknesses in work productivity and plan changes.

See Fig. 21-3 for an overview of time and motion advances over the past 40 years.

FACILITY DESIGN

Generally work flow problems can be solved readily if the team cooperates and financial and time resources are available to fill in equipment and training gaps. It is usually more difficult to solve facility design problems. They may involve major renovation, with plumbing and electrical changes, relocation of walls, and the subsequent need to redecorate. Such changes cost money both directly and indirectly. The indirect costs come from lost practice time while the facility is under renovation.

Leaving an inefficient facility as it is, however, has its costs as well. A poorly designed facility results in increased fatigue, loss of privacy, irritating noise, a feeling of crowding, traffic hazards in busy aisleways, and a sense of disorganization that affects the patients' view of the entire organization. Regardless of the quality of care being delivered once the patient has found his/her way to the proper treatment room, if the office is a designer's nightmare, the impression will be tainted.

The general guidelines for a well-designed dental facility include:

1. *Allow adequate space for heavily trafficked areas; conserve space in other areas.*
2. *Areas that are used by patients, such as treatment rooms, the reception desk, and rest rooms, should be located near the main entry so that patients do not need to travel great distances past areas that are not used by patients.*
3. *Noisy areas, such as the dental laboratory and central sterilization, should be located away from patient treatment and reception areas.*
4. *Areas used frequently by workers, such as sterilization or film processing, should be centrally located.*
5. *Less frequently used areas, such as the doctor's private office or the staff lounge,*

1940s

patient seated upright

clinician standing

no assistant at chairside

tray of instruments high over the patient's lap; at standing height

single-ended instruments

saliva-ejector for passive evacuation of oral fluids

cuspidor rinse procedure

slow-speed handpiece for all procedures

1950s

add: an assistant on the same side of chair as clinician, mixing materials and passing instruments

add: instrument pass copied from medical surgery (two-handed)

add: high speed handpiece and high volume evacuation

1960s-1980s

patient seated in supine position

seated operator/clinician (usually behind the patient's head)

seated assistant on opposite side of chair

contour chairs with easy adjustments

tray of instruments located behind patient

equipment located within reach of seated operator/assistant

tray, counters, and equipment low enough for seated access (2'' below flexed elbow)

double-ended instruments

standard instrument positions on the tray

one-handed instrument pass and retrieval

increased use of high volume evacuation; reduced use of cuspidor (often replaced with a funnel attachment to high volume suction)

use of more than one assistant for specific procedures

OUTCOMES: Less time per procedure and greater productivity; less fatigue for clinician, assistant, and patient; less physical strain on neck, arms, back, and legs; better contamination control

Fig. 21-3. Time and motion changes in dentistry.

should be located away from treatment areas.

6. *Rooms should be arranged so that staff and patient privacy are preserved.*

With these six guidelines in mind it is possible to review a floor plan and a study of traffic flow and generate modifications in the design, which can have significant impact on the utilization of time and energy.

Refer to Fig. 21-4 and begin an analysis of the location of each component and the overall design of the facility in terms of traffic flow. By using the six guidelines it is relatively simple to detect several traffic and space utilization problems.

The "frequently used" operatories are located near the back of the facility, whereas the laboratory, which requires little if any access to the source of patients, is located close to the reception area. Therefore patients are constantly ushered past the laboratory on their way to the appropriate operatory. The providers or other personnel have to pass by all the operatories and all the arriving patients as they move to the laboratory. And the noise usually generated by laboratory equipment can be quite fatiguing and annoying.

The sterilization area is located at the far end of the facility. Fortunately there are only three operatories that require supplies from that area. If there were more, the location of "central" sterilization would present quite a bottleneck by virtue of its remoteness and the narrow pathway in front of it, which would be a doubling-back point for people who received supplies to move back to an operatory. Also, its location across from the facility's private desk area could pose a serious distraction for personnel attempting to concentrate.

Then, of course, there is the reception area and the business area, which receive the heaviest traffic. The reception area has furniture lining the walls so that the patients sit and look at an open area. Persons sitting on the couch against the wall near the door may be in the awkward position of attempting to avoid tripping persons moving into the facility. People will be passing in front of them for as long as they are seated on that couch.

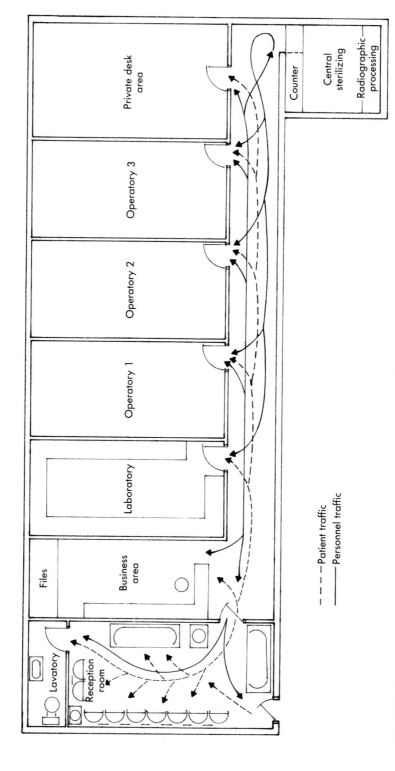

Fig. 21-4. Design of space is causing traffic problems.

There is little if any privacy or space for persons who need to concentrate on forms, records, and receipts.

Although the linear design of the facility severely limits the number of ways in which space can be utilized, several relatively simple changes in design could result in less annoying traffic and better access to the most heavily used areas. Consider the remodeling suggestions in Fig. 21-5. By simply changing the access to the lavatory and moving the locations of the private office area and laboratory, the traffic flow and noise control can be greatly improved. Plumbing and basic structures such as supporting walls and mechanical spaces can be left unaltered. All traffic must continue to flow up and down the same aisleway, but there should be fewer head-on collisions since personnel and patients do not need to encounter each other as often, now that their respective areas are more separate.

Personnel moving to the lab need not pass by all operatories and arriving patients. Patients moving to the private office area for case presentations and consultations need not travel the full length of the corridor. And it is no longer directly opposite the noise of the central sterilization area.

With even greater effort and cost, traffic flow can be enhanced even more significantly. Fig. 21-6 shows how two portals of entry can be made to the operatories by reducing the unused space at the ends of the operatories and by creating a second hallway for personnel traffic.

The business area now has a partitioned section for paperwork requiring concentration. Consultations can be scheduled for this area as well, allowing personnel to have a private area at the rear of the facility. And the reception area no longer has a hazardous or boring seating arrangement.

With relatively few modifications, the floor plan has created a more open environment, too. Instead of high walls and hinged doors, operatories are basically open on one side except for attractive, smooth-operating folding "walls" that can be closed to ensure privacy. These expanding walls allow easier access for handicapped patients and permit easier movement of equipment.

Fig. 21-7 depicts one of the facility's operatories before redesign. The storage area in the lower-left corner contains most of the supplies used for each dental appointment, but it is positioned too high for easy access by the seated assistant or operator. The one sink is located at the opposite corner of the room at standing height. The assistant and operator must stand in line to use it before the beginning of care. And then there will a squeeze play to fit into the corner space allotted to the seated assistant and operator. If it is necessary for the assistant to leave the operatory, there will be another scramble and squeeze. The storage under the counter in which the sink is located is accessible to the operator with a rather restricted swivel on the chair.

What is most obvious is the limited space allocated to the operating team. One probable reason this is such a common problem in facility design is that space is measured with the patient's chair in an upright position, rather than in the fully reclined position it will be in during the appointment. As the chair reclines, the center of activity is increasingly moved back from the site of the chair base, so what appears to be plenty of space is quickly lost as the operator, assistant, and instrument tray cart center around an area approximately 3 feet back from the chair base. The high intensity light, used to illuminate the oral cavity, is often positioned for use over the chairbase, making it a common problem that the light cannot reach to a point directly over the supine patient.

Even with slightly decreased square footage to allow for the second aisleway, it is possible to reposition equipment in the operatory to improve space utilization and access to equipment. See Fig. 21-8 for the improved design. Two sinks at "seated" height are installed to facilitate the team beginning procedures with minimal delay. Supply storage and counter tops are lowered and more accessible. More working area is provided for the seated team. The dental light is track mounted on the ceiling so that it can reach the mouth even when the patient is in the supine position. The patient enters from one door; the operating team enters from the other.

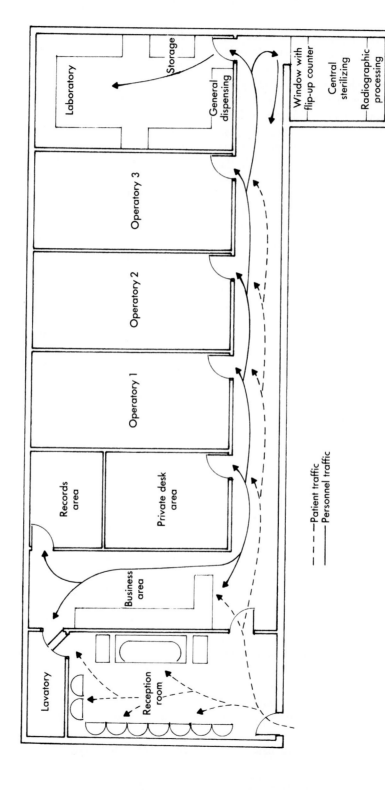

Fig. 21-5. Moderately improved traffic flow (simple modifications).

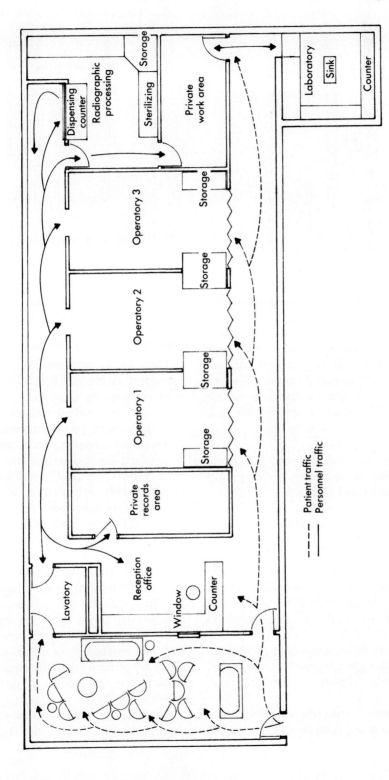

Fig. 21-6. Significantly improved traffic control (structural modifications).

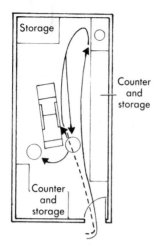

Fig. 21-7. Typical operatory unit.

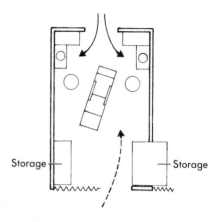

Fig. 21-8. Modified operatory unit.

With the improved floor plan and operatory design, the number of footsteps (and therefore time and energy) are reduced. People are less likely to be trying to occupy the same space at the same time. Concentration (and productivity) will improve as a result of increased privacy. And the relative positions of space should improve the comfort of the office. It will appear less cluttered, cramped, and busy, yet will be more productive.

Sound control may be better since the laboratory is away from the operatories. Folding walls that absorb sound rather than reflect it will also lessen noise.

Acoustical ceilings and carpeting on the floor (except in the laboratory and in operatories where mercury and nitrous oxide will be used) will reduce noise as well. Having background music masks sounds also; however, it is of little value if it creates a new kind of din or if it is so slow that it is soporific or so fast that it causes people to feel rushed.

There should be fewer instances of people running into each other and tripping over obstacles, thus reducing those elements of stress considerably.

In the operatory setting the complex movements of moving to and from the sink, twisting to reach, and stretching upward toward supplies are replaced by simpler swiveling motions.

ENVIRONMENTAL FACTORS

The color of the rooms can be brightened or modulated as needed. Studies indicate that yellows and oranges warm the atmosphere, bright red causes the blood pressure and anxiety to rise, and blues cause people to cool off and slow down. Green seems to provide the right element of comfort, but it soon becomes boring. Many color experts find that green used as a basic color is readily accepted when accented with red or orange. Darker colors are more depressing and conducive to uncleanliness, whereas pale colors are cheerier and offer an incentive for cleanliness.

The general rule is to use cool blues in sunlit rooms and warm yellows and orange in rooms with no natural light or where windows face north.

Colors can have a significant impact on the patient's perception of the practice and thus can affect their willingness to return. Colors can also affect the productivity of the team members, who become less productive if they feel bored, stressed, or cold.

Another environmental factor that affects productivity is overall room light. Dimly illuminated areas cause eyestrain, fatigue, and headache. The ratio of overall room light to the intense intraoral light should not exceed one to four. So it will not help to simply brighten the intraoral light to make up for low room lighting. This ratio should be kept in mind when removing fluorescent bulbs as an energy saving effort. Removing too much candlepower may greatly reduce efficiency as well as consumption of electricity.

Fluorescent lighting is the most commonly used source for work areas. An important factor to consider is that fluorescent lights flicker, sometimes nearly imperceptibly. Still, the flickering can cause considerable eyestrain and thus increase worker fatigue. When using fluorescent lights, two or more tubes that are phased to counterbalance the natural flickering should be used. This one simple change can result in significantly better performance, particularly in areas where there is a tendency for considerable glare (Roberts et al., 1977).

The temperature in the work area also affects performance. Air temperature, air movement, temperatures of surrounding surfaces (that is, walls, ceilings, floors, and machines), and the relative humidity in the area work together in creating the relative comfort of the personnel. The degree of discomfort can range from a vague annoyance to near agony, depending on the severity of the thermal regulation disturbance. Room temperature should be comfortable, the heat generated from nearby equipment should not be more than a few degrees different from the overall temperature in the room, air should be moving but not noticeably, and the humidity should be maintained at between 40% and 50%. Dropping below this percentage causes dehydration of the mucous membranes.

With even a rudimentary understanding of how to assess energy factors such as complexity of movements, frequency of movement, distance traveling, space needs, noise and color control, and proper illumination and temperature, it is possible to assess a health care facility and recommend modifications that can reduce stress and improve productivity. Such factors are of tremendous importance when any facility is being designed. Careful review of traffic patterns, accessibility of supplies, and equipment and space needs should precede construction, or the providers may find themselves in a shiny, new, miserably inefficient facility.

INFORMATION MANAGEMENT

The more complex an organization, the more information there is to gather, process, and report throughout the work group. In most organizations, managing information is a major task that is often supported by computers. Whether the information management system in the organization is accomplished manually or by computers, there are several components that will require managerial attention.

The most important source of information in a dental practice is the *dental record*. It contains the vital information regarding each individual—health status, dental history, treatment plans and outcomes, and often their financial history with the practice. Selecting a clear, thorough dental record is paramount in a dental practice. It must fit with the expectations of the clinicians and be comprehensible to more than one provider of care. All the dental records must fit into a filing and retrieval system that is logical and defies human error. Systems that combine color coding with a numeric or alphabetical system are less likely to camouflage misfiled charts.

Surrounding the main focus of dental care (the dental patient's individual record) are other information needs: *scheduling* (which patients are scheduled to appear at what time to see whom for how long in what treatment room for what procedure), *productivity* (how much of what services is produced in what amount of time by whom and with what quality), and *finances* (how much income was produced in what amount of time by whom with what direct and indirect costs and with what collection rate). Related to these main information needs are correspondence, inventory systems, accounting, tax reporting, recall systems, warranty and maintenance records, and clinical information (research reports, continuing education courses, journals, study club notes).

A manager's task is to ensure that each category of information is gathered according to a specific method. Some data should be obtained daily (finances, scheduling, productivity); some per appointment (patient record); and some as used (inventory) or on a weekly or monthly basis (clinical update). Data are then stored in raw form until they are needed; they are then assembled into reports directly related to the manager's needs. Some reports are routine while others are prepared only upon request. Reports should be reviewed before filing (a simple, but often broken rule). If the report contains information that requires action, it should be entered onto the next meeting agenda or otherwise handled by the appropriate person.

A computer can handle all of these information needs. Patient records, appointment schedules, recall schedules, financial reports, productivity reports, correspondence, inventory control, and even clinical information can be stored and processed by a computer into routine reporting. In some offices, members of the staff work with terminals that allow them to update information throughout the day. Computerized systems have cycles of reporting that describe the activity of a given time period. In some instances, activity is compared to that of a previous period.

Given the parameters of a patient's appointment needs (e.g., 45 minutes on a Tuesday or Thursday after 9 AM), the computer can search its appointment "book" for the next available place that fits the criteria and schedule the patient. It can produce a list of patients for confirmation, complete with telephone numbers. It can produce a day sheet for each provider or treatment room that shows the times, names, and procedures to be performed.

The manager is often the one to select the computer hardware (equipment) and software (the programs that make the hardware work the way you want it to). There are many computer systems

available for dental offices. Some have all of the features described above; some have only one or two features. The best way to begin evaluating computer systems is to identify what reports you prepare now that you must have and what reports and functions you would like to have. List all the management tasks you and your staff perform regularly (Bonner and McKenzie, 1986).

Visit other dental practices that have computerized systems. Listen to their comments about what works and what they wish they had. Sit down at a terminal and make a few entries if they will let you. See how difficult it is by testing how many key strokes are needed, how much prompting is on the screen, how easy is it to err, and how difficult is it to recover (Bonner and McKenzie, 1986).

Set aside at least a day to visit the commercial exhibits at a major regional or national dental meeting where the vendors can be found. Spend time with each vendor describing what you need and asking what they have. Take time for a demonstration. Gather up all the written information they have and identify which vendors provide a package that closely fits your needs within the general range of your financial resources. "Ballpark" prices are acceptable at this stage as long as you include hardware, software, supplies, and maintenance.

When the field is narrowed to two or three, zero in on costs, maintenance agreements on software and hardware, installation time, conversion plans and costs, and training for staff who will use the equipment. Some software packages include follow-up support which includes program corrections or replacements. Be certain you know how your vendors support you and what they charge. Negotiate and go with your best package. Be prepared for challenging times. Conversion from manual systems is not simple. When members of the staff decide they may like the manual system better, you can have another problem. And there will be bugs. No system is perfect, but most can improve dental practice management considerably by storing information, making it readily available, and by providing more reliable, regular reporting for evaluation and decision making.

MARKETING

Marketing is a dirty word for many members of the health professions (Perich, 1983). Mention the word, and they see neon signs, promises of painless dentistry, cut-rate dentures, green stamps, and a demeaning of the profession. This perception comes from the agelong injunction against advertising that was found in the professional's code of ethics until the late 1970s when the Federal Trade Commission outlawed prohibitions against advertising. Despite the change in the law and code and a gradual change in attitudes, many professionals still cringe at the mention of advertising and, by extension, marketing (Majewski and Shapiro, 1984).

Despite the professional's negative response to the word, successful professionals are successful marketers. Marketing is presenting one's goods and/or services (the whole package) for the public in such a way that people are drawn to the image, the attitude, the location, the convenience, the price, the quality, the cleanliness, and the long-term outcome. Marketing is the sum total of what a business person does to make what he/she has to offer match what the prospective clientele wants (Brown and Morley, 1986; Cooper and Maxwell, 1982; Farber, 1985).

For instance, a dentist who wants to attract blue-collar workers in the local neighborhood ensures that hours and fees are compatible with the work schedule and pricing expected by such a group. A dentist who wants to serve Medicaid patients locates where the Medicaid patients live and makes certain that the people know that Medicaid cards are welcome forms of payment. A dentist who wants to provide high-priced full mouth reconstruction sets up a practice that will attract and impress patients who have the money and inclination to undergo extensive dental care.

Regardless of the clientele expected, the smart marketer knows that smiling faces and warm attitudes bring patients back while cold, insulting manners drive people away. He/she also knows that accurate appointment management, care that maximizes patient comfort, cleanliness, and pleasing colors and sounds enhance a patient's perception of a practice.

Organizing the practice so that it runs smoothly is good marketing. Treating each person as if he/she were the only patient in the practice (and thus a cherished individual) also is good marketing. Remembering that it is not possible to practice dentistry unless there are patients to treat and income to pay the bills is also smart marketing. Thus, almost everything the manager does relates to marketing. From planning to communicating, from problem solving to advertising, the functions of a good manager relate to the image projected by the practice and thus to the practice's ability to attract and keep patients.

Advertising is one small piece of marketing, and even at that it does not have to be equated with neon lights and 6-inch ads in the newspaper. Advertising communicates to the public what the practice has to offer that is special. It is a simple translation of the practice's mission statement. The message could be read as attractiveness, good location, modern equipment and procedures, prevention emphasis, serving the handicapped, specializing in care for the elderly, low cost, comprehensive care, or any other theme that describes the practice accurately and that patients are looking for when they choose a practice.

Some dentists do advertise in newspapers and place large ads in the commercial phone directory, but for the most part they are "tasteful" and are worded so that other professionals are not insulted. A few, of course, step well beyond the bounds of propriety. The majority still take low-key approaches to advertising: giving volunteer presentations to community groups about dental health; supporting volunteer organizations by paying for printing, refreshments, etc.; or holding open houses. Some distribute coupons for free dental examinations. Others write columns about dental health in the neighborhood newspaper. The important point is that dentistry is learning to accept marketing and its benefits as "good words" (Press, 1984).

A manager may find him/herself in a practice where little attention has been paid to organized marketing. The practice has just floated along with the prevailing current, with no real effort to formulate a mission statement and no real effort to determine what the public is looking for in dental care. The manager can help move a practice so that it has a direction, a purpose, and ways of realizing its goals. The good manager can help the practice build a large, satisfied patient pool.

As with all of the essential functions of a manager, developing a marketing program has several steps: (1) research and analysis of both the practice and the environment so that an in-tune mission can be developed, (2) strategic planning to make the mission statement a reality, (3) development of services through updating, adding, and deleting services, (4) pricing evaluation and modification, (5) improved distribution or accessibility, perhaps including relocation, (6) advertising and public relations strategies, (7) evaluation and control of observed changes in the practice, (8) developing a continuing "closeness to the customer" that listens to their needs and invites their feedback, and (9) infusion of the "right attitudes" in the staff (how they go about their work and how they interact with patients) (Brown and Morley, 1986). These steps should be aimed at developing a match between what the dentist and staff want the practice to be and what the community is looking for. When a dentist happily offers what the public wants and makes them aware of where they can find it, the practice will flourish.

THE CONSULTANT'S ROLE

While a good manager should be well-versed and well-skilled in all the afore mentioned managerial functions, it is nearly impossible to be an expert in more than one or two areas. There will be times when the manager needs an expert in one or more areas and when attempting to be one him/herself is folly. The project is likely to fail, and getting it restarted, on the right track, is often met with resistance.

When such a project arises, it is time to find a competent consultant. The consultant's role should be to determine what the practice's needs are, to design a plan to help meet the needs, and to help the manager implement the plan. The manager therefore works very closely with the consultant and should look at the experience as an opportunity to learn more about a skill and to know how to take over the project and its ongoing implementation and evaluation once the consultant has left the project. It is never smart to turn over an entire project to a consultant. The manager will be left to pick up the pieces or to try and figure out what happened. An outsider never knows a practice's needs as well as the manager does, so the consultant needs the manager as much as the manager needs the consultant.

The manager should expect that the consultant will:

1. Conduct a needs assessment, however brief, to assess the practice's situation and needs.
2. Work closely with the manager to design and implement a plan that focuses on the needs.
3. Keep the manager informed of progress and roadblocks.
4. Ask for evaluation.
5. Maintain some contact past the end of the official project period to ensure continuity.

The consultant, in return, expects full cooperation and honesty, input of ideas and suggestions, a constructive evaluation, an agreed-upon reasonable fee, and an ending point for the project unless continuing consultation is arranged.

Selecting a consultant is no easier than selecting a dentist. It can be very difficult to find who you want; you need a person with the right skills and experience, who is easy to work with, and who charges reasonable fees. The person also has to be available—good consultants are often busy with several simultaneous projects. Places to start looking for consultants include other dentists who have had similar needs, a local university (the business or communications schools or the dental school), a local business consulting firm, or a firm that specializes in dental practice management. Leads come from word-of-mouth or from advertising. Check the references for each prospective consultant; call people who have worked with the consultants and used their services. Talk with the consultants to determine whether they speak the same language and are easy to communicate with.

Determine their fee structure, and draw up [...] ect contract that specifies what you want [...] much you expect it will cost. Negotiate a good agreement between you.

There are times when a consultant is one of the most important resources you will have. It is important to find a good one and to work well with that person. This ability rounds out the individual strengths of any one manager and brings fresh ideas and skills to the organization.

Review questions

1. Briefly describe the five steps in problem definition.
   a. *specify the feelings*
   b. *specify the events that bring about the feelings*
   c. *analyze the events to determine the sources*
   d. *work from the events backwards toward root of problem*
   e. *validate the hypothesis, consult w/ others, formulate the problem*

2. Once a problem is defined, the five steps in problem solving follow. List them.
   a. *list a variety of steps that could be taken*
   b. *analyze the likely outcomes of each alternative*
   c. *select an alternative, plan action*
   d. *implement the plan.*
   e. *monitor the outcomes*

3. Number each of the following examples of leadership style from most authoritarian (1) to most participative (7).

   5 "We've had a lot of problems with cancellations this week. I'd like you to give me some suggestions for what we can do. I'll make a decision using the best of your ideas."

   7 "We have $500 in the continuing education fund. I'd like you to decide how to spend it."

   1 "We have decided to close the practice for a week while the doctor is ill. You'll have paychecks sent for 50% of your regular earnings."

   4 "I've decided that in order to meet the patients' scheduling requests, we should close the office on Thursday and Friday and work 12-hour days on Monday, Tuesday, and Wednesday. I thought you might have some ideas for other ways to do it."

   6 "The doctor would like to use any one of these three patient record forms. The final decision is yours."

   2 "You are going to love the new film developing system we are buying. It does everything . . . ."

2 "From now on, George will be responsible for instrument cleaning and sterilization, Charlene will take over appointment control, and Martha will be the roving assistant. Questions?"

4. What four variables determine the amount of decision-making authority to extend to group members?

1) time 2) need for compliance 3) understanding of workers 4) control the managers should have over a decision.

5. What rule must be followed if the manager chooses a decision-making style based on the situation? *Inform workers the extent of their control.*

6. State six criteria for a well-designed dental office:
   a. *adequate space for heavy traffic areas*
   b. *tx area near reception area*
   c. *Lab away from tx + reception areas*
   d. *frequently used areas located centrally*
   e. *less frequently used areas away from tx areas*
   f. *pt + staff privacy assured*

7. List four primary management information systems that should exist in a dental office:
   a. *pt record*
   b. *scheduling*
   c. *productivity of info.*
   d. *financial info.*

8. Define marketing. *efforts to meet the wants + needs of public*
9. Define advertising. *part of marketing, describes our uniqueness*
10. Briefly describe the role of a consultant in the technical management of an organization.

GROUP ACTIVITIES

1. Form groups of three. One person in the group should identify a real or fictitious personal or school-related problem that needs solving. The other two group members should lead the person through each of the steps of problem definition and problem solving. Switch roles so that each of the triad has a problem that is analyzed. Allow 20 minutes per person. Discuss as a class how the problem analysis worked—its shortcomings and its usefulness.

2. Discuss how a program director might decide which of the following decisions should involve the input of (a) the faculty and/or (b) the students in the program. Recall the four criteria for selecting a decision-making style.
   a. Changes in the curriculum content
   b. New required books
   c. Major change in regulation uniform
   d. Whether to hold Saturday clinics
   e. Choice of space in new building
   f. Choice of office mates (faculty) or roommates (students)

3. List every step in the work flow followed when:
   a. Performing a head and neck examination.
   b. Exposing and developing a radiographic survey.
   c. Writing a research paper.

4. Use a movie camera to film a health care procedure exposing the film at one frame per second. Analyze the film for frequency and complexity of movement as well as for distance of movement. Institute motion economy measures and refilm the procedure. Compare the two films.

5. Select one of several geometric shapes (square, rectangle, circle, triangle) and design a dental office that has a reception room, rest rooms, doctor's office, staff lounge, sterilization center, four operatories, a business office, and a laboratory. The instructor should provide minimum dimensions for each component to be planned. Analyze the designs in groups of five using the criteria suggested in the text.

6. Review and critique four different computer information management systems designed for dental offices.

7. Scan the newspapers and other media for dental advertising. Critique each ad for the clarity of its message and how well that message is likely to attract new patients.

REFERENCES

Bonner, P.J., and McKenzie, S.A.: Computo-ease your dental practice, Tulsa, Okla., 1986, Penn Well Publishing Co.

Brown S.W., and Morley, A.P., Jr.: Marketing strategies for physicians, Oradell, N.J., 1986, Medical Economics Books.

Cooper, P.D., and Maxwell R.B., III: Marketing: entry points and pitfalls. In Spirn, S., and Benfer, D.W., editors: Issues in health care management, Rockville, Md., 1982, Aspen Systems Corp.

Cooper, T.M., and DiBiaggio, J.A.: Applied practice management: a strategy for stress control, St. Louis, 1979, The C.V. Mosby Co.

Farber, L.: Encyclopedia of practice and financial management, Oradell, N.J., 1985, Medical Economics Books.

Katz, D., and Kahn, R.L.: The social psychology of organizations, ed. 2, New York, 1978, John Wiley & Sons, Inc.

Kilpatrick, H.C.: Work simplification in dental practice, Philadelphia, 1974, W.B. Saunders Co.

Majewski, R.F., and Shapiro, I.A.: Attitudes of dentists and consumers toward advertising, J. Am. Dent. Assoc. **108:**345, 1984.

Perich, P.: The ethical marketing of dentistry: is it a misnomer? J. Am. Coll. Dent. **50**(2):12, 1983.

Press, B.H.: Ethics in the practice of dentistry. J. Am. Coll. Dent. **51**(1):9, 1984.

Roberts, D.I., Rosenbloom, D.T., and Curcio, F.B., editors: The dynamics of dental practice administration, Flushing, N.Y., 1977, Medical Examination Publishing Co., Inc.

Schein, E.: Process consultation: its role in organization development, Reading, Mass., 1969, Addison-Wesley Publishing Co., Inc.

Tannenbaum, R., and Schmidt, W.H. (1958): How to choose a leadership pattern. Reprinted in Spirn, S., and Benfer, D.W., editors: Issues in health care management, Rockville, Md., 1982, Aspen Systems Corp.

CHAPTER 22

People management skills

OBJECTIVES: The reader will be able to:

1. Explain how personnel management skills relate to other management skills.
2. List seven basic personnel management guidelines a good manager should follow.
3. Given examples of management practices, describe each as representative of Theory X, Theory Y, or Theory Z.
4. Explain each of eight leadership styles as a combination of emphasis on task and needs of people and explain how each is an effective or ineffective combination.
5. Describe the difference between active and reflective listening.
6. Given examples of talking and listening, label the "listening" response as active, reflective, or a response that closes down communication (i.e., one of the "dirty dozen").
7. Describe the impact good listening has on communication.
8. Explain the role of trust, empathy, and warmth in communication.
9. Describe the desirable and undesirable aspects of organization conflict.
10. Identify five typical ways of dealing with conflict.
11. Given examples of conflict situations, identify which conflict response style is being used.
12. Describe the positive and negative outcomes of each conflict response style.
13. Identify the typical signs of stress.
14. Explain how emotional stress and physical signs of disease are related.
15. List seven ways of reducing stress.
16. Explain the basis for deciding whether you *can* or *must* give feedback to another person.
17. List five guidelines for giving evaluative feedback to another person.
18. Explain the difference between passive, assertive, and aggressive styles of relating to others.
19. Define *work team,* contrasting it with "a number of individuals working in the same location."
20. Describe the manager's role in building and maintaining a productive work team.

ROLE OF PERSONNEL MANAGEMENT

It is difficult to shine as a manager when the people you are managing are unwilling to carry out the responsibilities you wish them to accept. No matter how clear you may be or how well-defined the objectives and work flow are, if you are unable to inspire the workers to comply, you are ineffective as a manager.

Up until the 1930s most management theory viewed workers as machines—one more necessary component in meeting work goals. People were expected to work to expected performance or they were fired. The general belief was that people generally did not wish to work hard and that their motivation was from external sources—threat or monetary reward. Most work at that time was unskilled. Since unskilled people were plentiful, management saw little reason to expend much energy on personnel. Management would simply look for a new worker if the current one was not performing as expected. McGregor (1960) described this approach as Theory X—an orientation that placed management emphasis on getting the task done.

McGregor contrasted this approach with Theory Y, where people were trusted and were believed to want to be productive. Managers whose tactics fit within Theory Y believed that workers had an internal need to fulfill through meaningful work as well as the external need for monetary compensation.

The development of Theory Y approaches to personnel management became important to industry when many jobs became more technical and it became very costly to replace workers. More emphasis was placed on the training and development of workers, and managers who also emphasized the integration of workers as contributors to the organization were able to reduce their turnover rates (Perrow, 1982; Katz and Kahn, 1978).

Theories X and Y are polar: either you care about the task or you care about the workers. Although there are organizations—including some dental offices—that are typical of one of the extremes, most are a mixture of both elements. Descriptions of a healthy balance between productivity concerns and people concerns are found in Theory Z, described by Ouchi in 1981. Theory Z is a productivity-oriented approach to organizational management that makes the most of worker input in the areas of objective setting, productivity monitoring, problem solving, and creative ideas.

Theory X, Y, and Z styles of management can be understood more clearly by showing those management strategies graphically (see Fig. 22-1). This diagram (Blake and Mouton's "managerial grid, 1964") shows how managers blend task and people emphasis. The diagram places task orientation (X) on the horizontal axis and people or relationships orientation on the vertical axis (Y).

The leader who functions in the upper-right quadrant emphasizes both people and task. Continuing clockwise on the graph reveals that the leader whose style fits in the lower-right quadrant shows high concern for task but low concern for people. The opposite is described for the upper left. Leadership in the lower-left shows neither task nor people concern.

One can be effective or ineffective regardless of the quadrant in which a leader's behavior falls. This dimension of the grid was added by Reddin (1964).

The plane of *ineffectiveness* is shown frontmost in the diagram. The leader who functions in the upper-left quadrant can be seen as a *missionary* or a "country club" leader who sacrifices task in favor of concern for people to the extent that the goals of the organization suffer considerably. Although the people in this group may have all their needs met, they may find that since the task has been ignored, they are without paying jobs when the organization files for bankruptcy.

Similarly, the person who emphasizes both people and task may function ineffectively by being the continual *compromiser,* going in the direction of the least resistance when two considerations conflict.

The *autocrat* makes all the decisions regardless of the needs of individuals involved and may generate considerable hostility. A resulting high turnover rate in personnel may jeopardize the high production the leader is seeking by being so authoritarian. Thus that person's leadership cannot be considered effective.

Finally, the *active deserter* is the leader in retreat who tries to avoid decisions and their related problems or who makes wishy-washy decisions, often too late to be effective.

The plane of *effectiveness* is shown behind the plane of ineffectiveness. In this plane the leader who emphasizes people but not task is known as the *developer*. This leader is willing to take time and perhaps sacrifice productivity for a short while to ensure that people are having their concerns and needs met adequately. Such a leader is willing to close down production long enough to hold an important staff meeting for workers to express their ideas and concerns and be fully informed of the direction of the organization. The goal is to develop the staff into thinking, contrib-

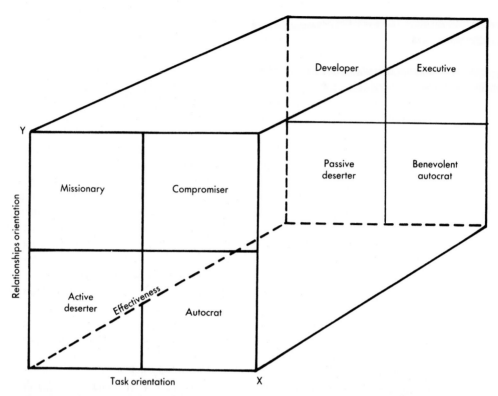

Fig. 22-1. The managerial grid places X and Y leader behaviors on two axes to show how the two combine to form four basic styles of leadership. The planes of effectiveness of leader style are shown with the plane of ineffectiveness in front and the plane of effectiveness in the rear. For each combination of degree of concern for task and for relationships, there is both an effective and ineffective style. (From Reddin, W.J.: Training Directors Journal **18**[7]:9, 1964. Copyright 1964, Training Directors Journal, American Society for Training and Development. Reprinted with permission. All rights reserved.)

uting members of the organization. This enhances their professional growth as well.

The *executive* functions with a high degree of concern for both task and people. This leader seeks out the input of the members, listens to their suggestions and concerns, and then balances them with the factors that affect cost-effectiveness and production. The executive's balancing is quite different from that of the compromiser. The executive controls the way in which factors are balanced without "caving in."

An effective leader who places higher value on task than on people is, known as the *benevolent*

autocrat. In this case decisions are made with task as the highest priority. However, this leader exhibits a certain fondness for the employees, similar to that of a demanding but caring parent. In other words, the benevolent autocrat makes the decision, but he/she is wise enough to inform the workers of the decision and exhibit some degree of warmth and support. The primary distinction between the executive or the developer and the benevolent autocrat is that both of the former recognize and respond to the *maintenance* needs of workers. The benevolent autocrat does not. The executive or developer grants input into decision making and considers how the organization and its planned changes affect its members. The benevolent autocrat assumes absolute control over the degree to which workers' concerns are voiced and acted on.

The *passive deserter* is not interested in task or relationships. The impact of this apathy on worker morale varies. There may be apparent cordial interest in people but only to muffle personnel problems. Employees may suffer without guidance, but others may develop skills and assume responsibility on their own and maintain the organization. The deserter can then retreat even further from the mainstream of activity as responsibilities are picked up by employees—at least until they discover or believe that they are being taken advantage of.

The most baffling style is that of the leader who falls close to the center of the grid. This person adopts styles that vary from situation to situation. At first, the flexibility seems desirable, but in actuality it is upsetting. The followers never know how the boss will respond.

Leaders do not typically adopt a particular style early in their careers and stay with it. Depending on their experiences with the people they manage and other influences, leaders may move from one style to another. Thus an autocrat who becomes good friends or forms a partnership with a developer may gradually seek more input from employees in decision making. It is just as likely that a developer who feels taken advantage of by callous employees may move to a much more controlling style.

Moving to a plane of ineffectiveness after years of success or simply retreating into the deserter role can be a sign of burnout.

The effective manager needs to know how to integrate task emphasis with people emphasis. Generally, prowess in this area does not come naturally. It is learned through observing well-skilled mentors, through study, and especially through practice with plenty of helpful feedback from co-workers and those being supervised. A few people are able to move smoothly into a managerial role and go about the business of giving instructions, listening to complaints and ideas, and looking out for the welfare of the workers with little fuss and few crises. Unfortunately, most people who find themselves in the position of manager (for instance, a dentist who wants to practice dentistry and wishes the business aspects of practice would go away) have almost no notion of how to manage the people they hire.

They ask themselves these questions: Should I be aloof since I'm the boss? Should I be buddy-buddy with the people I hire and try to be a close friend? Should I mother/father them? Will they accept me? Will they work if I ask them to? Will they try to tell me what to do? Will they be afraid to talk to me? Will they respect me? Will they talk (or worse yet, laugh) behind my back? How can I ask for their ideas without looking as though I'm incompetent for not having all the ideas?

Alternatively, some new managers just march ahead telling people what to do with little care for the response, blaming the employees for poor performance and for low commitment.

Where does a new manager start when faced with the prospect of supervising a group of people? There are at least seven important skills and attitude guidelines that apply to nearly all management interactions. They are integrally related, depending upon each other to support a sound managerial approach to working with people.

1. Maintain a genuine *respect* for the workers and their need for a sense of self-worth regardless of their age, education, job functions, appearance, habits, or abilities. This means treating every worker with the same adult-to-adult respect you would give to a highly successful, important person or at least to a peer (Metzger, 1981).

2. *Listen* to what each worker is saying—both in verbal and nonverbal expressions. Listen to what a worker says to you and what they say to each other as they work. Listen in meetings. Detect needs, problems, and progress by paying attention to what is happening among the workers (Metzger, 1981).

3. *Learn what motivates* each worker and the group as a whole. Ask what they want out of life; ask what they want out of their respective work roles. Help people see how their individual goals align with the organization's goals (Cooper and DiBiaggio, 1979; Deep, 1978).

4. *Treat workers fairly.* Avoid playing favorites. Everyone has personal preferences for some people over others; these preferences should not be obvious to the work group. Ascertain all the facts about a situation before taking punitive or congratulatory action.

5. *Respect confidences.* Do not discuss workers' problems (personal or professional) with other workers. Respect others' fears and concerns; show quiet understanding and compassion without taking responsibility for counseling and without excusing continual work-related shortfalls that may be due to those fears.

6. *Challenge people to grow.* Help people become better than they are by encouraging the acceptance of new responsibilities and educational opportunities. Encourage the group to set work objectives that cause them to stretch and learn and work vigorously, while ensuring that objectives are realistic. If you ask them to grow, support them in their efforts by providing guidance, helpful evaluation, and second chances.

7. Regularly (at least monthly) *ask for honest feedback* about your management skills. Listen to their responses and use that feedback to improve. Encourage the group to share responsibility for their own evaluation in terms of achieving work objectives, making it possible for people to openly discuss shortfalls and ways to improve.

The following vignettes describe a manager's attempts to supervise a team. After each is a brief discussion of what elements were present or lacking.

Example 1: A new dental associate has joined a large dental practice. Along with his well-equipped pair of treatment rooms, he is provided a well-trained chairside dental assistant who has worked in the practice for 10 years. She notices that the associate lacks good skills in passing instruments. Several times he has fumbled the instrument; his hand is not positioned correctly to receive the instrument safely. At the end of the second day of working together, the assistant mentions her observations to him and asks if they could spend a few extra minutes working out a more coordinated way of passing instruments. The associate turns beet red, announces that he is the doctor and she is the assistant and that she had better remember that. He adds, with fury, that it is "not his problem" and that she had better figure out a way of doing a better job.

Discussion: After years of dental school, the associate is finally away from constant evaluation by faculty and "is somebody." Here he finds himself being critiqued by a dental assistant. His reaction is understandable if not commendable.

The assistant is undoubtedly mortified by the dentist's reaction and will certainly be slow to make any other suggestions for work improvement in the future.

The associate is lacking a clear sense of respect for the assistant—he is preoccupied with his new-found position. Furthermore, he is unwilling to hear feedback, let alone eager to solicit it. He is letting his personal need for esteem get in the way of hearing the assistant's message. There is a filter working in his head that takes the assistant's message, "We need to work on better coordination for instrument passing," and distorts it to, "You don't know what you are doing. You aren't very important."

A manager needs to carefully listen to workers and set aside ego in order to learn what employees are thinking.

Example 2: A dental hygienist was promoted to manage a large dental clinic with 10 dentists, 14 hygienists, 20 dental assistants, and 4 clerical persons. The corporation that hired her stated that a critical part of her evaluation as a manager would be increased productivity and profit. In response she called a meeting of all members of the staff and gave each person a goal to increase productivity, income, or collections or to reduce costs, depending upon the responsibilities of the individual. Most of the goals were 60 to 70% above current achievement. Over the next several months, the workers seemed to be less productive! They avoided her, even though she had been one of them for 6 years as a practicing hygienist. She blamed it on their jealousy of her promotion and kept prodding them to produce more. When her 6-month evaluation occurred, she was fired for having hurt the practice morale and for having decreased profits.

Discussion: The hygienist's first mistake was setting the goals unilaterally. She simply announced them—apparently without any discussion or suggestions from the people who were expected to meet them. The workers felt no involvement or need to meet those goals. Also, in all probability, the goals were unreachable. If she had involved the workers, the goals may have been more realistic. Usually there is minimal motivation to achieve a goal that everyone knows is out of sight even if a mighty effort is made.

A second major mistake was not listening to the message the workers were giving her—alienation. If she was feeling the alienation, it was there. It was an error to assume it was jealousy. A wise manager would immediately call a meeting and ask for an honest, open discussion of the problem. A wise manager would listen to the feedback and alter the goals at that point—soliciting ideas and admitting error or misjudgment. The manager might have to stand firm on the need to improve productivity (and she certainly would not allow the group to usurp the manager's rightful role), but there would be a definite message of willingness to listen and then take action.

Example 3: A manager read a book about helping people stretch themselves to meet new goals and decided this was the perfect "cure" for a worker who had a poor self-image. The manager decided to put the fellow in charge of a subdivision of his department and to nurture him through his first few months of management. The manager explained to all the new supervisor's workers that their new supervisor had an image problem and that they should go easy on him, and that if they had problems they should come to him. He then put the man in charge with minimal direction and watched how he performed. Morale, productivity, and the new supervisor's self-image all worsened. Twenty percent of the workers resigned or were transferred to other departments. The new supervisor ended up in intensive psychological therapy. The manager threw away the book on helping people stretch themselves.

Discussion: Managers should not try to cure people

of psychological traits. They can offer feedback and suggestions if those traits are interfering with that person's work, but managers are not counselors whose job it is to treat such maladies. Also, the manager had no right to inform the workers of what he saw as the new supervisor's problems. Telling them to go easy on the new supervisor denied them the freedom to give direct feedback to him and it certainly undermined their impression of his ability to carry out the job. The new supervisor was stripped of three rights: the right to privacy, the right to openness and valuable information from workers, and the right to start with a clean slate.

The manager should have selected realistic "stretching" goals for people who are doing well in their jobs but who can probably do more and learn new skills. The workers should always be involved in identifying and setting those goals—they should be asked for their opinions and ideas.

LISTENING

Listening is the key ingredient in making any of the personnel management skills work (Metzger, 1981). It is certainly more than just hearing the words that people say. It is turning off one's "self-talk" that often runs on while someone else is trying to communicate. Self-talk is what we are saying to ourselves as we interpret, evaluate, and prepare to respond to another's message. It usually keeps us from really listening to what the other person is saying. It may help us be quick to reply or be well-defended against unwanted messages, but it is detrimental to clear communication.

When a person starts talking, he/she formulates an idea or thought, converts it into words, and says it. The listener hears the words, runs those words through a filter that represents that person's experience, and decodes the message (Deep, 1978; Metzger, 1981). Errors in communication occur when the speaker fails to choose accurate wording or expression for his/her thought. They occur if the message is not heard accurately—through hearing impairment, noise, or the interference of self-talk. They occur when the decoder runs the words through such a thick and cluttered filter that the real message is garbled, twisted, or simply ignored.

It is important for a good manager to take care to hear messages, to work hard to decode them accurately, and then to clarify that the meaning is accurate. Otherwise, costly failures to communicate can and will occur regularly.

Active listening (message clarification) is a skill a person can learn that helps ensure that decoding is occurring accurately. Clarifying a message helps the listener attend to the message and give it back to the speaker as directly and with as little filter-clutter as possible (Egan, 1976).

The content of a message can be clarified by reiterating the message in the listener's own words for the speaker to hear. The speaker can agree or disagree with the accuracy of the message and correct inaccuracies through restatement.

Example: A dentist says to her dental hygienist, "Please look at these radiographs. There is ledge calculus left on the distals of the last molars." The hygienist clarifies the message by saying, "So, when you looked at Ms. Swensen's radiographs you found areas where I missed calculus on the distals of the second molars." The dentist replies, "That's correct." If the hygienist had said, "You want me to retake these radiographs," (an obvious, but possible misinterpretation) the dentist could reply, "No, I want you to see the calculus you left on these teeth."

It may seem ridiculous to reiterate simple messages. For the most part, we do not spend our conversational time restating others' messages; we would sound like parrots if we did. However, when a message such as this one comes along it is best to make certain the interpreted message is accurate. Messages that trigger emotional responses (as the previous example might for the hygienist) or that are heavy with emotion from the sender are easily twisted in the defensive filters of the listener.

Also, listening for clarification helps the message sender know that you heard him/her correctly, and it is reassuring to know that a person has been heard correctly. In many instances, ac-

tive listening helps build a sense of trust between two people. Hearing a person reiterate a message can be an important indication of attentiveness and a valuing of one's efforts to reach out and communicate.

A further step into accurate listening is *reflective listening* (Egan, 1976). With this step the reiteration includes not only a restatement of the content of the message, but a statement about the emotion that is supporting the message (such as, anger, fear, joy, pride). The earlier example would have included reflective listening if the hygienist would have said, "It sounds like you are pretty disappointed about my missing that calculus." The dentist could have replied, "I *am* disappointed; in fact, I'm a bit angry about it." Or perhaps she would have said, "You sound pretty matter-of-fact about the leftover calculus. You don't sound angry at all." If she is correct in her assessment, the dentist might say, "Why should I be angry? Everyone misses calculus some of the time. Just make sure you get it off when she comes in for her restorative appointment next Tuesday."

Reflective listening lets the person know you are hearing the intent behind the content. Many messages are far more complex than the straightforward content or meaning of the words. There is voice inflection, speed of delivery, the message conveyed in the person's eyes, and body posture. A good listener attends to those messages as well and often will reflect back the "attitude" of the message as well as the content. A good listener is right on target with the content and the intent more often than not.

Being a good listener takes practice. It requires a conscious effort to respond to a person with sentences that begin with, "What I hear you saying is . . . ," "So you feel that . . . ," "You are telling me that . . . ," "You see it as . . . ," and other beginning phrases that force the listener into reiterating the speaker's message. Then comes the hard part: Active or reflective listening has to sound natural to be effective. The clarification or reflection has to be in the listener's own words; it cannot be an exact duplicate of what the speaker said.

Such listening skills are extremely valuable when trying to figure out what someone means when he/she is having trouble expressing it. They also are valuable when dealing with a person who is upset; hearing the listener rephrase one's concerns and problems is comforting—at least someone else understands what one is trying to say. Listening skills are valuable when receiving feedback and evaluative comments from supervisors, co-workers, and those being supervised. Good evaluation usually includes negative comments, otherwise the manager would not know where to improve. Most of the time those negative comments are difficult to listen to. The manager's first impulse may be to argue or defend his/her actions. Taking time to rephrase what the negative comments are helps the message sink in before reacting. It also helps the speaker know that an accurate message was received. Finally, it gives the speaker a chance to restate messages that were misinterpreted; there is less chance of carrying away distorted messages.

A good listener can attend to the real meaning of a message if he/she tries to "get inside" the other person's situation and feelings. This is called empathy—the ability to align with what the speaker is saying and feeling without criticism (Egan, 1976).

Warmth and respect for the speaker help the listener be a better interpreter of the messages (Egan, 1976). It may be difficult to feel great warmth for every person who speaks with you, but if you are able to find some aspect of that person that you admire or enjoy it helps to focus on that while listening to his/her statements. Respect was introduced earlier as a focal component of good management. This is particularly true when listening. Lack of warmth and respect and a failure to step (figuratively) into the speaker's shoes will be apparent to the speaker; he/she will be likely to stop talking and may be hesitant to bring up matters of importance again.

Most people unwittingly cut off speakers pre-maturely with their first response. There are several ways to do it. They are referred to as "the dirty dozen" (Egan, 1976), and they include:

1. Commanding, ordering, directing
2. Warning, admonishing, threatening
3. Exhorting, moralizing, preaching
4. Advising, giving suggestions, offering solutions
5. Lecturing, giving logical arguments
6. Judging, criticizing, disagreeing, blaming
7. Approving behaviors with praise, agreement
8. Name-calling, ridiculing, shaming
9. Interpreting, analyzing, diagnosing
10. Reassuring, consoling, supporting, sympathizing
11. Probing, questioning, interrogating
12. Withdrawing from, humoring, distracting

Add to these a most annoying habit of "one-upping" the speaker by having a much worse or much better situation to tell about. The response usually starts out, "You think that's bad? Well, when I was . . . ." The speaker is shut down or has to wait through a long story before being able to introduce a second sentence.

Whenever a person is approaching another with an important message and the "listener" responds with one of the dirty dozen or with a one-upper line instead of reiterating what the speaker was saying, the speaker is essentially cut off. If the listener uses active or reflective listening, the speaker will agree or clarify and usually continue with what is on his/her mind. There is almost always more to come.

LISTENING VERSUS SHUTTING OFF COMMUNICATION

Speaker: "I'm so worried lately about how well I'm doing. I'm losing a lot of sleep, and I can't seem to concentrate."

Good Listener: "It sounds like you are pretty upset. You are telling me that your performance is not what you'd like it to be and that worrying about that is costing you sleep and productive concentration."

Speaker in Response: "Yeah. I really am. Just last week when I was working on that big project, I . . ."

THE ARRAY OF POOR LISTENERS:

One-Upper: "You think that's bad? I've had a stomachache all week worrying about tomorrow."

Commanding, Ordering, Directing: "Take a sleeping pill and quit complaining."

Warning, Admonishing, Threatening: "Well, if you don't get yourself under control, you'll be in deeper trouble."

Exhorting, Moralizing, Preaching: "If only you wouldn't work so hard you'd be in a lot better shape."

Advising, Giving Suggestions, Offering Solutions: "Well, you could look at your schedule and see what things you could give up. Or you could take yoga. That helps."

Lecturing, Giving Logical Arguments: "You shouldn't feel that way. You are doing just fine. It's all in your head. Just count all the good things you do."

Judging, Criticizing, Disagreeing, Blaming: "Here you are doing so well and all you can do is complain and worry. It's your fault if you are losing sleep and not concentrating. You bring it on yourself."

Approving Behaviors with Praise, Agreement: "Yes, you really are having a hard time. It's hard to care so much and work so hard and try to keep it all together. I can see why you are worrying so much."

Name-Calling, Ridiculing, Shaming: "You are so stupid to worry like that."

Interpreting, Analyzing, Diagnosing: "You probably are under a lot of stress, and your body is trying to tell you that you are working too hard."

Reassuring, Consoling, Supporting, Sympathizing: "You poor thing. You try so hard and it seems like you just don't get the breaks to let you complete what you want."

Probing, Questioning, Interrogating: "How much sleep do you get each night? When do you have trouble concentrating? How long has this been going on?"

Withdrawing, Humoring, Distracting: "Well, look at this way: things could get worse. And they probably will."

Speaker Response: "Thanks a lot."

The listener shouldn't become a talker until the speaker has no more to say. Then it may be appropriate to ask, "Do you want suggestions from me?" if a problem has been presented. In a time of pain, the correct response may be comfort. In a time of uncertainty or complexity, it could be questioning that is appropriate. If the situation is one where the listener cannot become involved, it may be appropriate to withdraw.

CONFLICT MANAGEMENT

A skill that a manager relies upon when supervising people is conflict management. It occurs, in preferably small doses, almost every day. Conflict results when people are trying to align their personal and professional goals with the organization's and to fit them with other people's priorities and idiosyncrasies. A great deal of conflict can be avoided if the manager is a good planner, organizer, and so on, and has good technical management skills. Having the work place operate smoothly helps reduce unnecessary tension. But regardless of how smoothly the system functions, conflict will occur.

Conflict is not all bad. It can surface important ideas for alternative ways of doing things. It can point out weak links in how the work is performed. It can cause a person to decide that the work role he/she is in is inappropriate and bring about a shift in job responsibilities. It can point out to an individual that certain habits or idiosyncrasies are irritating to others. What is important about conflict is how it is handled (Appelbaum, 1981; Deep, 1978).

The first big decision concerning conflict is whether to handle it or not. A manager can watch a conflict brewing between two workers and opt to let them settle it. A hygienist and assistant may be battling over whose responsibility it is to develop the x-ray film. If the two workers can mutually set up guidelines that are likely to work, the manager's role may be nothing more than to let it happen and then to comment, "It sounds like you two have agreed upon a solution for sharing the task of developing x-ray film. Let's see if I have it straight. Whenever the stack of undeveloped film . . . ."

Note the active listening the manager uses. The manager clarifies what they decided and lets them both know what decision she thinks has been reached. If there is doubt or inaccuracy, it can be brought up by one of them at that time and settled. Such a strategy lets the workers know that the manager is on top of what is going on and approves of the decision reached in this case.

There are other times when the workers will not settle a conflict among themselves. It can fester and become a major distraction if left alone. In these cases it is up to the manager to call the people together and start listening to both sides. Avoiding the conflict is a short-term win for the manager since he/she does not have to work hard at being a listener and peacemaker; it is a long-term loss for the manager since the organization and the people involved will pay dearly for the continuing conflict. The manager's role in resolving conflict in this case is (1) to bring the situation out in the open for discussion, (2) to make sure that each of the people involved can fully explain the other person's perspectives as well as his/her own, (3) to ask for and help define a strategy agreeable to all people involved for settling the conflict, and (4) to monitor compliance with and the effectiveness of the solution.

There are several ways of dealing with conflict. *Accommodation* is living with the conflict, and hoping it will go away or smooth over. Other strategies include: *competition* where the stronger or more forceful of the parties in the conflict "wins"; *compromise* where both parties give up part of what they want through negotiation, with neither party fully satisfied with the result; *avoidance* where one or more of the parties leaves or avoids the situation by quitting, being ill a great deal of the time, or staying away from the troublesome person or situation as much as possible; and *collaboration* where the parties involved hammer out an agreement that is mutually satisfying and that does not require great sacrifice on anyone's part (Appelbaum, 1981).

The first four strategies have high human costs including the anger and reduced productivity that comes from "losing," the sense of dissatisfaction that comes from partial results, and the personal and organizational loss that comes from employee turnover or sick leave and lost opportunities for workers to communicate fully. Collaboration should be the aim of conflict resolution. It is not always possible to achieve, but it is the most satisfying result with the least human cost. In most instances collaboration provides a growing experience for the involved persons and can actually result in greater trust and teamwork. Collaboration does take time; it may require marathon sessions with the involved parties venting their frustrations and then slowly building an agreement that will work. A manager with finely tuned conflict management skills and good creativity can save an organization and its people considerable stress and distraction.

STRESS MANAGEMENT

Stress is an everyday fact in management. It is the body's response to demands or stressors placed upon it. There is stress involved in meeting demanding goals, in working with or for people who think differently, in following a tight schedule, in making up for ill or vacationing staff members, in working with scarce resources, and in a myriad of other factors. Just as conflict can be a good part of organizational life, stress can be good also. A modicum of stress gets people moving. It sharpens their awareness and drives them to perform well, to get the job done. Too much stress over extended periods of time is debilitating both to the organization's productivity and to the physical and mental well-being of the people under the intense, unrelenting stress (Dunlap, 1977; Selye, 1978).

When stressors continue to bombard a person, the body's natural defenses begin to work against the person rather than for him/her to save the person from an undesirable situation. The natural defenses involve hormonal releases that ready the body for "fight or flight." The body is poised for physical action, with adrenaline racing through the blood stream. Most workers would find fighting or fleeing self-destructive responses to the aggravations and demands of work; managers rarely advocate punching a co-worker, kicking the copy machine, or running screaming into the parking lot as appropriate responses to stress. Instead workers grimly contain themselves. The adrenaline is still pumping, but the body is not allowed to react and "burn off" those free-flowing hormones. Thus, blood pressure stays elevated, impaired inflammatory responses continue, and overall disease resistance decreases (Selye, 1978).

Poor adaptation to the stressors that exist in everyday life is a disease manifested in the body. Usually people can see it in one another without recognizing it in themselves.

People under stress sigh a lot. They complain of headaches. They are frequently ill—a handy response for those avoiding conflict, since they can call in sick and hope for sympathy from their adversaries. Their blood pressure is generally elevated; they perspire, especially on their hands and feet; and they may have trouble controlling their eating habits. They also often have indigestion and poor bowel function (either infrequent or continuous). Many stressed people are accident prone, forgetful, or generally poor workers despite their efforts and their beliefs that they are doing well. They sometimes may feel they are unable to catch a full breath; their voice often sounds shaky or uncertain. Sleep disorders often occur, either having an excessive need for sleep or an inability to sleep. Rising from a full night's sleep feeling exhausted is one symptom. Sexual urges are diminished. Stressed people often describe a continual feeling of foreboding (Appelbaum, 1981; Selye, 1978).

A stressed person will show a few of these signs in varying degrees of intensity. Rarely will a person have them all.

People under stress can actually dig their own graves if they ignore the signs of stress. Intense, persistent stress can lead to severe illness and death as the body gives way to the pressures placed upon it.

Since it is rarely possible for a person to avoid stress, recent attention has focused on ways of coping with it. Simple, but effective, methods for coping with stress include taking time to *exercise* vigorously. Aerobics, strength-building exercises, and companionship sports and physical activities should be a regular part of every week, with a balance of all three. Thus, a person might swim or run 3 days a week, lift weights 2 days a week, and play racquetball or some other companion sport the other 2 days. Many people describe a sense of well-being from feeling the body work effectively. Rather than feeling tired after such an effort, they describe a sense of vigor and increased energy when exercise is a regular part of their activities (Morse and Furst, 1979).

Other suggestions for coping with stress include frequent *meditation* breaks at various points during the day (early morning, at "coffee" break time, at the end of the work day, before sleeping), learning *biofeedback* skills that can enable the person to control blood pressure and the autonomic response, *hobbies,* and *good diet.* Avoiding caffeine and other stimulants, foods with high sugar content, and alcohol and other depressants is suggested. Leaving the table before feeling full is a related suggestion (Morse and Furst, 1979).

Recognizing and responding to stress in oneself and in others in the organization are important skills for the manager. Unrecognized, untempered stress hurts people. It also hurts the organization's productivity. The manager can encourage workers to talk about their jobs, their aspirations, their views of their productivity, the work problems they can't seem to overcome, and the solutions to these problems. Fixing the faults of the job is certainly an important contribution to reducing stress and a critical role of a good manager (Cooper and DiBiaggio, 1979; Huse, 1975). Many organizations are going further, offering aerobics sessions at lunchtime, providing nutritious snacks and beverages for break periods, discouraging smoking on the job and encouraging smokers to give up the habit, and providing or supporting alcohol and drug abuse counseling programs.

A person's actions to relieve stress and an organization's efforts to reduce job-related stress and encourage healthy ways of coping with stress can work together to minimize the burnout and ill-health that can occur in the modern work place (Phillips, 1982).

GIVING FEEDBACK AND EVALUATION

One of the more challenging functions of a manager that occurs on a daily basis is confronting a superior, a co-worker, or a person being supervised with feedback about how that person is doing. It is an easier task if the report is a positive one, where good performance is acknowledged. It is not easy when the performance leaves something to be desired. It is most difficult when that feedback is to be given to a superior in the organization. Let's assume for purposes of this initial discussion that the feedback is about undesirable performance.

How do you decide when to give feedback? When someone else's performance is, in your opinion, less than ideal an initial step is to determine whether you *can* or *must* give feedback to the person. There are times when you could offer the feedback because you think it might be helpful and because you think there is a chance the person will grow from hearing it. There are other times when it is your responsibility to tell someone what they could improve (such as when you are the manager) and when there will be a direct negative impact on you or on something you value if the person continues on his/her present course.

If giving feedback is your choice rather than your obligation, a basic rule to follow is to ask the person if he/she would like to hear what you have to say. "I'd like to talk with you about the way your report was written. Would you be willing to talk with me about it?"

The procedure is slightly different when it is your obligation to offer feedback. The request for a hearing can and should be more direct. "I need to talk with you about the way your report was written. How about if we meet in an hour?" In this case you are not implying that there is a way to avoid the discussion. To ignore one's obligation to provide feedback is a *passive,* no-win sit-uation that provides only the illusion of safety. Giving feedback is always risky; not giving feedback when it is obligatory invites doom.

There are several helpful guidelines for giving feedback once the right time and place are at hand. Begin by stating specifically what you see to be a problem and how you react to it. "When I read your report, I felt myself getting angry. It seems that several key pieces of information were missing that we need for making a good decision. The ones I noted were. . . . " Other examples of specific feedback are shown in box.

Format for Giving Feedback Effectively "When you (specify the behavior carefully) . . . , I feel (specify your reaction) . . . , because (give your reason and possible outcome)."

Examples:

"When you keep on working at those papers while I'm talking to you, I can feel myself getting angry, because it seems like I'm not important enough or don't have anything important enough to say for you to give me your full attention."

"When you come in a few minutes early and have everything prepared for the day, I feel really good about having hired you, because you make life a lot easier and you seem to really want to contribute to this practice."

"When you let the checks pile up for 3 weeks, I get really nervous and angry because they are not safe and they are not available to pay bills until they are deposited."

"When you are late for your appointment, I can feel my anxiety rise because I know I'll be behind for all my patients for the rest of the day."

"When you turn the music up loud, my head starts to hurt and I keep wondering how the others in the office are reacting, because not everyone likes that kind of music played that loudly."

After giving a direct statement of your concern, wait for the person's response. If that person is a good listener, he/she will probably clarify what you mean and how you feel. If he/she is not a good listener and feels threatened, a strong defensive, perhaps angry, retort may ensue. It is also possible that the person will crumble before your eyes. If the person's response is an emotional or defensive one, move into active, reflective listening. Make certain the person knows you understand what they are saying in response. Then restate your concerns, asking if he/she understands what you are saying. Ask for a rephrasing of what you mean, so that you are able to tell whether you were heard correctly. People hearing negative feedback have a very cluttered listening filter that often distorts an otherwise clear message in unusual, unpredictable ways.

After you are sure that the listener understands your concern, move to suggestions for how the behavior could be better. If the person is not someone you supervise, you might say, "I do wish you would modify the report to include some of these details. I think it will be more accurate and make it easier for us to make a good decision." If the person is someone you supervise, you could say "I'd like you to rewrite this report before Friday with these details included. I think it will improve the report's clarity and our ability to make a good decision." Make sure the listener understands what you are asking. Ideally you will obtain assent in both cases; but you should make certain it happens when you are functioning as a supervisor.

The general guidelines for offering constructive feedback to another person include: (1) making certain that the person has the power to change what you object to, (2) selecting the right time and place for giving feedback, (3) stating the feedback in clear, concrete terms, (4) assuring that the person has correctly understood your feedback, (5) offering specific suggestions for change, and (6) *always* taking into account the other person's needs.

Typically, feedback should be phrased in a "When you do . . . , I feel . . . , because . . ." or "When you do . . . , the following things happen . . . ." A key in successfully giving feedback is to combine this kind of phrasing with an understanding of how the person could feel when you deliver the message. It should always be straightforward, but it should also always be gentle.

The way in which the message is delivered is the difference between assertiveness and aggressiveness. When a person is assertive, he/she is ex-

pressing feelings and needs openly and directly in the hopes of bringing about a change in another person's behavior. Such a statement becomes aggressive when the speaker is trying to hurt or humble the other person or when he/she simply does not consider the other person's situation. Continuing with the previous example, the assertive person might say, "I know how hard you worked to get that report out on time and how much it means to you to have us decide in favor of your recommendation." If you have misjudged the motivation, you will likely hear about it, but an aggressive statement will certainly trigger anger and an argument. The aggressive person might say, "I know that you just want to sway the group to decide your way." Aggression masquerading as assertiveness hurts the listener and any possibility of constructive communication (Morton et al., 1981).

A good manager will not only have opportunities to give feedback, but will receive feedback as well. Teaching the people you supervise how to give constructive feedback to one another and to you can make accepting feedback easier. When receiving feedback, a simple rule is to clarify what is being said to you (listening), to discuss whether changes are possible, and then to come to some resolution. If workers know how to give and receive feedback, many behind-the-back complaints can be eliminated and productivity can improve.

Positive feedback can follow the same rules. Choose the right time and place, be specific and concrete, and take into account the needs of the listener. Ensure that the correct message is received by the listener; a worker may be so worried about receiving criticism that a clear, positive statement may be distorted into an unintended negative one!

TEAM BUILDING

Skills in listening, stress identification and reduction, conflict resolution, and giving and receiving feedback are the basis for team development. The manager is the group leader who helps individuals work together toward group goals in a coordinated, supportive manner. Thus the importance of all of these skills is obvious. The manager has to listen to the needs of the individuals and the tempo and tenor of the group as it works; to detect disgruntlement, conflict, work problems, fatigue, and stress; to bring people together in an open atmosphere to discuss what they need in order to feel successful, productive, and part of the organization's mission; to help people improve; and to learn what he/she needs to do in order to be a better manager.

A team is different from a group of individuals who happen to work in the same location. It is a coordinated group that shares common goals, that collectively contributes to the completion of high quality tasks, that watches out for each member in the group, that establishes norms of honesty and fairness within itself, and that has work roles and interpersonal roles established to keep the group humming along (Ducanis and Golin, 1979; Hare, 1976).

Work roles are established to a large extent by the manager as work assignments are made. Interpersonal roles usually emerge in the group. There is usually a person who attends to the personal needs of the group members (sending get-well cards; remembering birthdays; cheering up people on a rough day), another who watches the pace of the group and sets standards for performance, another who thinks through ideas and suggestions, someone who is the group clown or attention-getter, another person who likes to aggravate others, quiet people who keep to themselves, a leader

who emerges to be the spokesperson and liaison to the manager and other groups, and a variety of others. The group becomes a team when it recognizes the roles various people play and when the group learns to respond to those people in a healthy, open way. The members of the team support others' contributions to the work group and limit their ability to apply too much pressure or detract from the group's ability to function (Hare, 1976).

The manager needs to see those roles emerging in the group and to help the work team see them also. The group needs to have time to attend to its interpersonal needs as well as to getting the flow of work accomplished. The manager should watch how the group handles the contributions of individuals to the health of the group and provide a carefully chosen, brief comment in the group situation that alerts members to their progress as a team and to their needs to temper one another and listen to one another.

Good managers learn with experience and good guidance that being the boss doesn't mean being aloof or being buddy-buddy. They find acceptance from the group when they respect the workers; are well-skilled in basic and technical management; listen with accuracy, empathy, and a measure of warmth; reduce conflict and stress to productive levels; and look out for the team's welfare without becoming a surrogate parent. Good managers learn that managing people is perhaps the most challenging and rewarding aspect of their job.

Review questions

1. How do personnel management skills fit with the other basic and technical skills that a manager should possess?
2. Assume you are just beginning a position as a "people manager." What seven guidelines would you be wise to follow in beginning that job?
3. Below are three brief examples of managerial encounters. Identify whether the manager's action is that of a task-oriented Theory X manager, a people-oriented

Theory Y manager, or a Theory Z manager who combines task and people needs in a healthy balance:

a. A new chair-side assistant makes an error in selecting which restorative material the dentist requested. The dentist slams down the instruments and says: "I run a tight ship here; if you can't catch on, you'll have to get off." (Theory _____)

b. Appointment scheduling has been very slow over the holidays. Most days have only four or five patients scheduled. Unfortunately, the next month does not look much better. The manager is considering laying off two auxiliaries, both of whom will suffer a great deal if they lose their incomes. Instead he issues a challenge: if we can call sufficient numbers of recalls to fill the coming 2 weeks to 80% and can design a program to attract ten new patients with everyone working at it, no one will be laid off. (Theory _____)

c. A manager knows that a worker is not being very productive in what he does. He produces about 60% of what ought to occur. He has spoken with the worker several times, but little change has resulted. The manager just cannot bring himself to fire the employee. He encourages his superior to give the employee a promotion and move him to a different department where he will not longer bother the productivity. (Theory _____)

4. While it is not certain what the outcome of each of the above vignettes will be, it is possible to project what might happen. Identify each management style as effective or ineffective and state why; label each style according to the managerial grid described by Blake and Mouton as modified by Reddin.

5. Label each of the following "listening statements" as *active, reflective,* or a *dirty dozen* statement:

a. "I can tell that you are really upset about my being late again."

b. "You shouldn't feel that way. Your work is good."

c. "You're saying I should open the hinges on the scissors before I scrub them."

d. "What I hear you saying is that we have a different schedule starting in 1 month and that my shift will be . . ."

e. "You sure are excited about making our goal this month."

f. "Don't you tell me what to do."

g. "Why don't you lie down for a while. You'll feel better."

6. List the five typical ways of dealing with conflict.

7. How does emotional stress become expressed in physical signs?

8. What are six guidelines for giving feedback to a person?

9. What is the difference between passive behavior, aggressive behavior, and assertive behavior?

10. How is a work team or group different from a collection of people who happen to work at the same location?

GROUP ACTIVITIES

1. Describe experiences as a manager or as an employee where at least one of the seven basic personnel management guidelines was broken or was effectively used.

2. Examine your own leadership style, using a leadership survey that measures concern for task and for people. Plot the score on the managerial grid and discuss how accurate each student believes his/her score is. Solicit feedback from other students regarding their perceptions of the accuracy of the results.

3. In dyads practice active and reflective listening when a fellow student says each of the following:

   a. "You really seem to have all the difficult patients this semester. I wish I were as lucky."

   b. "I can't stand it when I study all night and the test asks me questions about things I've never heard of."

   c. "I love the way you told her off."

   d. "Perhaps someday I'll find as good a job as you have."

   e. "You have been working in this dental office for 6 months. Your work is unsatisfactory; tomorrow is your last day."

   f. "I've never worked with a hygienist before. Frankly I'm worried that you'll take over and want to change things. I want a hygientist but I don't want to make a lot of trouble for myself."

   g. "I don't care if you know how to give an oral exam, take blood pressure, and give good oral hygiene instructions. Can you scale a Class III in 20 minutes?"

   h. "I've never had a dentist ask me about my general health before. I just want my teeth checked. Would you please just do that for me and quit wasting time?"

4. Try different voice inflections and body language to express anger, sarcasm, joy, or concern in each of the previous sentences; see how the listener responds to those messages as well as to the words in the statements.

5. For a month- or semester-long project form groups of five and prepare a group presentation on one of the basic management skills, technical skills, or personnel skills. Record how the group of five forms, how leadership emerges, what norms develop, what roles are adopted, how the group controls and rewards itself, and what quality task was produced and why. Discuss the functioning of the group among the members.

6. Describe the characteristics, norms, leadership (formal and informal), and roles that exist in the whole group (class). Identify how the group developed and what makes it unique. Identify what *internal* and *external* forces exist that keep it from functioning well as a group and what helps it to do well. Specify what internal, group-support tasks the group performs.

7. Resurrect conflicts that have arisen in the class as a group since you started the program. What conflict management style was used? What was the result?

8. Complete a stress-identification survey. What signs of stress do individuals in the group identify? Discuss in groups of three the signs that were identified. Ask if the other two members in the group see additional signs of stress. Find out what individuals in the group are doing to relieve stress.

9. Identify five people (not in the group) to whom you would like to give feedback regarding a particularly annoying or especially positive behavior. Role play providing the feedback, using a classmate as a substitute subject. The person receiving the feedback should use good listening skills for practice and then at a second run-through respond with anger or misinterpretation.

   Evaluate the feedback in terms of asking to give the feedback (if it is a "can" situation), selecting the right time and place, being specific and concrete, taking into account the needs of the receiver, and the ability to respond to the receiver's response. Evaluate the verbal and nonverbal aspects of the feedback in terms of aggression versus assertion.

10. Observe when and how people listen with active or reflective listening. Observe what happens when one of the "dirty dozen" is used.

11. Try using active listening when a friend, a patient, an instructor, or another person begins a serious conversation.

REFERENCES

Appelbaum, S.H.: Stress management for health care professionals, Rockville, Md., 1981, Aspen Systems Corp.

Blake, R.R., and Mouton, J.S.: The managerial grid, Houston, 1964, Gulf Publishing Co.

Certo, S.C., and Doughterty, R.H. Organizational leadership, Dubuque, Iowa, 1975, Kendall/Hunt Publishing Co.

Cooper, T.M., and DiBiaggio, J.A.: Applied practice management: a strategy for stress control, St. Louis, 1979, The C.V. Mosby Co.

Deep, S.D.: Human relations in management, Encino, Calif., 1978, Glencoe Publishing Co., Inc.

Ducanis, A.J., and Golin, A.K.: The interdisciplinary health care team, Germantown, Md., 1979, Aspen Systems Corp.

Egan, G.: Interpersonal living, Monterey, Calif., 1976, Brooks/Cole Publishing Co.

Hare, A.P.: Handbook of small group research, ed. 2, New York, 1976, Free Press.

Huse, E.F.: Organization development and change, St. Paul, Minn., 1975, West Publishing Co.

Katz, D., and Kahn, R.L.: The social psychology of organizations, ed. 2, New York, 1978, John Wiley & Sons, Inc.

McGregor, D.: The human side of enterprise, New York, 1960, McGraw-Hill Book Co.

Metzger, N.: Communications. In Metzger, N., editor: Handbook of health care human resources management, Rockville, Md., 1981, Aspen Systems Corp.

Morse, D.R., and Furst, M.L.: Stress for success, New York, 1979, Van Nostrand Reinhold Co.

Morton, J.C., Rickey, C.A., and Kellett, M.: Building assertive skills: a practical guide for professional development for allied dental health providers, St. Louis, 1981, The C.V. Mosby Co.

Ouchi, W.G.: Theory Z, New York, 1981, Addison-Wesley Publishing Co.

Perrow, C.: The short and glorious history of organizational theory. In Spirn, S., and Benfer, D. W., editors: Issues in health care management, Rockville, Md., 1982, Aspen Systems Corp.

Phillips, E.L.: Stress, health and psychological problems in the major professions, New York, 1982, University Press of America, Inc.

Reddin, W.J.: The tri-dimensional grid, Training Directors Journal **18**(7):9, 1964.

Selye, H.: The stress of life, revised edition, New York, 1978, McGraw-Hill Book Co.

CHAPTER 23

Financial management in the 1980s

OBJECTIVES: The reader will be able to:

1. Identify at least five payment mechanisms related to the provision of health care.
2. Identify overhead costs in operating a health care facility.
3. Explain how each item of overhead is affected by the efficiency of the operation of providing health care.
4. List and explain four ways in which employees in a health care facility may receive remuneration for the services they provide.
5. Identify the advantages and disadvantages of each method of remuneration and select a method that is most compatible with his/her own personal goals.
6. Discuss a method that can be used to estimate the value of an auxiliary to a dental practice.
7. Summarize ways in which cost effectiveness and overall productivity can be measured in a health care delivery system.
8. List at least ten functions of a good financial manager.

Financial management of any business is essential to its longevity. No matter how skilled a person is in scheduling, evaluating, and people management, if the business does not take in more money than it spends to run the business, it will fail. Failures are not uncommon in a time of economic uncertainty, and a dental practice, where the owner carries significant debts from his/her dental education as well as new debts associated with opening a practice, is a candidate ripe for financial catastrophe if there is any mismanagement.

The vast majority of dental services delivered in the United States are provided by relatively small, privately owned dental practices. Most dentists are solo practitioners or are in a "space-sharing" arrangement with another dentist, where everything but the physical facility is a separate entity for each of the dentists (Anderson, What's Happening, 1984). Like any private business, if it expects to survive, a practice must bring in

enough revenue to pay expenses and provide an adequate return to the practice owner. In the past most dentists were able to survive without exerting much effort toward properly managing personnel and equipment and marketing the services they were prepared to offer. More recently the market for dental services has become much more competitive and, as a result, dentists are spending time and money to improve the quality of services delivered and reduce the cost of these services.

While the number of dental care providers and their scope of skills was the focus of the 1970s, cost containment in health care is the focus of the 1980s. This is true because the cost of health care (particular hospital and physician expenses) has increased at a pace even greater than the increase in consumer services in general. The cost of services in dentistry has risen at a more modest pace, following the overall rise in the consumer price index (Gowotka, 1985).

227

For dentists, the emphasis on cost comes from two major factors. One is an environment where demand for dental restorative treatment has declined. The second is the economic recession that occurred during the early 1980s, which kept people from seeking extensive dental treatment, particularly while they were unemployed and had no dental insurance benefits to enjoy.

As dentistry leaves the economic recession behind, its recovery is dependent upon the ability of the profession to switch from a restorative-intense mode of practice to a periodontal/prevention mode that better addresses the needs of the population. It also is dependent upon the ability of the practice organizations to operate cost-effectively and to draw additional numbers of patients to seek dental care.

This chapter is a primer on the economics of privately owned dental practice. The initial focus is on the source and methods for funding the delivery of dental care, followed by a breakdown of the major expenses of running a practice. A discussion of the terms under which dental auxiliaries are paid for their services and a section describing how an auxiliary can estimate the value of his/her labor to the practice follows.

PAYING FOR DENTAL CARE

While focusing on the funding of specific practice settings, it is important to identify who pays for health care and the terms under which the services are provided—two factors that have a significant impact on the care delivered and the financial success of the practice. Most dental care is paid for by the patients or families of patients who receive the care under a *fee-for-service* arrangement. These patients are billed for specific treatments and are generally expected to pay immediately or within 30 days after treatment if the patient is approved for credit. Granting credit to this type of patient can be an important factor in their acceptance of treatment. This is particularly true if the treatment is relatively expensive, such as crown and bridge restorations. However, it can and often does lead to complications because payment is delayed for a period of time and often

patients are slow in paying or do not make payments. Some practices write off as much as 10% of their total billings because of bills that are not collected. Obviously, collections from uninsured fee-for-service patients are a major concern to practice owners.

Dental insurance offered the first real alternative to paying cash for dental services. The trend grew slowly through the 1960s, with only 2.3% of the population having dental insurance. By 1981 it was 37.9%. By 1985 it was slightly less than half (Gotowka, 1985; Olsen, 1984).

The availability of dental insurance, primarily as an employee benefit, helped remove the financial barrier to dental care. Its availability has been an important factor in providing a sufficient patient pool for the growing number of dental health care providers who entered the profession in the 1970s. While the overall population has increased in size, contributing to the growth, a major contribution in growth is from people who did not see the dentist regularly but who are now doing so. According to the Institute of Medicine (1980), 60% of the population sees the dentist at least once every 2 years, an increase from 55% in the early 1960s.

The availability of insurance, however, does not place a cap on health care costs. In some ways it contributes to them since providers may be tempted to defraud the insurance carrier and since patients are less questioning about costs since a third party will pay the bill. The patient may not be paying directly, but the cost of insurance rises as health care costs spiral upward, and eventually the patient pays through fewer insurance benefits and higher copayments. Insurance companies have attempted to control costs by requiring copayments from the patients for more expensive care such as crown and bridge work (Olsen, 1984).

Dental insurance raises different concerns for the practice owner. The provider of care must be concerned about whether the care provided meets the guidelines and specifications of the carrier. Is the service covered under the policy? Is this particular family member included in the coverage?

Are the requests for payment reimbursement accurately and completely prepared? Does the carrier require that the patient records be examined prior to reimbursement for this type of procedure? And ultimately, how long will it take for the carrier to process the forms and actually complete the payment? Although ultimate reimbursement may be more certain when specific guidelines are followed, there are more involved and precise procedures that require additional personnel time. Great care must be taken both before and after the provision of care to ensure that *all* protocols are met. Otherwise, delays can be considerable, causing income to be slow in arriving.

Under several *government insurance* and *entitlement programs,* patients who are eligible due to physical or financial circumstances can have limited dental care coverage that pays at least a portion of the fees charged. The coverage amount is often far less than the customary fee charged, which discourages clinicians from accepting such patients since it may actually cost the practice money to treat them. This, in turn, makes it difficult for eligible patients to locate a dental practice that will accept them under the program and provide optimal care.

In accepting patients receiving assistance, it is important for the office personnel to review the government guidelines regarding what services are allowable and what dollar allotments are available for reimbursement for such services. There may be special restrictions that the patient is unaware of, which could cause embarrassment and perhaps nonpayment if those services are accepted by the patient and then cannot be funded by the government agency reviewing the procedures provided.

A classic and recurring example of procedures rarely funded by such agencies is orthodontic care. This aspect of dental care is still often viewed as primarily cosmetic by laypersons who write the laws to fund health services.

Preferred provider organizations (PPOs) have recently appeared as a way to deliver and reimburse health care. Such an organization solicits dental practices that meet certain standards of practice and that are willing to discount their usual fees or negotiate a specific fee schedule that is below customary levels. The provider is rewarded with a larger pool of patients and with faster claims reimbursement. The organization sells its program to purchasers of health benefits (usually for their employees), and eligible, enrolled persons select from the list of "preferred providers" for their medical and dental care. When one of the enrolled persons receives care from a dentist or physician, that provider bills the PPO for the discounted fee. Enrolled persons have the freedom to select a provider not associated with the organization, but usually they are then eligible for fewer "free" services or have higher copayments. The incentive is there for the person to select one of the efficient, quality providers on the list (Council on Dental Care Programs, 1983; Gable and Ermann, 1985).

One problem with PPOs is that they do not provide direct incentives for providers to control costs—overtreatment and insufficient emphasis on prevention are still quite possible. Practice review by the PPO could, however, add incentives since a practice's eligibility would be at risk if it was found to function outside acceptable parameters.

PPOs are relatively new—a phenomenon of the 1980s. Currently they serve less than 0.5% of the U.S. population for medical and dental care. But they have grown. In 1982, the American Hospital Association identified 33 PPOs; in 1984, they identified 115. The trend may continue, with greater numbers of dentists participating.

Health maintenance organizations (HMOs) and related *capitation* programs were introduced in the 1970s as a different way to pay for dental and medical care. Health care providers are reviewed by the HMO for specific standards of practice and join the HMO. They are paid an annual capitation fee for accepting a given number of patients who are enrolled in the HMO program. Thus, no matter if the patient presents only once for limited care or if he/she appears with extensive dental needs, the practice is paid a flat amount. The philosophy behind the HMO is that the providers are motivated to implement a strong preventive program so that the patients will need minimal costly reparative care. Opponents say that practitioners will simply undertreat the patients, regardless of their needs, and collect their annual capitation payment.

Capitation has grown in popularity, with many dentists accepting HMO enrollees for at least a portion of their patient pool. Quality reviews have been implemented to assure that patients are not undertreated. The general finding is that practitioners in HMOs do tend to spend greater effort on prevention than do their counterparts.

Capitation presents one major drawback for the dental practice. By agreeing to meet the dental needs of a specific group, the practice is assuming a considerable risk. If the patients demand a much higher level of services than the practice expected when it assessed the capitation fee and put an upper limit on enrollment, the practice is put in the position of either not providing the services demanded or providing the services at a significant financial loss. In either case its ability to deliver quality dental care at an affordable fee is called into question. In spite of the risk, many practices are choosing to provide care on a capitation basis, and this method of paying for services probably will become more popular in the coming decade.

During the 1970s growth in the number of people covered by dental insurance and capitation programs was a major factor in the expansion of demand for dental services. It is important to understand why this growth took place and its probable effect on the future. Before 1960 most health insurance covered the physician's fees and hospital costs associated with treating illness but did not cover the dentist's fee for treatment delivered in private practices. The reasons for excluding dentistry were simple: first, it was thought that patients *elected* to obtain dental care, and second, patients electing dental care utilized services on a regular basis and for a relatively small fee per patient visit. Thus it was thought that the cost of dental services was predictable and reasonably low and that families could easily budget for these

costs. At that time, a cost that occurred regularly and was relatively small did not qualify in the minds of insurers as a type of risk that private insurance companies would cover. A second reason was the ubiquitous nature of dental disease. If everyone who had dental disease sought care, the money paid would be substantial.

In spite of the stated barriers, private insurance companies began to market dental coverage plans in the late 1960s. Their primary customers were labor unions and employers who could provide dental coverage as a fringe benefit to union members or employees and their families. For the private insurance carriers the market for hospital and medical coverage had become saturated and offered little opportunity to expand business. Dental coverage was an ideal growth opportunity because the potential customers were the unions and companies who were already providing health coverage. Also, the effect of inflation on employee salaries encouraged workers to push for fringe benefits that did not increase their federal income tax liability. Instead of taking added compensation in dollars of which a good part went to the federal government as income tax, workers negotiated for fringe benefits such as dental coverage, which reduced their cost for dental care without adding to their taxes.

To cope with some of the negative economic consequences of funding dental coverage, the private insurance companies restricted their coverage by a variety of methods. For example, many policies required insured patients to pay the first $100 for dental fees charged in a given time period. Other policies required the patient to pay as much as 50% of the cost of dental treatment received. The $100 deductible meant that the insurance company did not have to pay for much of the regular, low-cost treatment that patients received. The 50% copayment meant that patients were responsible for paying a major portion of the fee for service, which discouraged them from overusing the covered benefits. Finally, the private carriers excluded coverage for treatment such as orthodontics, which was considered elective.

Treatments that contained a large patient elective component were predicted to be in much greater demand if the fees were covered by the company, which would lead to an overall increase in the cost of coverage. Thus to keep their policies marketable, insurance companies excluded these treatments from their coverage.

What kind of growth in private or government-funded dental health coverage can be expected over the next 10 years? Obviously, the answer to this question hinges on a variety of factors, including the level of inflation, possible changes in tax rates and the definition of what constitutes a fringe benefit, and finally, the general bargaining power of labor. Movement in any of these areas will affect growth in the dental insurance industry.

COST OF RUNNING A DENTAL PRACTICE

How is the income earned by a dental practice divided between the practice expenses and the income or profit to the owner-dentist? Generally, the term *practice overhead* refers to all practice expenses other than the income of the dentist. For example, employee salaries, equipment and facility cost, and the cost of insurance and supplies are expenses that must be paid if the dentist is to remain in practice and therefore are part of overhead expenses. In contrast, the net income of the owner-dentist includes the income that remains after all overhead expenses are paid. For this reason, accountants commonly refer to net income of dentists as residual income.

Figure 23-1 shows how the revenue earned by the average solo dentist in 1981 was distributed. The percentages are based on the data reported by 2,378 randomly chosen, independently practicing dentists for the 1981 calendar year. The graph shows that approximately 59.1% of the average practice income went to overhead while 40.9% went to the owner-dentist (American Dental Association, 1982). This represents an increase from 56.5% for overhead as reported in the 1976 ADA survey.

Dental Economics reported the results of a survey of dental practice activity for 1983. Nearly 30% of the 2,294 respondents reported that their incomes did not increase during that year; another 20.7% said their incomes increased by 5% or less (Anderson, What's Happening, 1984).

Most categories of expense remained basically unchanged from 1982 to 1983. Increases were noted in payroll taxes, laundry and cleaning costs, drug and operatory expenditures, and phone and utility costs (Anderson, 1984 Survey, 1984).

Salaries and benefits

In the category of personnel salaries, the upfront cost of paying the person is obvious. If a salaried person earns $300 each week, then that clearly is a cost of $300 to the practice. It may appear to be less than that to the employee, since the actual paycheck will be considerably less than $300. Amounts covering income tax (federal, state, and even local), Social Security, and other payments are deducted by the employer before the check is written to the employee. The usual guideline is that a person works 1 day per week "for the government" (20% of effort) and this amount is deducted from the check. However, it is important to understand that it is not the employer who is keeping that 20% deduction. The employer deducts it from the paycheck and forwards it to the government.

In addition to the obvious gross salary amount that the employer pays the employee, there is another less obvious 10% to 25% or more of the salary that the employer is paying. Social Security deductions from paychecks are matched by the employer. In other words, if $30 is subtracted from a person's weekly paycheck to pay for Social Security, the employer must pay $30 of the practice's income too, so that a total of $60 is sent to the government for the Social Security benefits of that employee each week. Worker compensation and unemployment insurance are also costs subtracted from the practice income.

Other benefits included in the 10% to 25% of gross salary suggested here include money spent for health or life insurance that the employer pays

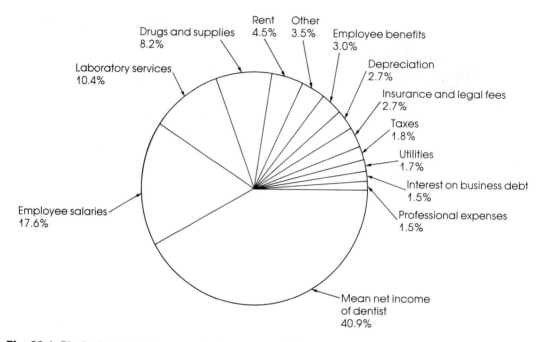

Fig. 23-1. Distribution of earned revenue for the average solo dentist in 1981 (American Dental Association, 1982).

for the employee. It may include the cost of free health care in the facility (which costs the practice lost income dollars since no other patient can be receiving care during that time and since it may cost the practice the amount of related laboratory services paid for by the practice). Lab coats or uniform service may be provided to the staff person, costing additional weekly dollars. And factored into the weekly salary is the cost that the practice will incur if that employee loses days because of illness or bereavement or when the employee attends professional meetings or takes a vacation. The cost of replacing the person on the days he/she is away from the office is absorbed by the practice while the "missing" employee's salary is continued. If no replacement is hired for those days, the working power of that person is lost, reducing the efficiency and subsequently the overall productivity of the practice on those days.

The percentage of additional cost to the employer for benefits will of course vary with the benefits the employer is offering. Some employ-

ers may have a profit-sharing plan. Some offer a retirement plan in which money set aside by the employee is matched by the employer, at least in part. So the cost-conscious employer should be aware of the actual costs involved in the employment of an individual as well as the amount listed on the period paycheck.

As gathered from the *Dental Economics* survey, overall employment of auxiliaries rose from 1982 to 1983. However, expenditures for salaries did not rise and the percentage of dentists employing hygienists dropped from 63.6% to 51.2%. Dentists may be moving to a greater percentage of part-time help at lower pay and foregoing dental hygiene services in their offices (Anderson, Staff Salaries, 1984).

Facility cost and maintenance

For the typical dental practice, the salaries and benefits paid to personnel make up the largest component of overhead costs. This is even more the case in practices that employ dental auxiliaries who assist in four-handed dentistry or do expanded functions. Next to personnel costs, the cost of laboratory services and then the cost of renting or owning and maintaining an office space take up the highest portion of overhead. Rent in a commercial building is usually based on the number of square feet utilized, ranging from as little as $8 to $30 or more per square foot per year. The actual rental price will depend on the location and the type of utilities and maintenance services that are included in the lease. If the rent were set at $10 per square foot per year, a typical practice occupying 1200 square feet would run $12,000 a year. The same practice located in a fashionable urban office building may rent for $20 per square foot per year, or $24,000. These figures make it apparent why it is important to use space effectively and why employers may be reluctant to expand the facility space before it is certain that the added space will generate additional income.

Related to the size of the facility and the number of usable operatories is the cost of utilities. The cost of lighting and water can be considerable to a commercial enterprise. The rates may be higher than they are for residential areas. Of course, adequate lighting and readily available water are necessary for most health services; what is important to remember is that they are expensive and should be conserved wherever possible. Perhaps this is one of the reasons the flushing cuspidor is rapidly disappearing from the practice of dentistry.

Equipment and supplies

Although it represents a significant expense, the cost of using, repairing, and maintaining dental equipment accounts for a relatively small portion of total overhead. The purchase price is only one factor in the overall cost of equipment. Most of the newer equipment is more reliable and requires less repair and maintenance expense. Furthermore, federal income tax policy encourages dentists to write off the depreciation expense of equipment before the expense actually occurs, a factor that further reduces the out-of-pocket cost of using equipment. When all aspects of equip-

ment costs are considered, it may well be that over the last decade, equipment costs have actually declined in comparison with the cost of dental treatment and the cost of employee services. If the cost of equipment relative to labor costs continues to decline, employers will tend to favor purchasing equipment (such as an automatic processor for radiographic film, an automated instrument sterilizer, or a computer) rather than hiring more personnel as a means of expanding their practices.

Insurance

As in any business, the dentist who owns and manages a dental practice faces the remote possibility that a disaster or lawsuit will result in a major financial loss. Fire, for example, could completely destroy valuable property and dental records, or a patient may sue and successfully recover for damages resulting from dental malpractice. To protect themselves against these risks, dentists buy insurance policies that cover their financial losses if and when these events do occur.

In recent years the premiums paid for medical malpractice insurance have risen sharply. A rise in the frequency of malpractice actions has caused insurance companies to increase medical malpractice policy premiums substantially. Solo dental general practitioners spent an average of $659 on professional liability insurance in 1981. Solo dental specialists spent an average of $1,132. These numbers reflect a recent, continuing rise in the cost of such insurance due to the increased number and severity of malpractice claims in the profession (American Dental Association, 1982).

Although fire, theft, and personal liability insurance do not relate to actual delivery of care, nearly all dental practices maintain insurance against these risks. They are roughly twice as expensive as malpractice coverage (American Dental Association, 1982).

Other expenses

Even with the ethical restrictions against advertising lifted, dentists responding to the *Dental Economics* 1983 survey reported minimal expenditures for advertising. More than 50% of dentists practicing solo, sharing space, and in partnership arrangements reported having spent no money on advertising. Group practices typically spent less than $1,000 for the year (Anderson, 1984 Survey, 1984).

REMUNERATION FOR HEALTH CARE PROVIDERS

Currently it is widely believed that only a licensed dentist has the experience and training necessary to diagnose and prescribe treatment. Dental practice acts in every licensing jurisdiction in the United States except Colorado (Colorado, 1986) prohibit licensed dental hygienists and qualified dental auxiliaries from supervising the treatment of patients. These professionally trained health care providers are generally required to work as agents of a licensed supervising dentist. Although not specifically stated in most acts, this commonly means that hygienists or dental auxiliaries must become employees of a dentist to practice their professions.

One may put aside the question of how this law affects the general level of oral health. Yet such a law clearly has a direct impact on the salary levels and the terms under which auxiliaries

work. Since licensed dentists for the most part still have the only legal access to patients, they ultimately determine the number of jobs that exist for auxiliaries.

Over the last 20 years, total compensation for dental hygienists, including money income and benefits, has not increased enough to keep up with inflation. (See Table 4.) At the same time the number of licensed hygienists and trained auxiliaries available to work in dentistry has increased dramatically, partly as a result of expanded facilities for training these professionals. It is easy and accurate to conclude that the compensation for hygienists and certified assistants is more a function of their availability than of their contribution to the practice. Both groups are highly vulnerable to changes in market conditions. If patient demand declines, dentists can adjust by substituting their own labor for that of hygienists or other auxiliaries. When patient demand is high, dentists can hire assistants who are not trained or certified to work as auxiliaries. As a result hygienists and certified dental assistants are in a poor position to benefit from growth and are more vulnerable in periods of little or negative growth in demand for dentistry.

It appears that the solution may lie in part in

Table 4. Salary trends in dental hygiene adjusted for inflation 1965–1984

Year	Estimated gross income*	Gross income annually+	Applied CPI (The worth of the U.S. dollar)	Adjusted annual income	Change in purchasing power**
1965	$20/day	$ 5,200	1.06	$ 5,512	+$ 312
1967	$50/day	$13,000	1.00	$13,000	—
1969	$60/day	$15,600	.91	$14,196	+$1,196
1971	$65/day	$16,900	.82	$13,858	+$ 858
1973	$65/day	$16,900	.75	$12,675	−$ 325
1975	$65/day	$16,900	.62	$10,478	−$2,522
1977	$70/day	$18,200	.55	$10,010	−$2,990
1979	$70/day	$18,200	.46	$ 8,372	−$4,628
1981	$80/day	$20,800	.41	$ 8,528	−$4,472
1982	$80/day	$20,800	.37	$ 7,696	−$5,304
1984	$97/day	$25,220	.34	$ 8,575	−$4,425

*Estimated income based on anecdotal information corroborated by survey data in various regions. No reliable national data are available.

+Based on 5 days/week over 52 weeks.

**Compares purchasing power to 1967 base.

educating the dental assistants and hygienists. The educational emphasis is on determining their worth in the practice. The individual should ask the following questions: How do my efforts contribute to the productivity of the practice? What effect would my absence have on its productivity? What percentage of this productivity should I share with my employer based on overhead costs and his/her personal income needs? The ultimate questions may be: What level of income is minimum survival wages for me? What level am I willing to accept?

This is a new approach to income for women who for years believed they had to settle for whatever was offered. Dental assistants' assertiveness in requesting a living wage was uncommon, and it was easy enough for the employer to refuse to increase the salary because there was always another high school graduate looking for a job who could fill the position after a period of on-the-job training. Assertiveness for dental hygienists was a bit easier some years ago because they had almost all the ''cards.'' After accepting a position at a reasonable salary, they may have discovered that frequent raises were a myth. Many moved on to other jobs, since the only way a raise could be had was to change jobs. Hygienists often acquired the stigma of being job-hoppers or prima donnas who were only interested in money and were somewhat lacking in commitment. Dental assistants, strapped with low salaries regardless of where they worked, developed an understandable resentment toward well-paid dental hygienists. Dental hygienists often did not display an appreciation for the effort expended by the assistant and undervalued the assistant's contribution. Hygienists were loners in their own operatories, keeping their own hours.

The stabilized salaries that dental hygienists now earn because of underutilization of dental hygienists in dentistry and the new assertiveness that dental assistants have acquired have begun a trend to equalize the salaries the two workers earn. One element that has precipitated this change is the delegation of additional functions to dental assistants. Once a dental assistant is trained to perform expanded functions, it costs the dentists a good deal more to change personnel. Retraining takes time. And in states where the EFDAs must be formally prepared and certified or licensed, the same scarcity that kept salaries for the dental hygienist high has caused a similar rise in the salary of the dental assistant.

A 1984 survey of dental assistants showed that 35% earn between $12,500 and $17,500, 30% earn between $10,000 and $12,500, and 24% earn under $10,000. Only 7% earn more than $17,500. Hourly pay rates for 53% of dental assistants fall between $5 and $7 (Results, 1985).

A 1984 survey of dental hygienists showed that approximately 76% of the responding ADHA members were paid by the hour or were on a daily salary. The mean daily rate was $97 or $25,220 per year, with slightly higher amounts paid to hygienists working in specialty practices. Of those working on commission, 47.3% reported working for 50–54% commission. An additional 16.1% reported earning 60–64% commission (Richards, 1985). Data regarding daily salaries are confirmed by the results of the *Dental Economics* survey (Anderson, Staff Salaries, 1984).

While there is still a discrepancy between dental assistants and dental hygienists, this differential of 30% is less than that frequently encountered in the mid-1960s, when dental assistants were earning minimum wage ($1/hr) or less and dental hygienists were earning $4–5 per hour or more.

Regardless of the social or environmental forces that are affecting auxiliary compensation, a knowledge of the basic method dentists use for paying auxiliaries can be helpful in negotiating an agreement with an employer (Table 5). Probably the most common method of remuneration, especially for the dental assistant, is straight *salary*. A predictable weekly wage is paid to the person for having appeared for work and for having performed as the employer expected or contracted for. Usually this arrangement allows for continued salary even if the person is ill or on vacation.

There may or may not be fringe benefits in addition to this, depending on the individual arrangement with the employer. At the time of the employment interview or after the person has been offered a position in the practice, the employer and employee agree on the wage and the fringe benefits. They continue until the person is granted an increase or until the work relationship ceases.

An alternative approach is to be paid a *commission* for services provided. This method is relatively common among dental hygienists who work part-time. Hygienists earn a certain percentage of gross receipts for the day. Or they receive a certain percentage of the fee of each procedure. For instance, there might be 50% commission on prophylaxes provided, but only a 30% commission on radiographic surveys exposed. Generally speaking, the daily take-home pay for the dental hygienist on commission is higher than that of the salaried person. However, if a patient cancels or if the hygienist is ill or wishes to attend a professional meeting, no income is generated for the employer or the hygienist during those nonproductive times. Fringe benefits are not as likely to be provided for the commissioned worker as for the salaried person.

Being on commission has from time to time been regarded among some hygienists as disreputable. The logic behind this belief is that the hygienist on commission must be in a tremendously tenuous position ethically if each procedure performed is viewed as a money-making procedure. Some believe that the commissioned hygienist probably envisions dollar signs in the eyes of each patient and undoubtedly rushes through procedures so that more patient procedures (more dollars) could be realized. The salaried hygienist was viewed as more ethical since he/she was guaran-

Table 5. Methods of remuneration

Method	Risk level	Potential income level	Fringe benefits	Method of calculation
Straight salary	Lowest	Usually lowest	Often provided; includes illness and bereavement days, vacation	Fixed amount each pay period regardless of number of services delivered
Salary plus commission	Slightly higher	Slightly higher	Few included in most employment settings; little or no allotment made for days lost due to illness, vacation, etc.	Fixed amount (low) regardless of services delivered; percentage of billable services is added; amount fluctuates with productivity
Commission	High	High	Few if any included; no allowance for days lost	Amount earned is a percentage of billable services delivered; amount varies with productivity
Independent contracting	Highest	Highest	None, except those provided to all staff by virtue of incorporation of the practice	Collect all income from billable services; pay overhead costs to employer of persons providing services, rent, etc.; amount fluctuates with productivity and economy of resources

teed the same salary regardless of how much was accomplished. Those in favor of commission argued that the employer-dentist's income rises and falls with patient visits, and this is not taken as a sure sign of lowered ethics.

Now that salaried hygienists' incomes have stabilized and those of hygienists on commission increase with higher patient fees (assuming that the hygienist's percentage is the same or greater and that typical hygiene service fees have increased with inflation), commission is viewed with less disdain. It is a more attractive financial arrangement that is not causally related to unethical practices.

Employer-dentists seeking greater productivity and more accountability on the part of the hygienist have opted for the commission approach. Many hygienists have found this approach to be rewarding not only financially but in terms of assuming additional responsibility in the success of the practice.

A third system, which combines salary and commission, is more palatable among those persons who have attacked commissions and some of those commissioned hygienists who have suffered financially from winter blizzards closing down practices on their workdays. *Salary plus commission* ensures the hygienist a minimum wage. Perhaps the guaranteed minimum is $60 per day, substantially lower than the usual gross earnings for a hygienist but certainly better than nothing at all. The hygienist is then paid, in addition, a certain portion of the daily receipts that may exceed the baseline salary. In other words, if the hygienist were to calculate earnings on the basis of 40% of the daily income of $400, the hygienist would earn $160 for the day. However, what if the receipts of one day were only $100? Despite the fact that 40% of $100 is $40, the hygienist would earn the guaranteed minimum of $60. This procedure is a more secure approach to income since there will never be a time when the hygienist is without income. However, usually this procedure is accompanied by a lower percentage of earnings. The risk factor (no income) associated with straight commission is usually counterbalanced by

the substantially higher take-home pay on the days appointments are full and the procedures provided are many.

It is important to find out the actual amount charged for dental hygiene procedures in a given practice and to establish the amount of overhead that is associated with the charge. In some practices, dental hygiene fees are surprising low—perhaps to encourage patients to return for regular recall visits so that more expensive treatment needs can be identified. Also, dental hygiene overhead is usually very low, since few expendable supplies are used per appointment. Assuming a high patient fee or accepting statements about the outrageous overhead for dental hygiene appointments can distort break-even analyses.

In one study in Kentucky, dental hygienists' production accounted for 24.7% of total dental practice production but only 14.7% of total gross billings for the practices. Mean hourly billings for dental hygiene procedures were $25.47; when materials costs were deducted, the billings were $24.32. In this study, dental hygiene fees are low in comparison to dental billings and so are direct materials costs for most procedures (Bader et al., 1984).

There is one other system that is probably more prevalent than organized dentistry or dental auxiliaries realize. There are some auxiliary practitioners who operate as *independent contractors* within the confines of a dental practice. The patients seen by the hygienist are sometimes considered his/her own, with referrals made to the dentist in the office as needed. The hygienist receives all the income from daily receipts and pays the dentist for a share of the rent, utilities, insurance, and other overhead. In this instance the auxiliary has full responsibility for financial success. This is only one step away from a hygienist hiring a dentist to perform dental work for the patients for which he/she provides preventive services. It does require, however, a willingness to expend capital to establish a practice and to establish continuing responsibility for the practice and the personnel employed by the hygienist.

Each state law must be carefully examined to

determine if a dental hygienist would be precluded from practicing this way. The law in most instances simply requires that the dentist supervise the dental hygienist, which in most definitions is interpreted to mean that the dentist is physically present in the dental facility or has given orders for the care to be delivered by the hygienist when the dentist is not present at the time services are delivered.

The particular method of remuneration that the auxiliary selects should be based on the individual's goals. If the auxiliary would rather not worry a great deal about whether or not a patient arrives for an appointment and would rather have a predictable, albeit smaller, wage, then salary is the method of choice. It is particularly helpful for personnel who have just graduated and who have not yet built up any reasonable speed in delivering services.

The experienced practitioner might find commission or salary plus commission more attractive, particularly if he/she rarely needs sick days and is able to save sufficient money to finance vacations and professional trips. Surely the commission route does foster a sense of fiscal responsibility that many auxiliaries currently lack.

Evaluating the financial contribution to the practice

An auxiliary can estimate his/her contribution to the practice by applying what is known in business circles as break-even analysis. This analysis is commonly used by managers who are deciding whether it is financially feasible to hire another employee or buy additional equipment. For the auxiliary, the first step is to determine how much additional overhead the practice would incur if he/she were hired. This includes the salary and fringe benefits plus the cost of added space or equipment required to accommodate the new employee. Step two is to estimate the average fee charged by the practice for each dental or hygiene visit. It is usually easier to estimate the fees charged for the average hygiene visit because it consists of the fees for a prophylaxis, x-rays, and an oral examination. For dental visits, the average

fee can be obtained by dividing total billings by the number of patient visits. This information may not be easy to obtain. However, asking about the fees charged per patient visit on the employment interview can provide this type of helpful information. The final step in break-even analysis is simply to divide the added overhead cost by the fee charged per patient visit. This gives the number of patient visits necessary to pay for the added overhead and allow the employer to break even. If the addition of the new employee increases the number of patient visits above the break-even number, the revenue from these visits results in added income to the owner.

An example may better illustrate break-even analysis. A hygienist agrees to treat recall patients for 50% of the total bills charged. If the dentist charges $50 for a hygiene visit, $25 would go to the hygienist and $25 to the owner-dentist. An additional $70 per day in facility and equipment costs is added to overhead to accommodate the hygienist. By dividing $25 into $70, the hygienist calculates that the owner-dentist can break even if he/she sees three recalls per day. If the hygienist sees an average of ten patients per day, he/she would earn $250 in commissions. The owner-dentist would cover the $70 in overhead and earn an extra $180 in income.

MEASUREMENT OF COST-EFFECTIVENESS

Cost-effectiveness can be assessed in two different and, it is hoped, complementary ways. One is to assess the number of procedures performed as compared to the outlay of resources. The second is to assess the actual quality of the procedures or "health effectiveness" of what was provided in relation to the resources expended. Dentistry probably does better in assessing itself in terms of the production efficiency. With a little help in time and motion management, most practices could improve the efficiency with which resources are allocated. But it takes far more skill to definitively demonstrate that health has significantly improved as a result of dental care. The fact that nearly everyone has some form of dental disease is the proof of this. Any periodontist who hourly faces the questions, "How could I have this periodontal disease you describe, when I have faithfully visited my dentist every 6 months for the last 20 years? What went wrong?" has a reasonable idea how effective or efficient dentistry has been in eliminating dental disease.

Do dental hygienists assess themselves in terms of plaque-free, sound teeth remaining in the dentition? Or do they assess their performance in terms of the number of calculus-free surfaces and bright shiny teeth at the end of each prophylaxis? What of the public health dentist or dental hygienist, or the public health physician or nurse? Have they really significantly affected the health of the population? Or can they simply say that they were able to carry out several educational programs within the state budget provided? Although there is considerable value in assessing efficiency in terms of the number of treatments delivered, the bigger challenge lies in assessing how the health of the people changes as a result of the providers' efforts.

ROLE OF THE MANAGER IN FINANCIAL WELL-BEING

All the issues surrounding the financing of dental care should be studied and monitored by a good financial manager in dental services delivery. Each change has an eventual direct impact on the well-being of a practice.

A good manager watches the finances of the dental practice carefully, preparing and following a budget that looks at the difference between essential spending and elective spending. The manager balances income against expenses and projects where and how additional spending can draw additional income (e.g., advertising draws new patients; hiring a dental hygienist generates income and frees the dentist to perform procedures that bring a bigger financial return, given sufficient patients).

Other skills the manager needs include the ability to purchase services and supplies wisely, to recognize quality in goods and services and balance that quality against cost, to prepare income statements and break-even analyses, to prepare tax information for filing, to identify good investments, and to plan and work toward increased financial stability.

Dentistry can be a rewarding career and a stable business if it is properly managed. Financial management is an essential aspect of its continued well-being.

Review questions

1. List five financial arrangements used to pay for the care delivered by dental care practices.
2. List five categories of overhead costs incurred by a dental care practice.
3. What is the distinction between overhead cost and the owner's residual income?
4. If a practice is operated inefficiently so that fewer patients are seen, how would that affect overhead and income?
5. Is the gross salary of the personnel in the office the total cost of employing those persons in the facility?
6. List four ways in which employees in a health care facility may receive remuneration for the services they provide.
7. What are the two outcomes that provide a basis for assessing the efficiency of a dental practice?
8. How many patient visits at $38 per visit does a hygienist need to have per day, with

overhead costs of $95 on 50% commission, (a) for the dentist to break even and (b) for the hygienist to earn more than $120 per day?

9. List ten functions of a good financial manager.

GROUP ACTIVITIES

1. Review the dental and medical benefits of four insurance carriers who reimburse for such services. Assess what services are covered, what the companies' policies are with regard to determining how much is reimbursed, and whether a mechanism for assessing the necessity and quality of the service exists.
2. Review the prospects for growth in the market for dental services in the 1980s and 1990s. What new type of practice organizations do you expect to thrive during this period?
3. Examine the socialized health care systems of four countries. Read descriptions of the effectiveness of the care delivered in those countries and the impact the socialization has on the health of the public and on the esteem of the health professions.
4. Interview several dental auxiliaries regarding the methods by which they are paid. Ask them why they have chosen those methods of remuneration as opposed to others that could be followed.
5. Debate the statement, "A hygienist who works on commission will not last long in practice before his/her ethical principles will be compromised and patients will be no more than dollar signs." Is this true of dentists who practice on a fee-for-service basis?

REFERENCES

American Dental Association: Survey of dental practice, Chicago, 1982.

American Hospital Association: Hospital statistics, Chicago, 1982.

American Hospital Association: Hospital statistics, Chicago, 1984.

Anderson, P.E.: 1984 survey looks at changes in dentists' office costs, Dental Economics **74**(1): 64, 1984.

Anderson, P.E.: Staff salaries level or down for 1983, Dental Economics **74**(2):46, 1984.

Anderson, P.E.: What's happening to the middle income dentist? Dental Economics **74**(9): 34, 1984.

Bader, J.D., Kaplan, A.L., Lange, K.W., and Mullins, M.R.: Production and economic contributions of dental hygienists. J. Public Health Dent. **44**:28,1984.

Colorado State Senate Bill No. 2, Signed into law, May 16, 1986.

Council on Dental Care Programs: Preferred provider organizations and dentistry, J. Am. Dent. Assoc. **107**:76, 1983.

Gabel, J.,and Ermann, D.: Preferred provider organizations: performance, problems, and promise, Health Aff. **4**(1):24, 1985.

Gowotka, T.D.: Economic growth of the dental profession: comparisons with other health care sectors, J. Am. Dent. Assoc. **110**:179, 1985.

Institute of Medicine, Division of Health Care Services: Public policy options for better dental health, Washington, D.C., 1980, National Academy Press.

Olsen, E.D.: Dental insurance, a successful model facing new challenges, J. Dent. Educ. **48**:591, 1984.

Results of ADAA Salary Survey, The Dental Assistant **54**(1):7, 1985.

Richards, C.: Who are we? An update based on 1984 data, Dent. Hyg. **59**(3):121, 1985.

CHAPTER 24

Integrating prevention in dental practice

OBJECTIVES: The reader will be able to:

1. Briefly describe the primary objective of a prevention-oriented health care delivery setting.
2. Outline three reasons for emphasizing prevention in dental practice.
3. Contrast a prevention-oriented practice with a traditional approach to health care delivery.
4. Outline the clinical and educational procedures that could be included in a prevention-oriented practice.
5. Explain four approaches for making a prevention-oriented practice financially viable.

People in health care periodically rediscover the concept of prevention of disease. Despite the fact that the health providers of ancient times described approaches to caring for patients that emphasized the control of disease and the establishment of a personal hygiene routine that would prevent disease, the literature over the ages has contained a series of ''new'' messages regarding prevention.

Despite periodic resurgences of preventive dentistry, clinicians seem to return to the ''nuts and bolts'' of dentistry, which usually means a return to a *treatment* emphasis. Newer and more effective ways to repair the damage caused by disease receive greater attention than do new ways to convince people to take responsibility for daily oral hygiene.

PRIORITIES AND OBJECTIVES IN PREVENTION

In some ways the return to treatment-oriented approaches is understandable. When a restoration is placed or when surgery is completed, the clinician can stand back and point to a job well done. That special treatment requires skilled hands, extensive knowledge, awareness of new materials and procedures, and an exacting approach to accomplish a task. It results in something tangible; the results of prevention provide delayed satisfaction and are less tangible. Outstanding skills in patient therapy were rewarded in professional school; skills in prevention were rarely acknowledged and then only as an adjunct to what really counts—treatment. Usually difficult treatment procedures command a higher fee than do preventive procedures so an emphasis on extensive treatment carries a greater financial reward for the clinician as well. Finally, for many years patients were believed to undervalue their ability to prevent dental disease. Therefore, clinicians saw little possibility of success in developing a patient pool that would seek, value, and pay for prevention.

Many of those beliefs and circumstances are being challenged by current and predicted changes in the population and in the composition of the dental profession.

The primary objective of a preventive practice is to put oneself out of business—out of the treatment business, that is. If all the patients are effective in their prevention regimens, little if any disease will occur. This objective fits well with the ethical mandate of a health care profession. A health care profession should want healthy people—not increasing numbers of diseased ones. This is a noble and worthy goal toward which to strive. It was a safe goal, because no one believed it could possibly happen.

And then it did happen. The fluoride that had been added to drinking water, toothpaste, and oral rinses, in combination with professional applications of fluoride, reduced the caries prevalence dramatically. By the early 1980s, 37% of children 17 years of age and younger had no dental caries (Miller et al., 1981). Dentists noticed that their young patients were getting good dental checkups requiring minimal restorative treatment. Older patients' dental problems were less decay-related. For some dentists, outstanding restorative skills were being used less frequently. For clinicians lacking the ability to carve out a new future in dentistry, it looked as though they would be put out of business.

Added to this was the growing number of dentists in private practice. The number of dentists increased from 98,680 in 1970 to 118,300 in 1979, due mainly to increased enrollment in existing dental schools and an increase in the number of schools (Gowotka, 1985). Thus competition for patients was greater, and when a dentist did attract new patients, he/she discovered that they had less need for extensive dental care.

Concomitant with the decrease in dental caries has arisen a new health emphasis among the general public. People are interested in preventing high blood pressure, heart disease, cancer, and other general health maladies that can be avoided by changes in diet, exercise, and other habits. Depending upon which surveys you read, between 30% and 50% of American households have at least one family member who is consciously selecting healthful foods, limiting food intake, exercising regularly, avoiding cigarette smoke, and in general taking good care of his/her overall physical well-being (Miller, 1985).

Thus, having prevention of dental disease as the major emphasis of a dental practice has more than an altruistic rationale. Certainly, the main reason for emphasizing prevention should be that it improves health and saves people from costly, uncomfortable, time-consuming treatment. However, an important second reason is that it fits with the needs and wants of a growing percentage of the population. People want prevention as a part of their general health; they should have ready access to it for their dental health as well. The third reason is that it can help a dental office find financial and professional renewal. Instead of offering ''dinosaur'' dental service, the practice can offer a ''new'' kind of care that values healthy teeth and supporting tissue situated in a healthy body.

DEFINING A PREVENTIVE PRACTICE

The way of the future does not seem to be in restorative care. It can perhaps be found in periodontal care, since nearly every adult has some form of periodontal disease. Clinicians can shift some of their emphasis and expertise in diagnosing, treating, and preventing periodontal disease. It can be found in a practice that focuses on prevention in every area, emphasizing a broad range of preventive services designed to promote oral health.

What do you do in a preventive practice? Clinicians emphasize thorough assessment of the person's dental health. They stress helping the patient learn to assume responsibility for the daily maintenance of their oral and general health. Time is spent teaching preventive procedures and showing how daily care can ward off slowly advancing dental disease. In-office treatments are explained as ways to ready the teeth and soft tissue for effective home care. Repairing disease still occurs, but it is repositioned attitudinally in the importance of what happens in the practice. Practices similar to what is described here do exist; many are thriving. These practices provide alternatives to the scale-and-polish, drill-and-fill nature that characterized practices in an era of plentiful dental caries and minimal attention to real prevention.

While every practice has to assess what procedures it will emphasize in its preventive approach, a list could include: a guided self-assessment of oral conditions and characteristics while the oral examination is occurring; a complete head and neck examination; a thorough medical history and blood pressure screening; nutritional assessment and dietary counseling; tobacco-use counseling; oral cancer self-examination procedures; plaque and gingivitis assessments; procedures and agents for improving oral hygiene; periodontal instrumentation and monitoring; fluoride therapy; sealant application; preventive orthodontics; and finally, restorative and surgical procedures. Again, the importance is how various procedures are emphasized and explained to the patient. How each clinician conveys and lives prevention is just as important.

The dental hygienist plays an important role in the development of a preventive practice. Hygienists were "invented" to be the prevention specialists with special functions in teaching oral hygiene to patients and preparing the teeth (the oral prophylaxis) so that they could be cleaned on a daily basis by the patient. Through all the historic ups and downs of prevention, the dental hygienist consistently has been learning about and providing preventive services.

Hygienists see themselves as health promoters with a strong role in that area both currently and in the future. They see prevention as very important—for general health as well as for dental health. Furthermore they practice health promotion for themselves. In comparison with the general public, a greater percentage of hygienists have quit smoking or have never smoked, wear seatbelts, have their blood pressure checked, and exercise vigorously at least three times per week (Holcomb et al., 1985).

Thus, any dental practice that intends to call itself preventive and make a cultural shift should include a dental hygienist to help make the transition. With preventive values already in place, structuring appointment sequences and preventive activities is easier to do and to promote to the patients in the practice and to the other clinicians.

FINANCING PREVENTION

The biggest roadblock to creating a fully prevention-oriented practice is the belief that it is not financially possible. Altruism is fine, but the care that is delivered in the practice still must pay the bills and generate a reasonable income for the clinicians.

In some ways, it may be the dedicated hygienist who at least historically caused prevention to be a money "loser" for the practice. Most hygienists have rarely specified a separate fee for patient education. Typically, it has been an integral part of the prophylaxis appointment. Patients became accustomed to having it as a part of the package, with a toothbrush and a new sample roll of floss included for good measure.

With the advent of dentistry's new awareness of prevention, charging a fee for the sixteenth-revised-edition of the prevention approach became nearly impossible. It is not easy to begin charging a fee for what has been "free."

Also, during the double-digit inflation of the 1970s and again when dental offices were having difficulty keeping their appointment books full during the recession of the early 1980s, many dentists decided to stabilize the fees charged for preventive care. Recall procedures, including the oral prophylaxis, were used as "loss leaders" to bring patients back into the practice so that dental needs requiring more costly treatment could be identified and treated. Thus, patients have come to think of prevention as not very valuable and not very expensive.

This approach needs to be turned around. The concept of a *series* of prevention appointments that address all the prevention needs of a given patient needs to become essential, and it needs to acquire new value that is worth paying for.

Most practices, including brand new ones, will

need to ease themselves and their patients into the idea of valuing prevention and paying for it. Introducing new preventive procedures to patients over time, carefully explaining their relationship to sustained oral health, and pointing out that the alternative is expensive repair later on can shift a patient into preventive thinking. As mentioned earlier, this scenario may be less difficult with a population that already has changed its life-style to be health conscious and that sees itself as capable of controlling the incidence of certain kinds of disease.

Making prevention pay is not a new challenge in dentistry. When prevention was revived in the 1960s and the American Society for Preventive Dentistry existed, many practices experimented with ways to make prevention work. Their experiments with payment alternatives took mainly three paths: charging noticeably higher fees and justifying those fees, burying the cost of prevention in other more treatment-oriented procedures (such as scaling and root planing), and selling a form of in-house "insurance" to the patients.

Clinicians following the first option made prevention new and special to justify higher fees. New gadgetry was introduced, with specially colored (red) sinks separate from the dental operatory so that a dental hygienist or control therapist could have a more clearly distinct opportunity to discuss prevention. Multiple appointments to measure plaque and hemorrhage indices for patients were introduced, with a fee specifically attached for all the attention. Some practitioners recommended charging high fees because it caused the patient to "realize the importance of" the control appointments. It was not uncommon to find a fee of $250 to $500 attached to such a sequence of care.

It may be easily argued that it is far better to pay hundreds of dollars to keep one's teeth rather than hundreds of dollars to lose them. However, it did become an ethical issue among providers whether such high fees could be justified for a procedure that used minimal supplies, very little

space, little time, and the services of an auxiliary, who in some instances had little or no formal preparation in controlling dental disease.

A second approach was to bury patient education in the cost of other procedures, such as the oral prophylaxis or the oral examination appointment. Instead of charging for only the actual scaling and polishing or for the actual oral examination, a charge was assessed for the time and supplies used in the control portion of the appointment. In other words, patient education was not really specified as a separate cost item, but there was some dollar allotment in the total fee to cover its being provided for the patient. This causes the business manager to begrudge prevention's inclusion in the daily schedule a good deal less. It is no longer a "free" service. During the high inflation years, increasing fees to reflect that added factor was a realistic solution to the problem, since fees were rising anyway. Burying the patient education fee also makes it a good deal easier to obtain third-party reimbursement for the procedure. Health insurance carriers will often cover the cost of the oral prophylaxis but are wary of covering such nebulous procedures as "control appointments." It is far too easy to fake such delivery of care, and the third-party payment system has difficulty being certain that prevention has any measurable impact on the patient's health.

A third approach to receiving a fee for prevention is to sell the patient dental "insurance" or a "guarantee" based on their continued participation in a control program in the office. In other words, the dentist charges a substantial fee for the oral examination, oral prophylaxis, and control sequence. The patient is informed that if he/she returns for frequent assessment of oral health conditions and if the oral hygiene index indicates that plaque is being regularly removed, then the dentist will provide at little or no cost any restorative or other therapeutic work necessary once control has been established. So the patient may pay for initial restorative and other therapy, but as long as the patient is under control and follows the recommended sequence and interval of control appointments, no cost will be incurred if additional disease appears. The dentist in this case is saying that he/she believes in prevention and is "guaranteeing" that the practice of prevention will indeed prevent dental disease. The patient has the added bonus of pleasant dental visits and a much greater likelihood of keeping his/her teeth for a lifetime.

This system does have its loopholes. The patient can feverishly brush and floss just before the control appointment, placing the control therapist in an awkward position with regard to accusing the patient of playing the system. Specific, defensible, observable criteria must be spelled out in advance for the patient regarding how compliance will be measured. The oral hygiene index or other measures to be used should be explained in detail, so the patient is aware of how prevention of disease can be measured. The patient needs tools to self-assess progress between the control visits, also, so that the recall visits are minimally authoritarian in nature. The visits should be an objective verification of how well the patient wishes to practice control and comply with the insurance arrangement. The visits can provide additional instruction and motivation for the patient, if the assessment indicates that less than adequate efforts (or at least results) are evident.

This strategy is in many ways what capitation programs, such as health maintenance organizations (HMOs), were designed to create. Under an HMO, the owner of the practice is paid yearly a certain amount per person enrolled in the capitation program to provide the care the person needs. In this case it is the owner (usually the clinician) as well as the patient who stand to gain from prevention. A strong emphasis on prevention, it is believed, will improve the health of the patients so that they need fewer expensive, time-consuming procedures that will earn no additional money for the clinicians. The clinicians are motivated to help the patients stay healthy and minimize the number of treatment hours per enrollee.

A fourth alternative, one that has become more of a possibility since increasing numbers of patients have dental insurance, is the prospect of having third-party payers fully reimburse preventive care and continue a policy of hefty copayments and deductibles for restorative and surgical care. The problem in having this be accepted completely is the difficulty of measuring what preventive measures were used and how effective each was in improving an individual patient's oral health. The area is ripe for fraud. Still, procedures that establish reasonable fees that show the value for prevention and mechanisms that track what services were provided should be established if prevention is to acquire its necessary position in dental care.

While each of these methods has been tried in practices and a few probably persist with varying degrees of success, none of these methods has been carefully researched as a viable alternative for paying for comprehensive preventive care. Such research is necessary, with alternative models clearly defined and tested, not only in terms of provider and patient acceptance but also in terms of clinical changes in the prevalence of disease. We have the data to show that caries prevalence has been successfully diminished through community and dental-practice methods and recommendations. We need similar data for periodontal disease, oral cancer, orthodontic care, and other oral diseases that can be addressed through prevention.

In the meantime, dentistry can attract patients with a new message that fits with the growing interest in health promotion and self-help. It can retool the kinds of health care provided to focus on prevention of a wide range of oral maladies. Individual practices can find suitable ways to make prevention pay—in terms of improved health for patients and a reasonable financial return for those who design and deliver the preventive care. It is undoubtedly a direction for the future, and for many it spells success in the present.

Review questions

1. What is the primary objective of a preventive practice?
2. What are three reasons for emphasizing prevention in a dental practice?
3. List five preventive procedures that could be included in a preventive dental practice.
4. Briefly outline four approaches for making a prevention-oriented practice financially viable.

GROUP ACTIVITIES

1. Ask a panel of hygienists and dentists to describe how they charge for prevention, patients' reactions to paying for prevention, and what they see as the positive and negative aspects of a strong preventive program.
2. Assemble a list of factors that could have contributed to the decline in caries prevalence in North America. Specify which factors are community, education, or mass media based and which are related to the prevention efforts of individual dental practices. Substantiate opinions with facts wherever possible.
3. Outline the incremental steps a traditional practice could take in shifting toward a prevention-oriented practice.
4. Invite a representative from a third-party payer organization to discuss how prevention is reimbursed (if at all) and how fraud could be perpetrated by practitioners if prevention were fully funded. Design a system that eliminates fraud in implementing prevention.
5. Describe in detail all those features that characterize a truly prevention-oriented practice.
6. Design a program for promoting a prevention-oriented dental practice.

REFERENCES

Gowotka, T.D.: Economic growth of the dental profession: comparisons with other health care sectors, J. Am. Dent. Assoc. **110:**179, 1985.

Holcomb, J.D., Mullen, P.D., Fasser, C.E., Smith, Q., Martin, J.B., Parks, L.A., and Wente, S.M.: Health behaviors and beliefs of four allied health professions regarding health promotion and disease prevention, J. Allied Health **14:**373, 1985.

Miller, A.J., Brunnel, J.A., and Carlos, J.P.: The prevalence of dental caries in United States children 1979–80, The National Dental Caries Prevalence Survey, National Caries Program, National Institute of Dental Research, NIH Publication No. 82-2245, 1981.

Miller, R.: America's changing diet, FDA Consumer, **19**(8):4, 1985.

PART SIX

Planning for greater responsibility for direct patient care dental auxiliaries

There is no single solution to the problems of improving health care. The answer, or at least the point of change, will probably result from a confluence of solutions. As incremental changes fit together, perhaps the larger picture of a logical system of care that measurably improves the health of the people will form.

The forces that have been identified in the early portions of this text encompass the primary sources of influence on change. The educational system, credentialing agencies, the state and federal governments, consumers, and professional organizations will help shape whatever stasis or change health care delivery realizes in the years ahead.

Primary to those forces is the concept of professional responsibility, which in its various interpretations defines what each professional holds onto and works toward when grappling with the problems of providing better care to more people in a more patient-centered system. Professional responsibility has been cited as the reason for not fully utilizing available auxiliaries. It has been identified as the reason for spending a year or more providing care in a remote rural area despite the attractions of the metropolitan areas, so people who usually have no access to care may have the services available to them. Likewise it has been cited as the stimulus for improved patterns of individual practice and as the reason for closing down experimental programs.

Whatever value system underlies a person's professional responsibility, it probably is the single greatest source of influence on the future.

CHAPTER 25

Prospects for a changing profession

OBJECTIVES: The reader will be able to:

1. List the four key issues that have driven the changes in dentistry since the 1960s.
2. Identify the key issue of the 1960s, 1970s, the early 1980s, and the late 1980s.
3. Explain four major steps dental hygiene will need to complete before being prepared as an organized profession for independent practice.
4. Explain three major steps dentistry will need to take in attracting a new patient base.
5. Explain the rationale behind differing views of the future of dentistry and dental hygiene in the coming five years.

The four key issues that have driven the changes in dentistry since the 1960s are those of access to care, cost, quality, and resource allocation. The poor oral health of the country spurred the development of entitlement programs and the discussion of national health insurance programs that would enable all citizens to have access to health care regardless of ability to pay. The major issues at that time were breaking down barriers so that people could have access to care. While there were major efforts in the areas of cost, quality, and resource allocation, those efforts were tied to efforts to bring dental care to the public.

The 1970s was an era of developing health care providers—both in numbers and in a variety of skills. It was an era of experimentation with expanded functions and a time during which educational programs to prepare dentists and dental auxiliaries grew in number and in enrollment.

The inflationary spiral of the early 1980s and the failure of national health insurance to materialize refocused our attention. The emphasis during that time was on cost containment, as health care costs outpaced the consumer price index for goods and services. Numerous plans appeared to reestablish how health care is paid for. It was a time of dwindling patient pools for many dentists as their numbers increased and as high unemployment relegated dental care to "luxury" status until families were able to return to work and have their union benefits reinstated.

The emphasis of the late 1980s appears to be on issues of quality, the legal issues surrounding resource allocation, and a new twist to access to care.

Dentistry is making inroads in ways to assess the quality of dental care. Third-party payers and practice networks are interested in how they can ensure that the care provided meets high standards. Increased litigation by consumers against health care providers, including dentists, shows the public's growing willingness to demand quality care and seek legal restitution if dissatisfied.

The primary resource allocation issue seems to be the degree of supervision that will be required for dental hygienists and denturists to provide care for the public. Denturists have made inroads in establishing themselves in state laws as recognized direct patient care providers—with their own governing law and dental board in some

249

states. Dental hygienists are pushing for less supervision, challenging the restraint of trade that the current laws place upon them. The coming years will probably see continuing debate and movement toward greater legal freedom for both groups. As periodontal disease emerges as the dental disease to be conquered in the coming decade, the efforts for greater practice freedom for dental hygienists should acquire energy and the attention of policymakers. The argument is that people should have ready access to a dental hygienist for preventive care and initial therapy for periodontal disease without having to go through a dentist.

Access to dental hygienists is the consumer side of the access issue that has emerged in the late 1980s. But the more compelling access issue is the access dentists would like to have to that segment of the population that does not regularly seek dental care. This group has periodontal disease, and it has unrestored caries and areas where teeth have been lost and not replaced. This segment of the population needs dental care; dentists need to see this segment of the population in order to provide the restorative care that has comprised the vast majority of the services dentists provide in practice. Attracting this group can mean the difference between a marginal practice (in terms of busyness) and a flourishing one. This issue will spawn debate about the ethics, legality, and practicality of various marketing strategies, including advertising, networking, capitation programs, and pricing. It will tend to emphasize dentistry as a business.

BEFORE DENTAL HYGIENE WILL BE INDEPENDENT . . .

Dental hygiene as a profession—as an organized group—needs to complete several important tasks before it can accept independent practice with grace. Individuals within the profession are ready now and have been for several years to establish their own businesses and provide dental hygiene care to consumers seeking such services. Readiness within the whole group is another matter.

Dental hygienists seem more willing to discuss independent practice than they did in the early 1980s, when it was spoken of only in hushed tones and even then with a strong sense of guilt. It was a sacred taboo. Now it is discussed openly in large groups of hygienists, and the majority of people in the room are willing to fight for its approval. However, an important step in the direction of obtaining independent practice is communicating among hygienists what the movement means, why it is important, and why many hygienists believe it is important to have it as an alternative. The profession's members need to see it as an alternative for those who are inclined and able to practice in this new mode. They should not see it as the only choice when it becomes legal. So the first major task is consensus seeking among dental hygienists—helping every hygienist be able to discuss the issues objectively, explaining why it is an important alternative for hygienists and what continued strict supervision clauses mean to hygienists and the population seeking dental hygiene care.

A second task is preparing realistic standards for permitting hygienists to become independent practitioners. This includes defining educational attainment, practice experience, and licensing mechanisms for this alternative. It could mean establishing two tiers of dental hygiene. It could mean establishing baccalaureate education as the minimum entry for dental hygiene licensure. It could mean a required residency for hygienists. The preferred strata should be discussed, defined, and ready to be put into effect at the time independent practice is more widely legalized.

Self-regulation is the challenge of the third task. Hygienists earning their practice independence may also be acquiring dental hygiene practice acts regulated by state boards of dental hygiene. The profession has acquired considerable experience in the ways of dental regulation since the majority of states have dental hygienist members on their boards. The collective experience and wisdom of the profession should be pooled in defining the scope of function of a dental hygiene board that would enforce the dental hygiene laws and evaluate candidates for dental hygiene licensure. In addition, dental hygienists should define what standards should be met in dental hygiene education programs and begin evaluating programs for their ability to meet those standards. Eventually dental hygiene may be accrediting its own programs rather than relying upon the American Dental Association.

Dental hygiene needs to establish a sound research base. It can do this by defining the scope of practice of dental hygiene—beginning by defining a dental hygiene diagnosis taxonomy. Such a taxonomy can help focus clinical research efforts to establish the validity of those terms and concepts and then establish research-based assessment procedures and treatment protocols. Dental hygiene needs to develop a body of knowledge that supports the content of clinical education and clinical practice. The questions that arise from the limitations of knowledge should drive the inquisitive minds of dental hygiene researchers to seek new knowledge. This effort can be in consort with dental research, particularly periodontal research. Recent years have witnessed the emergence of important contributions to the literature that support the efficacy and the importance of traditional dental hygiene functions in preventing periodontal disease and maintaining periodontal health after treatment. This knowledge should be assembled in a coherent way to establish the vital nature of dental hygiene practice—whether it is delivered in a dentist's office, in public schools and clinics, in community sites and institutions, or in independent dental hygiene practices.

BEFORE DENTISTRY WILL HAVE ACCESS TO THE PUBLIC . . .

Dentistry needs to reassess its priorities. The members of the profession need to blend changes in the dental health care needs of the public with their own needs for professional self-esteem and financial success. Dentists who want to perpetuate dentistry as it was practiced in the 1950s or even the 1970s may find that patients are no longer

seeking their care. The emphasis is shifting in the public's eye from caries to periodontal disease. Thus, a "good dental checkup" may no longer refer to "no cavities." It will refer to healthy gums. Dentists who look only at the teeth will find less work that needs to be done, and they will be missing an opportunity to help people maintain healthy supporting tissues and to provide a needed service.

Dentists need to redefine how they value the oral prophylaxis and initial periodontal therapy. It can no longer be the "loss leader" that keeps the patients coming back so that more costly restorative work can be identified. Periodontal care and prevention will probably emerge as the backbone of a dental practice in the 1990s; thus it must carry value—including financial value.

Dentists need to learn how to attract patients into their practices and retain them in their patient pool. They need to be better business managers and personnel managers so that highly skilled staff are retained, income exceeds costs, and patients' needs are always seen as the highest priority in the practice. The stereotype of the dentist will need to change from a well-intentioned, well-educated mechanic to a genuinely interested people-person who is interested in the well-being of each individual. Dentists need to learn to be lovable.

Finally, dentists need to learn to work with dental hygienists. If dental hygienists are employees in a dental practice, they need to be seen and treated as important team members who contribute to the daily income of the practice and to the goodwill value of the practice because of their relationships with the patients. If the hygienists are independent practitioners, dentists need to see them as important conduits for new patients—patients who were able to muster the courage to make an appointment with a prevention specialist but who couldn't face the prospect of a dental drill. Hygienists may be able to help patients move from total dental neglect to prevention and initial periodontal treatment and maintenance to an appointment with a dentist. Such a cooperative effort should diminish dentists' fears that hygienists are potential competitors for patients.

CONCLUSION

No one knows for certain what dentistry will be like in the coming decade, nor what actual issues will emerge for debate, public policy, and action. The certainty with which policies were made in the 1960s and 1970s has in some instances created rather than solved problems. Each new trend, whether it comes from within the professions or from the society, highlights a new issue and new debate. Ultimately, professional responsibility and a stronger sense of cooperation among all the groups looking for better ways for dental care to reach people should bring new problems and issues into perspective and help forge new directions.

Review questions

1. What are the four key issues that have prompted the changes in the dental care system over the past 20 years?
2. How was each of those key issues emphasized during the 1960s, the 1970s, the early 1980s, and the late 1980s?
3. List four major steps dental hygiene will need to take before being prepared to accept independent practice as a recognized practice alternative
4. Briefly describe three major steps dentistry will need to take before being able to attract and maintain a new segment of the population as their patient base

GROUP ACTIVITIES

1. Read the chapter by this title in the earlier two editions of this book. Discuss as a group how visions of the future have changed over a 10-year period. How does the way the chapters were written reflect the key issues of those times?
2. Invite local leaders in dentistry and dental hygiene to discuss their respective views of the issues facing the professions, how their differences in opinion are shaping dentistry/dental hygiene in the future, and what steps they see as necessary for dentistry's, dental hygiene's, and the public's needs to come together in harmony. Use your listening and conflict resolution skills as the leaders speak. Note how well they listen to each other. Identify their points of greatest difference and project how they might come to a collaborative solution.
3. Follow the ADA news and the Legislation & Litigation pages in the *Journal of the American Dental Association* for changes in dental practice acts and policies regarding alternative methods for delivering care and reimbursing for services.

CHAPTER 26

Attitudes, beliefs, perception, and change

OBJECTIVES: The reader will be able to:

1. Analyze the symbols traditionally associated with health care providers in various roles in terms of how they create stereotypical mind sets or expectations in the observer.
2. Assess traditional symbols regarding their impact on the flexibility and growth of the health care profession associated with those symbols.
3. Develop "objective observation skills" that enable the observer to look past traditional *symbols* to those *signs* that are justifiable in terms of what is observable.

This chapter is composed primarily of photographs of health care providers and their patients. Each shows a dental hygienist, a dental assistant, a dentist, or a student who is preparing for one of those three roles, functioning in some capacity within the scope of his/her practice. Typically, a person viewing these photographs arrives at snap conclusions about what role the provider is playing. A picture of a white-uniformed woman wearing a white cap with a lavender stripe signals "dental hygienist" to those who are familiar with the profession. Those who are not may conclude that she is a nurse. If she is in a dental office, the person may place her in the category of a dental assistant. A man providing dental care is most often labeled "dentist." A person in a lab coat, regardless of the person's sex, is often viewed to be in a position directive of or superior to the uniformed person. A care provider in street clothes may be mistaken for a patient.

The labeling is related primarily to attire (uniform, lab coat, street clothes) and secondarily to sex (men as dentists and women as support personnel). People feel less secure about labeling when the symbols are mixed, such as when a woman wears a lab coat or when a provider of care wears no symbols to distinguish him/herself as a provider of care.

Before sex role stereotypes can be broken down, they must be analyzed for their sources and for the impact they have on a profession if they continue to be used. As stated in previous chapters, most auxiliaries in dentistry are women. Most dentists are men. Because people see this so consistently, they begin to *assume* that a woman health care provider is an auxiliary and a man is the primary deliverer of care. Male nurses and hygienists and female dentists and physicians can no doubt recount numerous episodes of role confusion on the part of people encountering them for the first time. There are no doubt instances of patients reluctant to receive care from a provider who does not match their preconceived notion of what that person should be.

This includes preconceived notions regarding age, race, or other individual characteristics. A student 50 years of age in a class of dental hygienists may be mistaken for a faculty member. A faculty member 25 years of age may be mistaken for a student. Regardless of the *actual* role and skill of the person providing care, the patient may sometimes feel more comfortable in receiv-

253

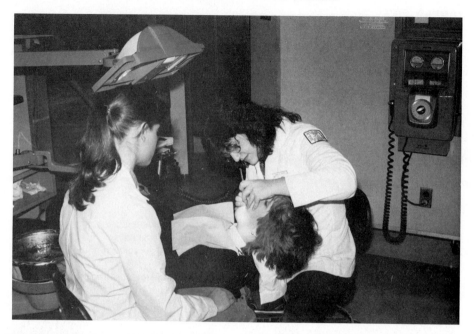

Fig. 26-1. Instructor teaching dental student? Dental hygienist with a chairside assistant? Dentist explaining care to an interested family member? On the basis of what is observable in the photograph, what conclusions can be drawn about the persons involved in the activity?

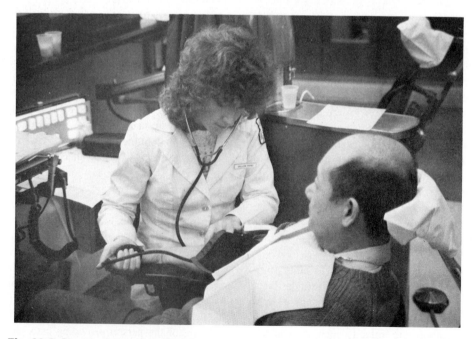

Fig. 26-2. Physician? Nurse? Dentist? Dental auxiliary? What symbols (present or absent) influence judgments regarding who this person is?

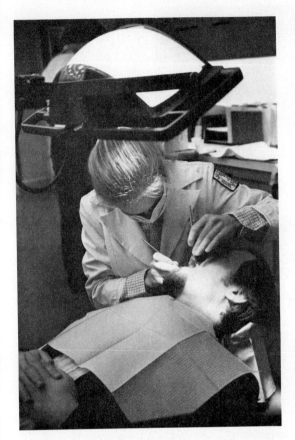

Fig. 26-3. What is your initial judgment? Is this a hygenist or dentist? What beliefs have shaped your judgments?

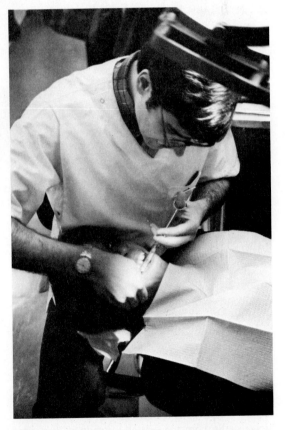

Fig. 26-4. Is this a dentist giving local anesthesia? Or is it a dental hygienist? How do sex role stereotypes contribute to assumptions?

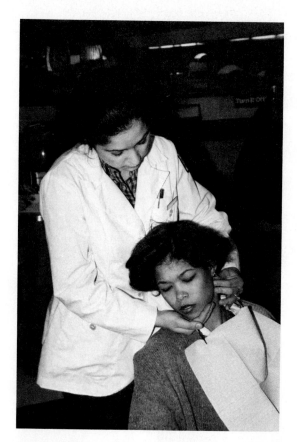

Fig. 26-5. Is this woman a dentist? Is she a dental hygienist? Is she an EFDA trained to perform the head and neck examination? Again, based on what can be objectively observed in the photograph, what conclusions are justified?

ing care from someone whom he/she would *expect* to have the role and skill.

These expectations become more serious when a potential employer has them and when a fully qualified person is denied employment on the basis of his/her inability to match those expectations. Admission to educational programs may be denied for these same reasons. Federal law has attempted to halt this kind of discrimination both in employment and admissions practices.

However, it is not possible to "legislate away" a person's prejudices and assumptions. Modification usually comes about as a result of continued bombardment by encounters with persons who do not fit the mold prejudice has created. Continued

references in education to male hygienists and female dentists is one way. Employment practices that favor members of "minorities" is another way. However, this may be difficult to accomplish if the educators designing materials and the employers themselves have prejudicial approaches to role delineation. Where should or can change begin?

Perhaps the best place to begin is with whomever is willing to learn to strip away traditional symbols and focus on objective observation. This exercise involves evaluating each "encounter" with minimal reliance on preconceived notions. Instead of concluding what a person's role or function is on the basis of symbols, the person

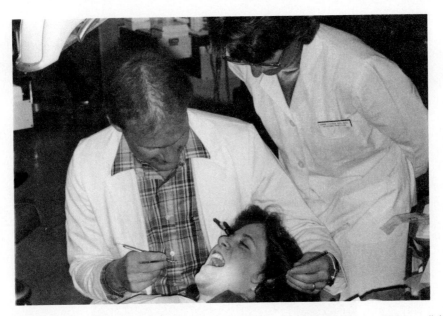

Fig. 26-6. Is this an instructor hovering over a student? A dentist teaching an EFDA a clinical procedure? What can you learn from the traditional symbols? How can you be misled?

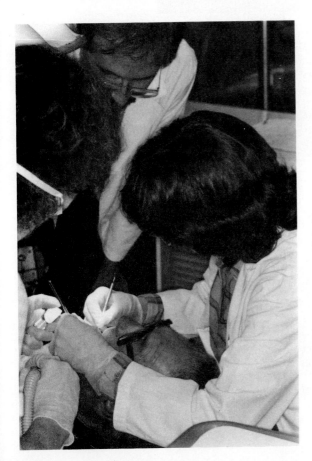

Fig. 26-7. A hygienist being observed by an employer? A dentist being observed by a student? What roles do you expect each person has?

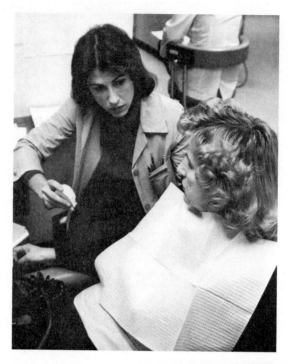

Fig. 26-8. Dentist presenting a treatment plan to a patient? Dental hygienist giving oral health instructions to a patient? What symbols trigger assumptions or expectations about the person providing care?

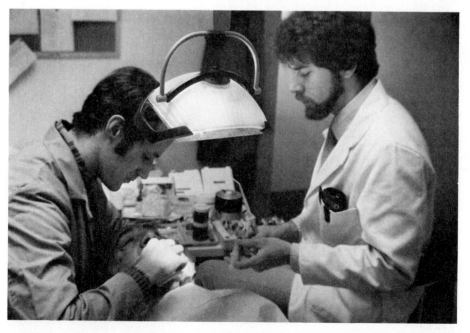

Fig. 26-9. Dental student learning from a master clinician? Dental assistant at chairside with a dentist? Dental assistant at chairside with a dental hygienist? What was your first conclusion? Why?

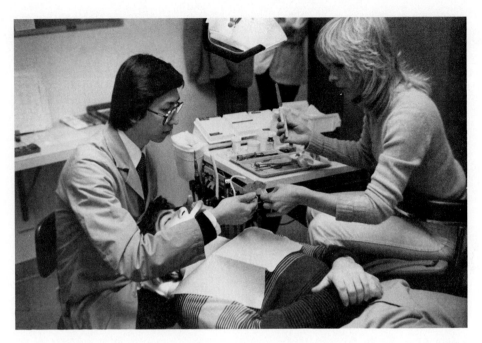

Fig. 26-10. Dental auxiliary assisting a dentist? Two dental students learning from each other? Or is this an instructor helping and observing a dental student? How do typical occurrences keep individuals from considering an array of alternatives?

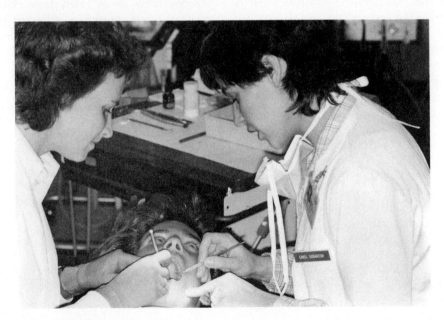

Fig. 26-11. Two EFDAs working together? An instructor teaching a dental hygienist? An instructor teaching a dental student?

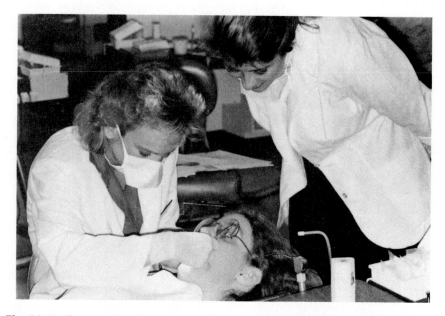

Fig. 26-12. Two dental students? Two auxiliaries? Are sex role stereotypes difficult to expel?

assumes as little as possible and rather investigates what the reality of the situation is. It is merely a scientific approach to role delineation. Although it is obvious that any preconceived notions people have had may be reinforced by what they learn (since men and women, for the most part, do still often fall into traditional role patterns), at least the mind can begin to practice separating out fact or objective observation from assumption.

If this skill of objective observation is not developed, there is little way in which people can begin to break down their prejudices. There is little way of knowing how many decisions regarding role delineation or expansion of function have been based on the usual sex, age, or race of the group or person rather than on the education or skill of the person. What seems important is to separate those issues. They have clear implications regarding manpower utilization if they are intermingled in the minds of educators, employers, providers of care, and patients.

GROUP ACTIVITIES

1. Discuss responses to questions posed regarding each of the photos in this chapter.
2. Debate the statement, "Before dental hygienists or assistants are fully recognized as providers of care and not just support personnel for dentists, they will have to abandon their traditional symbols that are associated with subservience."
3. Return to Chapter 1 and repeat the values clarification exercise. Discuss any changes in perception that are apparent in the group.

Values clarification statements

Dentistry is practiced nearly the same today as it was 20 years ago.

Dentists should be free to hire and fire people at will without interference from state or government laws protecting workers.

Dentistry has always "taken care" of dental auxiliaries.

No licensing jurisdiction recognizes dental hygienists who have had no formal education.

You don't need formal education to be a dental hygienist.

You don't need formal education to be a dental assistant.

Dentists learn how to work with dental auxiliaries while they are in dental school.

Dentists receive good preparation in practice management in most dental schools.

Management skills are not learned. You come by those skills naturally.

As long as a dentist practices good dentistry, there is little need to worry about business management.

High turnover of auxiliaries is to be expected. Dental auxiliaries are not very career oriented.

Most dental auxiliaries practice only a few years and then drop out of the work force for good.

Most dentists employ dental hygienists.

The number of dentists employing dental hygienists rose during the late 1970s and early 1980s.

The prevalence of dental caries has decreased dramatically among children in the United States in recent years.

Most dentists spend the majority of their time treating restorative needs and very little on periodontal needs.

Dental hygiene is an ideal profession for a person who plans a lifelong career.

Auxiliaries should unionize to improve working conditions and benefits.

There are too many dental hygienists in certain parts of the country.

Dental hygiene and dental assisting are best suited to women.

Unionization would deprofessionalize auxiliary practice.

Dentists have no reason to unionize.

Assistants stay in practice longer than hygienists.

Dental hygienists spend most of their time performing prophylaxes.

Hygienists who receive a commission tend to be more dollar-oriented.

Hygienists should work under the direct supervision of a dentist.

Dental hygienists in community programs should be free to provide clinical services without a dentist physically present.

Dental hygienists should be free to practice independently if they wish, making appropriate referrals to dentists.

A dental hygienist needs a chair-side assistant to function most efficiently and economically.

An expanded function dental auxiliary is another term for a traditional hygienist with added skills and knowledge.

Hygienists should always remember that their primary role is to prevent disease.

The white uniform is an important symbol of dental auxiliaries that should be retained.

A dental auxiliary must have and maintain good oral health.

The most important aspects of a dental hygienist's expertise are problem-solving and decision-making skills.

The most important aspects of a dental auxiliary's expertise is the ability to communicate effectively with patients.

A dental auxiliary is a decision maker.

A dental auxiliary implements the dentist's decisions.

A dental hygienist should wear a white uniform and cap.

A dental auxiliary should participate in continuing education.

Dental auxiliary practice should be regulated by dentists.

Dental hygiene should be regulated by dental hygienists.

Many hygienists do not stay in practice long because they are unchallenged.

Hygienists remain in practice a long time because of their commitment to oral health.

Auxiliaries remain in practice a long time because of their excellent working conditions.

Auxiliaries have excellent opportunities for personal growth and career advancement.

Auxiliaries leave practice because of the lack of opportunity for personal growth and career advancement.

A higher percentage of dental hygienists follow good general health prevention practices than found in the general population.

Dental students learn as much about practicing prevention as do dental hygiene students.

Just because a woman gets married and has a family does not mean she automatically gives up her career.

Both partners in a marriage should share in child care and in opportunities for career growth.

Dental hygiene and dentistry have a good communication pattern between them on the major issues.

Dentists should be required to have continuing ed-

ucation each year to retain licensure for practice.

A large percentage of dentists are inadequate clinicians.

Marketing a dental practice is an unnecessary and unprofessional activity.

Advertising dentistry makes it unprofessional.

Marketing dentistry can be an ethical activity that lets people know what kind of practice is available for them.

No licensed profession should be regulated by another licensed profession.

In general, dentists are pushing for tighter supervision of dental hygienists rather than less restrictive supervision.

A dental hygienist working independently can be an important source (for dentists) of patients who have been reluctant to receive treatment.

Patients fully appreciate the knowledge and skill of dental auxiliaries.

Patients prefer to receive care from dentists rather than from auxiliaries.

Auxiliaries are legally responsible for the quality of care they provide.

Hygienists are fully capable of assuming responsibility for the quality of care they provide.

Dental auxiliaries are not fully appreciated by most dentists.

Dentists are not fully appreciated by most dental auxiliaries.

Auxiliaries are receptive to suggestions for change and improvement.

Hygienists are prima donnas.

The best aspect of dental hygiene is its economic stability.

The best part of clinical practice of dental hygiene is the sense of completion when a prophylaxis is finished.

Hygienists really are more technically oriented than people-oriented, despite their protests to the contrary.

It is easy to get into a rut when practicing dental hygiene.

The clinical skills of a dental hygienist are not sophisticated.

Dental assisting is a high-status profession.

Men will not become dental auxiliaries because they need more money to support a family. Women do not need as much money as men.

A dental auxiliary needs a full complement of basic sciences to be competent clinically.

Dental hygiene is an excellent profession for a woman until she gets married but is quite unrewarding as a lifelong career.

Dental hygiene and assisting change slowly because practitioners are so isolated in various practice settings.

Dental hygiene and assisting change slowly because practitioners are reluctant to change traditions.

Dental hygiene and assisting change slowly because they are regulated by dentists.

Dental hygienists and dental assistants should ally themselves if the dental team is to function more effectively.

Dental hygienists and other auxiliaries should remain relatively independent of each other if they are to maintain their roles in the dental team.

There will always be a dental auxiliary known as the "dental hygienist."

If dental hygiene or assisting loses its prestige, I will leave it.

If dental auxiliaries become more assertive, dentistry will crush us.

If the preventive orientation of dental hygiene is lessened, the profession will be lost.

Future research discoveries in the control of dental disease will put hygienists out of business.

Dentistry will always be a viable profession.

Dental hygiene will always be a viable profession.

Dental assisting will always be a viable profession if it changes with the health needs of the public.

Dental auxiliaries learn cooperation skills rather than competitiveness in dental auxiliary programs.

Dental auxiliaries learn competitive rather than cooperative skills in school.

Auxiliaries need to have most intraoral procedures evaluated by a dentist.

Assistants for the most part are pleased with the relationships they have with their employers.

Most dental hygienists function to the maximum in terms of their ability to accept responsibility and perform complete clinical services.

Dental hygiene functions could fairly easily be expanded to be important components of most dental specialties.

A dental auxiliary is limited to general practice settings because of limited education and skill.

Most hygienists could not function adequately in a periodontics practice without additional training by a periodontist.

An orthodontics practice could find little use for a dental hygienist.

I would be reluctant to learn new clinical procedures through continuing education.

I would like to stay in one employment situation for as long as I can—even for a lifetime.

The adventure of change would make me want to change employment situations at least every 5 years.

A raise in salary is the primary reason I would want to change employment situations.

Hygienists are not able to assess the level of quality of dental care provided by a dentist.

There are areas of responsibility in which the dental team leader should be the dental auxiliary.

The leader of the dental team always is the dentist.

As long as there are many people with dental diseases, dental hygienists are needed.

There are not too many hygienists in some parts of the country; there are only too few mechanisms for people to receive the care hygienists could provide.

I would feel most comfortable practicing in an upper middle class dental practice.

Dental auxiliaries should be expected to learn to provide emergency care requiring administration of drugs.

The dental auxiliary's main goal is to provide service to dentistry.

The auxiliary's main goal is to provide service to patients.

The traditionally subservient role of women has

accounted for many of dental auxiliaries' problems in relationship to dentistry.

If dental auxiliaries want more responsibility, they should go back to dental school and learn to be dentists.

The practice of dental hygienists is in most instances intellectually and emotionally rewarding.

The practice of dental assisting is in most instances intellectually and emotionally rewarding.

The dental patient is a member of the dental team.

The dental patient in most instances does not care to be much involved in treatment planning.

The only reason most hygienists didn't become dentists is because they didn't want the additional responsibility.

Male dental hygienists are more assertive than female hygienists.

Auxiliaries need the security of a daily routine.

Auxiliaries are not paid well enough for what they do.

Direct patient care auxiliaries should be free to work on salary or commission.

Working on commission does not necessarily lead to lower clinical standards.

A hygienist's attire really is unrelated to his/her professionalism.

Dental hygienists need to change their image to be more closely associated with the concept of total patient care.

Dental hygiene should remain primarily interested in the education of patients in preventing dental disease.

Dental auxiliaries have always been oriented toward both therapy and prevention.

Some dental auxiliaries should be legally able to practice with no direct dental supervision.

Dental hygienists should be able to practice in schools, hospitals, and nursing homes, providing a full range of preventive and therapeutic services.

Dental hygienists should be able to practice in county and state health department programs providing a full range of preventive and therapeutic services.

Variety in dental hygiene lies in the wide range of skills its members can provide for patients.

Variety in dental hygiene lies in the wide range of practice settings from which its members may select.

Variety in dental hygiene lies in the number of patients for whom care is provided.

Dental assistants are generally overworked.

Dental hygienists earn unreasonably large amounts of money compared to what their level of expertise is.

Dental assistants generally earn reasonable salaries in return for their expertise and effort.

Dental auxiliaries generally have low salaries.

Auxiliaries should have a complete understanding of the costs of operating a health care delivery setting.

Dentists are overpaid for what they do.

Dental assistants are underpaid for what they can do.

Auxiliaries receive salary increases regularly in most private practice settings.

Fringe benefits for dental auxiliaries are excellent.

Auxiliaries generally have a ceiling on their salaries that rarely is raised despite length of service or quality of performance.

Most dental auxiliaries are content with their financial rewards.

Dental hygienists' skills can be learned through on-the-job training.

Dental hygienists' skills require formal education.

Dental auxiliaries should be licensed by the state to practice.

Dental auxiliaries need no legal regulation (licensure or certification) to practice.

Dental hygienists should be required to have continuing education each year to retain licensure for practice.

Dental hygienists do not need mandatory continuing education to retain licensure, since voluntary systems work as well.

Dental auxiliaries should be members of their professional organization.

There is little reason why dental auxiliaries should join their professional organization.

Student membership meetings and projects are

good preparation for local membership responsibilities in ADHA, ADAA, or ADA.

Student membership meetings and projects are poor preparation for ultimate professional membership responsibilities.

Dental assisting skills can be learned through on-the-job training.

Dental assisting skills require formal education.

Local component activities of professional associations should be mostly social.

Local component activities of professional associations should be mostly scientific/educational sessions.

Local component activities of professional associations should be mostly political/business sessions concerned with the role of the profession.

A large percentage of dental hygienists are inadequate clinicians.

People change their prevention routines for the better as a result of the efforts of dental hygienists.

Dental auxiliary practice should attract persons of all age groups into its ranks.

Dental auxiliary practice should primarily attract people into its ranks in the age range of 18 to 22 years.

Graduates of 2-year auxiliary programs have only a skeleton education for clinical practice.

Graduates of 2-year programs are not prepared to practice in sites other than private practice.

Graduates of 2-year programs are not as clinically competent as graduates of 4-year programs.

Graduates of 4-year dental hygiene programs in most instances are better able to make decisions regarding patient care.

Graduates of 4-year dental hygiene programs in most instances have higher status in the eyes of employers.

Graduates of 2-year programs are clinically competent for most community clinical practice settings as well as for private practice in dental hygiene.

For most dental hygiene functions, 2-year graduates are as well prepared as 4-year graduates.

The source of professional leadership lies mostly with 4-year and master's degree graduates.

The source of professional leadership lies with 2-year and 4-year graduates.

The main source of leadership for the dental assisting profession lies in dentistry.

Dental assisting should rely on dentistry for its leadership.

Dental auxiliaries should ally themselves with other health professions for strength.

Dental auxiliaries should ally themselves with other health professions to capitalize on scientific/educational events and sessions of mutual interest.

Dental auxiliaries should ally themselves with other health professions to create a health care delivery team that extends beyond dentistry.

Dental hygiene has much in common with nursing.

Dental hygiene is a unique health profession with little in common with other health providers.

Dental hygiene and traditional dental assisting have much in common.

Expanded function assistants and dental hygienists have a great deal in common.

EFDAs should not perform the oral prophylaxis.

EFDAs should not perform patient education procedures.

Dental assistants can easily learn clinical skills currently delegated only to dental hygienists.

Dentistry has tried to unify dental auxiliaries.

Dentistry has responded favorably to auxiliaries' efforts to modify their own future roles.

The fact that auxiliaries are almost exclusively women and dentists are almost exclusively men has little effect on the roles each have in decision making for the dental team.

EFDAs should have formal education.

EFDAs should be licensed.

Dentists are not interested in hiring auxiliaries over 40 years of age.

Age is of little importance to most dentists when hiring auxiliaries.

Dentists would probably prefer to hire women as employees.

The best feature of dentistry is its prestige.

The best feature of dentistry is its flexibility.

The best feature of dentistry is its pay.

The best feature of dentistry is its independence.

The dental assisting organization (ADAA) provides little leadership for the profession to change.

The dental assisting organization (ADAA) provides a primary source of leadership for changes in the profession.

Dentistry is a rewarding lifelong career.

Dental assisting is a rewarding lifelong career.

The term *auxiliary* is an appropriate title for an assistant or hygienist who provides direct patient care.

Allied health professionals in dentistry is a better term than *auxiliary* in describing dental care providers who are not dentists.

The rewards of a lifetime career in auxiliary practice are mostly related to service to people.

Dentists choose their career primarily because it affords them independence.

An ideal employer would be a hygienist who has gone on to become a dentist.

I would be unwilling to work for a woman.

I would be eager to work for a woman dentist.

Dental hygienists' salaries have kept up with inflation.

Dental hygienists' salaries have risen little in the past 10 years and have not kept up with inflation.

Some dentists dismiss dental auxiliaries to hire a less-experienced person for less money.

Dentistry and dental hygiene are coprofessions.

The financial security of dentistry is threatened by the prospect of dental hygienists working independently.

Dentistry for the most part supports independent practice for hygienists.

Dental hygiene should be regulated by state boards of dental hygienists rather than by a board of dentists.

It costs the dentist money to employ a hygienist.

The dentist receives income from the work of an employee-hygienist.

I am aware of my rights in the employer-employee relationship.

I wish I were aware of my rights as an employee.

I trust that my employer will take care of me.

I am interested in having an opportunity to practice as an independent contractor in a dentist's office or to own my own practice.

Some auxiliaries enjoy being treated like "girls."

If I think of myself as a woman rather than as a girl and reject being called a girl, I seem to get more professional and personal respect.

If a dentist insists that an auxiliary perform an illegal procedure, the dentist has the *full* responsibility.

Dental hygienists are a basically happy, fulfilled group.

Dental hygienists seem rigid in their ways.

Dental hygienists are as eager to change themselves as they are their patients.

Dental hygienists like things carefully defined and uniform.

Dental hygienists are suspicious of change that affects them.

Hygienists should be willing to change the name of their profession and their self-image to meet a changed need in dental health care delivery.

Dental hygiene is a therapeutically oriented profession.

Dental hygiene has a strong tradition that should be maintained.

A good dental hygienist will work him/herself out of a "job" by having the patients prevent dental disease.

Decision making and working for a dentist are incompatible roles for a dental auxiliary.

A dental hygienist has the skill to diagnose caries.

A dental hygienist educated to perform gingival recontouring or place a restoration cannot be expected to do as well as a dentist.

A dentist and a dental auxiliary who have been given equivalent education to perform a given skill should be able to do equally well.

A patient sees the dental hygienist as the "person who cleans my teeth."

Dental hygienists soon drop patient education from their scope of practice after graduation.

Dental auxiliary programs emphasize total patient care more than mastering individual clinical skills.

Dental auxiliary programs emphasize clinical expertise that is not needed in practice.

Dental hygienists are full members of the dental team.

Dental assistants are full members of the dental team.

A dental practice that does not have a hygienist is missing an important team member.

A dental hygienist can and should be able to supervise other auxiliaries in a practice setting.

The best feature about dental assisting is its prestige.

The best feature about dental assisting is its flexibility.

The best feature about dental assisting is the pay.

The best feature about dental hygiene is the pay.

A dental hygienist often believes he/she is separate from the dental team.

Current dental practice does not permit a dental hygienist to perform all the services learned in school.

Dental hygiene is a relatively static profession.

The dental hygiene organization (ADHA) provides little leadership for the profession to change.

The dental hygiene organization (ADHA) is a primary source of leadership for changes in the profession.

Dental hygiene should expand its scope of responsibility in practice.

Dental hygiene should stay as it is.

Dental hygienists should be women.

When I think "dentist," I think "man."

When I think "dental auxiliary," I think "woman."

When I think "dental auxiliary," I think "girl."

Male dental auxiliaries cannot provide the same caring service that women can.

Male dental auxiliaries can be just as caring as their female counterparts.

Dentists view auxiliaries as subservient.

The idea of a dental hygienist practicing without a dentist on the premises is frightening or at least makes me uncomfortable.

An auxiliary usually is hired largely on the basis of appearance.

Dental hygienists should be the group to examine candidates for dental hygiene licensure.

Dental hygiene is a widely recognized health profession.

Dental hygiene is more of a vocation than a profession.

The oral prophylaxis is the most important function of the dental hygienist.

Patient education is the most important function of the dental auxiliary.

Answers to review questions

Chapter 2

1. Alfred C. Fones
2. Irene Newman
3. A preventive role in which the profession removed calcareous deposits (oral prophylaxis), performed oral examinations, and provided patient education. The role developed primarily in public school systems in the East.
4. The preparation and placement of restorations, extraction of deciduous teeth, pulp capping, diagnosis, treatment planning.
5. a. Placement of amalgam and tooth-colored restorations
   b. Preparation of teeth and placement of restorations, local anesthesia, periodontal functions including surgery on soft tissues.
6. The caries prevalence in the United States and in most developed countries has dropped dramatically so that the demand for restorative care has diminished. In contrast, prevalence of periodontal disease has not decreased. It affects nearly all adults in all countries. It is more likely that periodontal functions will be delegated than restorative functions as a result of this change.
7. The trend toward independent practice for dental hygienists.

Chapter 3

1. Dentistry is moving from a cottage industry with a large number of solo practitioners to a delivery system that includes a wider range of practice settings, including group practices, franchise and retail dental practices, and hospital sites. It previously operated on a fee-for-service payment system; now insurance and capitation programs are far more prevalent. Access to dental care is blocked by cost, attitude, and geographic distribution factors. There is no formal widespread system of peer review, although as a greater percentage of dental procedures are reimbursed through insurance programs, dentists are more frequently reviewed for appropriateness of care and outcome of care. Dentists typically use few auxiliaries, with limited delegation of expanded functions.

2. The prediction of increased demand for care in the 1960s and 1970s.
3. a. Carnegie Commission Report of 1970.
   b. Survey of Dentistry, 1961.
4. The ADA has acknowledged that services *can* be delegated to auxiliaries, but they question whether they *should* be. Position statements of the late 1970s indicate that dentistry has adopted a more conservative view of auxiliary utilization, essentially reversing its position of the 1960s and early 1970s.
5. a. Acceptance of professional advertising changed the nature of how dentistry is explained to consumers.
   b. Dentistry became available in retail stores targeting that segment of the population that does not routinely receive dental care, and dental franchises opened capitalizing on their ability to market and manage effectively.
   c. The increased numbers of dentists and the change in dental disease increased competition among dentists for patients.
   d. The economy of the early 1980s and the competition for patients caused dentists, insurance companies, and employers offering dental benefits to focus upon cost containment.
   e. The decrease in caries prevalence affected the mix of services a dentist could provide and made delegation of restorative functions to dental auxiliaries less likely.
6. A dentist is paid a set amount for each enrollee in the health maintenance organization (HMO) that appears for dental care. Thus there is a predictable annual capitation payment made to the dentist, upon which he/she can rely in addition to fee-for-service collections made from non-HMO patients. The drawback is that the patients may require extensive dental care that exceeds the capitation amount.

   A dentist who joins a preferred provider organization (PPO) has access to a pool of patients who are enrolled in the plan, thus increasing the patient base. Each service provided the PPO patients is reimbursed by the PPO at a discounted fee. There is a risk that the discounted fee is so low that little net income is derived from offering the service.

Chapter 4

1. Together accreditation and credentialing provide methods for ensuring the quality of care delivered to the public. They also serve as a control over the growth and direction of the professions.
2. License
3. Certification
4. Dentistry is only recently increasing its reliance on third-party payment reimbursement and has had little reason to be "excepted" by such payers. Therefore they have not been active until recently in accreditation of practices by any group that might specify *certified* personnel.

5. With the rapidly growing allied health movement of the 1960s, numerous categories of workers were created, each with its own certifying process. No comprehensive plan was followed.

6. Except in Colorado, hygenists may not own their own practices and may not compete with dentists or have direct access to the public to provide care. Hygienists must be able to find a position with a supervising dentist in order to work.

7. An administrative ruling by the Federal Trade Commission calling the supervision clauses a restraint of trade; a judicial overturn if tested in the courts; a legislative change in the laws which would eliminate the clauses.

8. Enforcing the dental law; approving candidates for licensure; approving dental hygiene programs within the state.

Chapter 5

1. The consumer movement; third-party payers
2. Cost, access, quality
3. External reviewers, sometimes including consumers, review patient records to evaluate patient assessment techniques used and to match them against the subsequent diagnosis and treatment. They ensure that treatment was actually performed. In addition, audits can match the number of procedures a clinician performs against national norms to determine "outliers" who should be investigated in greater depth.
4. A small peer group includes clinicians who determine the clinical criteria that will be used and then observe one another during patient procedures to determine whether those agreed-upon criteria are followed. The group discusses discrepancies and prescribes changes. Such groups are voluntary and are not yet connected to third-party payer systems of review.

Chapter 6

Case 1

1. Not necessarily
2. If the dentist is employed in a federal clinic, he/she is obligated to provide care to eligible persons; if the provider is in the midst of providing care, he/she must complete the treatment agreed to; if the patient is enrolled as a subscriber to a prepaid dental plan with which the provider has a contractual arrangement, the dentist must accept the patient for care.

Case 2

The duty to commence treatment within a reasonable time

Case 3
1. Yes
2. Breach of the duty to protect the patient from hazards in the office
3. The patient may sue for negligence charging that the "reasonably prudent man" would clear the patient's pathway of such obstacles; the provider could claim contributory negligence on the part of the patient as a defense.

Case 4
1. Yes
2. Duty to complete treatment that has begun; the patient has been abandoned.
3. Agent
4. The hygienist and the hospital (and perhaps an intermediate dental supervisor)

Case 5
1. Secure written permission from the patients to use the photographs and models; omit patient names from the display unless specifically allowed, in writing, by the patients.
2. Duty to protect the patient's right to privacy
3. Patient could sue for breach of contract or invasion of privacy (if harm resulted to the patient as a result of the display) or sue under quasi contract grounds for reasonable compensation. (The loss in this case assumes a contract exists if a person earns money from the use of another's picture.) (See Chapter 7 for further discussion of contracts, including quasi contracts.)
4. Yes
5. The patient has a right to privacy, and the dental hygienist has a duty to protect that right.

Case 6
1. Yes
2. Duty to pay a reasonable fee
3. Dentist can sue for breach of this duty to recover payment.
4. The patient may attempt proceedings charging negligence.

Case 7
1. Yes
2. Duty to perform only those services agreed to
3. Patient may charge technical assault or battery. However, recovery will be minimal unless the patient can show some significant harm.

Case 8

1. Yes
2. Breach of duty to satisfy the patient *if* satisfaction (or a given result) is promised and breach of duty to obtain informed consent regarding the possible outcome of treatment
3. A health professional is not expected to guarantee his/her results, but if he/she does promise or guarantee a result, the law holds him/her to that promise as a matter of contract; the provider is expected to inform the patient of outcome before commencing treatment.
4. The patient can charge breach of contract.
5. The dental hygienist will suffer time and anguish in court, a tarnished reputation and financial loss (especially if he has no personal liability insurance).

Case 9

1. Yes
2. Not necessarily. A reasonably prudent dentist could fracture a root tip. The fracture *in itself* is not proof of negligence.
3. The dentist breached the duty to keep the patient informed.
4. Yes, the dentist could have told the patient about the fracture and suggested they wait to remove it.
5. The patient may bring a breach of contract charge since the duty to keep the patient informed is a contractual matter, or the patient may bring a negligence charge since she suffered so much harm as a result of a breach of professional duty.

Case 10

1. Yes, if she can prove that she was not given "reasonable care" by not having the benefits of plaque control information.
2. The question will be: "Would the reasonably prudent dental hygienist and dentist in that locality have done more in plaque control?" An interesting note is that if the patient can prove that plaque control programs are an integral part of dental hygiene programs and that licensing procedures include examination of skills in plaque control, the patient may be able to use a regional or national standard in proving negligence on the part of the dental hygienist.

Case 11

1. Yes
2. Duty to protect the safety of the patient
3. The patient will probably sue both the dentist (invoking *respondeat superior*) and the dental assistant (since he actually performed the harmful act).

4. The assistant's behavior will be measured against "the reasonably prudent dental assistant" and an educated assistant at that. Whether a person is certified, licensed, or not, if he/she sets himself up as having the skills to perform his/her services correctly, the individual is held to the standards of the qualified person. The dentist is liable because of the agency relationship, but he/she may also be measured against "the reasonably prudent dentist" for not ensuring that the person responsible for sterilization is performing that service correctly.

Chapter 7

1. Consensual, contractual
2. a. Oral
   b. Written
3. An implied contract relies on the consenting *actions* of the patient and health care provider. No oral or written agreement is made.
4. a. True
   b. True
   c. True
   d. True. Often a patient does not pay because he/she is dissatisfied with the care. The suit for nonpayment brings that dissatisfaction to the surface in the form of a countersuit.

Chapter 8

1. Negligence is the commission of an act that the reasonably prudent person would not have performed or the omission of an act that the reasonably prudent person would have performed.
2. Whether or not the reasonably prudent person in that profession and under the same circumstances would have performed similarly, according to defined standards of practice.
3. a. Duty is owed to a person (a contract exists).
   b. There is a breach of that duty.
   c. The person has been injured or harmed.
   d. The breach of the duty is the proximate cause of the harm.
4. The patient "contributed" his own ignorance or action to the situation, "contributing" to the harm.
5. The "proximate cause" is the factor that can be directly and causally related to the harm.
6. False or at least unlikely; check the state law for the exact provision.
7. False; definitive performance criteria are now more commonly used.
8. False; all providers of care *are* responsible for their actions.

Chapter 9

1. Technical battery
2. A person in a contract does not perform as agreed to.
3. In technical battery, some procedure *not* agreed to *is* performed, rather than some agreed-to procedure not being performed.
4. a. Negligence
   b. Technical battery
5. Express
6. a. Could be upheld
   b. Could be upheld
   c. Not likely to be upheld
7. Provide minimal damages awards.

Chapter 10

1. Contracts and fees may be implied or expressed (verbal or written).
2. It is based on what is customary locally, on the scope of the procedure and the skill of the operator, on overhead costs, and on the ability of the patient to pay.
3. He may countersue, charging malpractice.
4. a. Accurate, coherent, quality radiographs
   b. A medical history
   c. Care is related to need
   d. Progress of health is discernible
5. *Res gestae*
6. Admission against interest
7. False

Chapter 11

1. True
2. False; criminal law is an act committed against society by virtue of a violation of an enacted state or federal law or case law.
3. True; case law is another source.
4. False; dental practice acts are written and enacted by the legislature.
5. True
6. False; in a closed practice act, all regulations are contained in the enacted law. In an open practice act, some modifying or clarifying clauses may be made by the state board in the form of rules and regulations.
7. False; it is to protect the public. It also limits entry to the profession, which many view as a form of professional protection.
8. Criminal law

9. Civil law
10. Civil *and* criminal law; the patient can sue the assistant and dentist. The state can prosecute the assistant and dentist.
11. Criminal law

Chapter 12

1. a. False; behaviorists see ethical problems as a matter of not having ''learned'' the appropriate behavior. A systematically applied program of positive and negative reinforcement, and perhaps punishment, will in their view change the person's behavior.
   b. False; although humanists may be atheistic, many are theistic, believing that a part of the deity resides in each of us.
   c. True
   d. True
   e. False; Eastern philosophies differ in that they place greater emphasis on the Cosmos.
2. 1. d.
   2. c.
   3. b.
   4. e.
   5. a and d; some people would add b and c as well.
5. A bill of rights expresses what a person, in this case a patient, can expect. Behavior that ensures that those rights will be maintained is inferred from the document. So the health care provider is expected to read the rights to which the patient is entitled and then act accordingly.
6. a. Obedience-punishment
   b. Näive hedonistic and instrumental
   c. Good boy–nice girl
   d. Law and order
   e. Social contract
   f. Universal ethical principle
7. a. False; all people pass through the stages, but many people stop at an early stage.
   b. False; it should be to promote the professional covenant to provide service, ensuring its availability and using all of one's resources to meet the needs of one's patients with humility.
   c. False; Nash disagrees with paternalism.

Chapter 13

1. Compare your five principles with the 1975 code in the previous chapter. Save your written suggestions for inclusion in group discussion.

2. a. Practitioners sometimes bill for services that were not performed, provide unneeded services, or otherwise submit incorrect information to third-party payers to secure more reimbursement than they or their patients are entitled to.

   b. Many people believe that there is an ethical responsibility to provide services to people who either because of geographical location or economic status have been unable to secure health care. This places a considerable burden on health care providers who would not normally select the geographical locations in which the unmet need exists and because the present state of the economy makes it extremely difficult to attempt to provide care for patients who cannot pay.

   c. Advertising is now an ethically and legally allowable practice for the health professions. However, the nature of the advertisements and the growth of large franchise dental practices cause many professionals to believe that the profession is in a decline.

   d. Some practitioners will not provide health care services for people on public assistance. They may have preconceived notions of the needs of those persons and therefore may discriminate against them by refusing them care. The situation is compounded by the fact that reimbursement for such services may be a great deal lower than the usual fee for care; thus the dentist takes a loss.

   e. Some believe that it is unethical to tell patients that the care they have received is poor. However, patients rely on the health care professionals to be fully informed of their dental needs.

Chapter 14

1. Private dental offices
2. Scope of practice can be broadened; financial goals and security are often better in other employment sites.
3. Independent contracting (independent practice depending upon legal status), hospitals, centers for the physically and mentally handicapped, long-term care facilities, hospices, programs for the homebound or for the homeless, and many others.
4. Management and planning, marketing, research, teaching, and an array yet to be developed.
5. Establishing a firm foundation in clinical practice, advanced education, accepting employment opportunities that gradually lead toward a career goal by offering additional experiences and developing new skills.

Chapter 15

1. a. Salary
   b. Fringe benefits
   c. Location

d. Security
e. Opportunity for advancement
f. Role/responsibility
g. Variety of services that can be provided
h. Personnel relationships
i. Working environment
j. Need of the people
3. A form similar to that shown in Tables 6 and 7 will probably meet one's needs.
4. Either the calculator needs new batteries or the health care provider ought to be more honest with him/herself regarding the weighting of factors.

Chapter 16

1. A resume is often the first contact between an applicant and a potential employer. If well-prepared, it can assist the reviewer in identifying how a person's qualifications match with the available position. It can lead to an interview.
2. a. Name, address, telephone
   b. Educational background
   c. Licensure or certification status
   d. Work experience
   e. Research, publication, continuing education
   f. Goals statement or brief autobiography.
3. Age, sex, race, creed, or national origin.
4. Employment responsibilities directly applicable to the position being applied for may be described in a brief line or two below the appropriate employment experience entry. The purpose of the description is to point out to the prospective employer how previous experience qualifies the person for the intended position. It is important that such entries be worded to enhance the value of the various work experiences and that they not crowd or clutter the resume.

Chapter 17

1. The interview provides a potential employer and an applicant an opportunity to meet and evaluate each other to determine whether the characteristics of the available person match the requirements of the available position.
2. a. By self-assessing job qualifications such as education and work experience.
   b. By self-assessing personal strengths and weaknesses and describing how weaknesses can be overcome.
   c. By anticipating the interests, expectations, and attitudes of the interviewer and adapting the identified qualifications to those interests, expectations, and attitudes.

    d. By organizing key points and practicing (especially with a mirror).

3. a. Introduction
   b. Candidate's background
   c. Matching of the candidate with the position
   d. Closure

4. True

5. False; it should be tactfully corrected.

6. False; it is important that the applicant offer any key items of information for the interviewer even though the interviewer has not asked.

7. False; the interviewer may be assessing the applicant's response to an unstructured encounter.

8. False; it should be the applicant's role to become the highlight of the interviewer's day.

9. False; it may contain additional information and even another expression of interest in the position.

10. a. Draft key questions from the resume or application.
    b. Develop a trust relationship through active listening and a genuine interest in the applicant's statements.
    c. Withhold key information about desired characteristics until their presence or absence in the applicant is determined.
    d. Use follow-up probing questions to learn more about the applicant's experiences, attitudes, and beliefs.
    e. Assess each item of information and each insight for a match with the job description and requirements.

Chapter 18

1. An employment contract is the set of terms to which the employer and employee agree with regard to role, working conditions, salary, fringe benefits, and other relevant factors. It can be oral or written; sometimes it is even implied.

2. A written employment contract specifies the terms agreed to and creates a more permanent record so that the terms do not change at the whim of either party and so that it is more likely the terms will be followed.

3. a. Title and basic functions to be performed
   b. Hours to be worked; days to be worked
   c. Amount of remuneration and its method of calculation
   d. Schedule or review for raises
   e. Method of review (evaluation) for raises and continued employment
   (Others include fringe benefits, opportunities for professional advancement, methods by which the employment contract may be severed, and specific expectations with regard to the employment situation that are not covered above.)

4. Collective bargaining is the process representatives of the union and the employer

utilize to formulate and agree on policy and procedure with regard to the employment of union personnel.

5. a. Teachers—American Federation of Teachers, National Education Association

   b. Nurses—American Nurses Association (its constituent bargaining units)

6. Dental care delivery is primarily a cottage industry with individual dentists providing care at scattered sites with few numbers of auxiliaries at each site.

7. a. Initial loss of employment

   b. Adversary relationship with dentistry

   c. High dollar cost of collective bargaining

Chapter 19

1. A person entering employment encounters a variety of events that can result in substantial loss unless there is some source of money to pay for the unexpected costs.

2. An insurance company assesses the likelihood that the need for benefit payment will occur and covers only those persons for whom there is a probability that a claim will not be filed or for whom there will be a considerable delay before a benefit will be collected. The idea is to collect more premiums than there are claims paid out. Also, the premiums collected are invested so that the dollars earn money.

3. a. Malpractice

   b. Health

   c. Disability

   d. Life

   e. Retirement

   f. Personal liability

   g. Household/personal property

4. a. A patient charging a tort or breach of contract may win the case.

   b. Hospital, physician's costs, and medications may be high if illness strikes.

   c. If the ill person cannot work, some income will be needed.

   d. The person may be leaving dependent persons without an income and with cost of the funeral.

   e. To continue living, there will have to be some income after retirement.

   f. A person harmed by the insured's negligence will need damages covered.

   g. An apartment or house and its contents may be destroyed and need replacement.

5. a. Amount of coverage

   b. Special exempting clauses

   c. Deductible or copayment clauses

Chapter 20

1. Planning is an integral part of organizational effectiveness. It helps the organization determine future needs, activities, and outcomes. It is deciding in advance what must

be done in the future.

2. a. Mission
   b. Goal
   c. Objective
   d. Goal
   e. Objective
   f. Goal (but could be a mission depending on the nature of the organization)
   g. Mission

3. a. Identifying a complete sequence of tasks.
   b. Specifying contingency plans for each step.
   d. Assembling the appropriate staff; making assignments.
   e. Ensuring the availability and organization of resources.
   f. Using appropriate, established lines of communication.
   g. Specifying when activity and outcome reports are necessary.
   h. Establishing tracking methods for task completion and outcome measurement.
   i. Delegating authority for decision making to people who carry responsibility for various aspects of the plan.

4. Directing

5. Fishbone

6. a. Call the meeting
   b. Set a time and place
   c. Invite the right people
   d. Describe the purpose and list an agenda
   e. Start the meeting on time

7. Even though a person may have good management skills, it will be difficult for a manager to help and direct the workers if he/she is not technically aware of the intricacies of their work; credibility relies upon good technical skills.

Chapter 21

1. a. Specify the feelings.
   b. Specify the events that bring about the feelings.
   c. Analyze the events to determine the sources.
   d. Work from the events backward to the roots and nature of the problem.
   e. Validate the hypotheses; consult with others; formulate the problem.

2. a. List a variety of steps that could be taken.
   b. Analyze the likely outcomes of each alternative.
   c. Select alternative; plan action.
   d. Implement the plan.
   e. Monitor the outcomes.

3. 5, 7, 1, 4, 6, 2, 3

4. a. Time
   b. Need for compliance
   c. Understanding of workers
   d. Control the manager should have over a decision
5. Inform the workers of the extent of their control on each decision they are considering.
6. a. Adequate space for heavily trafficked areas.
   b. Treatment areas near the reception area.
   c. Noisy areas (laboratory) away from treatment and reception areas.
   d. Areas used frequently by workers should be centrally located (sterilization).
   e. Less frequently used areas (doctor's office; lounge) should be away from treatment areas.
   f. Patient and staff privacy should be assured.
7. a. Patient record
   b. Scheduling
   c. Productivity information
   d. Financial information
8. Marketing is the continuing effort of a business to provide goods/services that fit with its mission and that meet the wants and needs of the public seeking those goods/services.
9. Advertising is one component of marketing. It brings to the public the message of what makes a business with its goods/services special or unique.
10. Since no manager can be an expert in all aspects of management, it may be appropriate to hire a consultant on a short-term basis to assist the manager in needs assessment and for planning and implementing a project that the business requires.

Chapter 22

1. A good manager needs to have good personnel management skills in order to obtain the cooperation and energy of the workers to fulfill the work that needs to be accomplished. Outstanding skills in organizing, directing, and so on are worthless if the people will not do the work as directed, on time, and with quality.
2. Seven helpful guidelines in managing people are:
   a. Respect their words and their needs.
   b. Listen to what the workers are saying.
   c. Learn what motivates each of them individually and as a group.
   d. Treat them fairly.
   e. Respect confidences.
   f. Challenge people to grow.
   g. Ask for honest feedback regularly.
3. a. Theory X
   b. Theory Z
   c. Theory Y

4. a. Ineffective; strong task orientation without feeling for the needs of the worker, unlikely this manager is benevolent; autocratic style.
   b. Effective; can probably muster the workers to meet the task needs (scheduling more patients) while helping each person retain employment; executive style.
   c. Ineffective; there are times when task needs should be set aside (briefly) to meet the needs of workers, but obtaining a promotion for a poor worker is ultimately costly in most cases; missionary style.
5. a. Reflective
   b. Dirty dozen
   c. Active
   d. Active
   e. Reflective
   f. Dirty dozen
   g. Dirty dozen.
6. Avoidance, collaboration, accommodation, compromise, competition
7. When the blood levels of hormones typically associated with the "fight or flight response" rise and are not mediated by physical action—fighting or fleeing—they actually work against the body causing high blood pressure, susceptibility to illness, digestive problems, and difficulty in sleeping among other signs.
8. a. Make certain the person has the power to change what you object to.
   b. Select the right time and place.
   c. State the feedback in clear, concrete terms.
   d. Offer specific suggestions for change.
   e. Take into account the needs of the other person.
   f. Assure that the person has correctly understood what you have said.
9. Passive behavior does nothing to change the situation—it is an accommodating approach to conflict; aggressive behavior hurts the other person—it does not take into account the needs of the other; assertive behavior states the needs for change but does not seek to harm the other person and it accounts for the needs of the other.
10. A work team is a coordinated group that shares common goals, that collectively contributes to the completion of high quality tasks, that watches out for each member in the group, that establishes norms of honesty and fairness within itself, and that has work roles and interpersonal roles established to keep the group functioning. Individuals simply working at the same site do not share these characteristics.

Chapter 23

1. Fee for service; insurance; government insurance and entitlement programs; preferred provider organizations; capitation programs.
2. Employee compensation; facility costs; equipment costs; supplies and laboratory fees; insurance.

3. Overhead represents out-of-pocket expense to the owner; it is the cost of doing business. Residual income is what is left for the owner after all overhead is covered.
4. Rent and salary costs continue while income drops.
5. No; Social Security is matched by the employer and other fringe benefits should be calculated.
6. Salary; commission; salary plus commission; accept full income of services provided and pay employer for overhead incurred.
7. Number and type of treatments delivered; health outcomes.
8. a. Five visits per day
   b. At least seven visits per day
9. a. Studying and monitoring the issues surrounding dental care financing
   b. Preparing and following a budget
   c. Balancing income against expenses
   d. Projecting ways to draw additional income
   e. Purchasing wisely
   f. Balancing cost and quality
   g. Preparing income statements and breakeven analyses
   h. Preparing tax information for filing
   i. Identifying good investments
   j. Planning and working toward increased financial stability

Chapter 24

1. The primary objective is to put oneself out of business—the treatment business that is. If a preventive program is really working, patients will remain healthy and require little dental treatment.
2. a. There is less dental decay to treat, previously the mainstay of a dental practice.
   b. Prevention fits well within the ethical mandate of a health profession to promote health rather than to repair disease.
   c. The public seems ready to value prevention as the critical component of dental care, given the public's readiness to adopt preventive regimens for general health.
3. a. Guided self-assessment
   b. Thorough medical history and head and neck examination
   c. Occlusal sealants
   d. Nutritional assessments and dietary counseling
   e. Preventive orthodontics
      (and many others)
4. a. Charge large amounts for preventive care, hoping to shift the values from expensive treatment to expensive but worthwhile prevention.
   b. Bury the cost in treatment-related charges.
   c. Provide an in-house insurance or guarantee program where patients who show

consistent compliance with a preventive regimen have whatever disease that occurs treated for very low cost or no cost at all.

d. Encourage third-party payers to value prevention and devise acceptable ways to determine that preventive care was delivered and that it is an effective health measure worthy of reimbursement.

Chapter 25

1. Access to care; cost; quality; and resource allocation

2. During the 1960s, access to care was the major issue since large parts of the population had no access to care and oral health in general was very poor. In the 1970s, resource allocation was the focus as the numbers of providers grew and experimental programs looked at ways to delegate functions to auxiliaries. The economic recession of the 1980s and the failure of national health insurance to be made law brought a greater focus on the cost of care. Efforts were made to contain costs, including alternative delivery systems and payment mechanisms. The late 1980s appears to be dominated by issues of quality as third-party payers, practice networks, and consumers are interested in receiving high quality, appropriate care. It also is a time for looking at resource allocation, but with a different twist: the movement toward independent practice for dental hygienists. Dentistry is increasingly interested in drawing in new population groups who need restorative care.

3. Dental hygiene needs to ensure clear communication among the profession's members regarding the need for independent practice and why it should be an alternative; realistic standards for licensure for independent practice need to be defined; hygienists need to be able to self-regulate licensure and accreditation of educational programs; and dental hygiene needs to establish a sound research base so that a growing body of knowledge regarding dental hygiene care can be established.

4. Dentistry needs to shift from a restorative emphasis to a prevention/periodontics emphasis in order to meet the expectations and the health care needs of the current population; dentists need to learn how to attract patients into their practices and retain them in the pool; and dentists need to learn to work with dental hygienists regardless of whether it is an employee/employer relationship or a referral relationship, where the hygienist is a conduit for bringing new patients into the practice.

Index

Italicized page numbers refer to illustrations; *t* refers to tables.